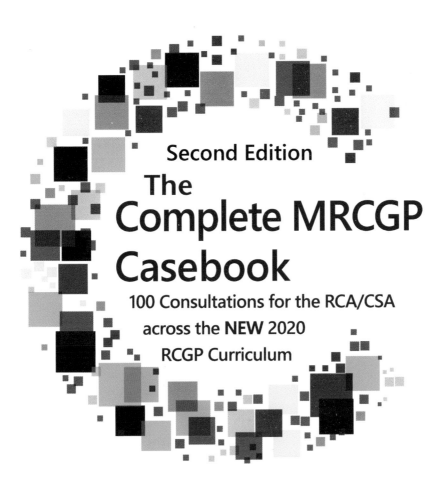

Second Edition

The
Complete MRCGP
Casebook

100 Consultations for the RCA/CSA

across the **NEW** 2020

RCGP Curriculum

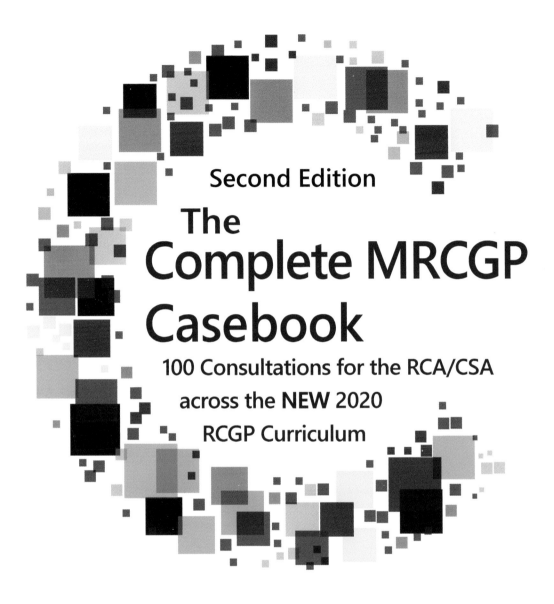

Second Edition

The
Complete MRCGP
Casebook

100 Consultations for the RCA/CSA

across the **NEW** 2020

RCGP Curriculum

Emily Blount • Helen Kirby-Blount • Liz Moulton

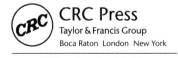

CRC Press

Taylor & Francis Group

Boca Raton London New York

CRC Press is an imprint of the
Taylor & Francis Group, an **informa** business

2nd edition published 2022
by CRC Press
2 Park Square, Milton Park, Abingdon, Oxon, OX14 4RN

and by CRC Press
6000 Broken Sound Parkway NW, Suite 300, Boca Raton, FL 33487-2742

© 2022 Taylor & Francis Group, LLC

First edition published by CRC Press 2017

CRC Press is an imprint of Informa UK Limited

The right of Emily Blount, Helen Kirby-Blount, and Liz Moulton to be identified as authors of this work has been asserted by them in accordance with sections 77 and 78 of the Copyright, Designs and Patents Act 1988.

This book contains information obtained from authentic and highly regarded sources. While all reasonable efforts have been made to publish reliable data and information, neither the author[s] nor the publisher can accept any legal responsibility or liability for any errors or omissions that may be made. The publishers wish to make clear that any views or opinions expressed in this book by individual editors, authors or contributors are personal to them and do not necessarily reflect the views/opinions of the publishers. The information or guidance contained in this book is intended for use by medical, scientific or health-care professionals and is provided strictly as a supplement to the medical or other professional's own judgement, their knowledge of the patient's medical history, relevant manufacturer's instructions and the appropriate best practice guidelines. Because of the rapid advances in medical science, any information or advice on dosages, procedures or diagnoses should be independently verified. The reader is strongly urged to consult the relevant national drug formulary and the drug companies' and device or material manufacturers' printed instructions, and their websites, before administering or utilizing any of the drugs, devices or materials mentioned in this book. This book does not indicate whether a particular treatment is appropriate or suitable for a particular individual. Ultimately it is the sole responsibility of the medical professional to make his or her own professional judgements, so as to advise and treat patients appropriately. The authors and publishers have also attempted to trace the copyright holders of all material reproduced in this publication and apologize to copyright holders if permission to publish in this form has not been obtained. If any copyright material has not been acknowledged please write and let us know so we may rectify in any future reprint.

British Library Cataloguing-in-Publication Data
A catalogue record for this book is available from the British Library

ISBN: 9780367627669 (hbk)
ISBN: 9781003110729 (ebk)

DOI: 10.1201/9781003110729

Typeset in Minion Pro
by Evolution Design & Digital Ltd (Kent)

Dedication

This book is dedicated to our wonderful family, the many children that have appeared in our lives since we began writing the first edition and our cherished friends who know who they are. We thank you for all your love and devoted support.

Contents

Chapters 2–21   100 Cases, Aligned to the NEW 2020 RCGP Curriculum, Clinical and Life Stages Topics

Chapter 22   Examination Checklists

Preface

The Complete MRCGP Casebook will help you with your exam preparation whether you are submitting recorded consultations, or preparing for a simulated surgery, or a mixture of both. We provide examples of how to demonstrate skills in 100 cases across the new RCGP curriculum within the exam marking scheme.

The example consultations may give you ideas on how to develop your consultation skills and meet the challenge of managing the presenting problem safely and effectively within 10–12 minutes. Our Learning Points provide a summary of guidance or a discussion around the topic.

The challenge of the RCGP clinical and consultation skills exam is to be able to synthesise 10 years of medical education competently, sensitively, quickly and safely, to manage any medical problem presented by any patient who walks through the door or picks up the phone. This is also the challenge faced every day by busy GPs in clinical practice. To help show you what can be achieved, the Casebook breaks down the consultation into elements; important building blocks of the consultation which encourage demonstration of all the skills across the marking domains.

The more you practise these skills, the more likely it is that they will, both consciously and unconsciously, become an integral part of your consultation toolkit. When under exam pressure, remember that these elements are grouped into our FOCUS Consultation Model, an easy to remember acronym.

Whatever consultation model(s) you use, we strongly advise that you use your own style for authenticity, have a fluid approach and adapt to meet the needs of each individual consultation. When you meet a new acquaintance or a friend in any setting, demonstrating courtesy and respect for that person and showing a genuine curiosity and interest in their life will enable rapport, storytelling and conversation to come naturally – there is no need to follow a rigid formula.

We appreciate that some readers may have specialist knowledge in particular areas and may well approach some problems differently. The authors are conscientious generalists and this is reflected in our approach to the cases. We hope you find our example consultations helpful – but would remind you that there are many ways to deliver a good consultation, and to pass your final RCGP assessment!

The Learning Points for each case also extract information from the relevant resources or guidance, and we strongly advise always referring to the full text of the most up-to-date guidelines.

See our website www.completeMRCGP.co.uk for the Link Hub and further resources. Look out for dates for exam preparation courses created and run by the authors and examiners.

You may also wish to look at *The Naked Consultation: A Practical Guide to Primary Care Consultation Skills* which will help you develop and hone your consultation skills further.

When role playing cases, we encourage the doctor to remember this:

'Common things are common … But what mustn't I miss?'

Finally, the responsibility of making frequent and fast decisions while holding risk, the urge to always get it right (with the fear of getting it wrong), the pressure to not waste NHS resources, whilst managing complexity, with a high patient load and the medico-legal need to document it all within too little time can feel overwhelming. However, take every opportunity to remember your own loved ones and just do your best for the person looking to you for help. Keep faith in general practice and remember the unique, professional and supportive work ethos we share.

We wish you all the best.

Emily, Helen and Liz

Acknowledgements

Dr Rachel Ruddock, Dr Richard Wood, Dr Ros Lloyd-Rout and Dr Lynnette Peterson who helped to brainstorm this book and whose voices and wise words are hidden within.

Author Biographies

Dr Emily Blount

MBBS (merit) DRCOG DFSRH MRCGP

Emily graduated from Newcastle University in 2008. After working in Auckland, New Zealand, she completed the Oxford GP training scheme and CSA exam in 2014, scoring in the top 3% of candidates. Emily is a GP in Oxford, an Oxford GP Training Programme Director, a GP facilitator at Oxford's 'Dragon's Den' workshops, an Examiner for GP Recruitment, a GP Appraiser and, above all, a mother of two children.

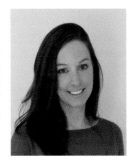

Dr Helen Kirby-Blount

MB ChB (hons) DRCOG MRCGP PGCME

Helen graduated from Manchester University in 2009. She is a GP partner and trainer in Retford and a Training Programme Director for Doncaster and Bassetlaw scheme. She sat the CSA exam in 2013 and facilitates teaching sessions for the RCGP consultation skills exams for her local GP trainees and trainers in Health Education England (HEE) Yorkshire and Humber. Helen created the FOCUS Consultation Model. In her 'spare time' she is a busy mother to her two daughters and loves all things 'sport'.

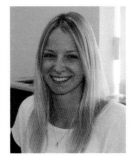

Dr Liz Moulton

MBE MB ChB DRCOG FRCGP MMEd (distinction)

A GP trainer for 30 years, with a wealth of experience of preparing candidates for the MRCGP, Liz has also undertaken most roles within HEE Yorkshire and Humber and was Deputy Director of Postgraduate GP Education. Liz was a GP advisor to Leeds Health Authority and to the Department of Health. She currently works as a freelance GP and appraiser as well as working for the RCGP practice support unit. Liz is the author of *The Naked Consultation*.

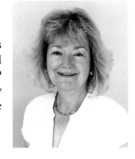

The Complete MRCGP Casebook

100 cases covering all the RCGP 2020 clinical curriculum topics

100 cases
- 100 paired role play cards so no need to pass around a book!
- Seamlessly aligned with the new 2020 RCGP curriculum.
- Five cases for each module of the curriculum.
- Includes even the 'difficult' modules: neurodevelopmental and genomic medicine cases.
- Helps build confidence that you are on the right track.

Example answers
- For every case.
- Example consultations written in prose, word for word – how we would do it.
- See how it can be done… in 10–12 minutes!
- How to give quick and jargon-free explanations.

Easy-to-use generic feedback cards
- Marking schemes can be hard to follow if you are not a trained examiner. We have a single easy-to-use marking scheme and tick lists for each consultation example.

Guideline summaries
- For every case.
- Revision cards and up-to-date guidelines.
- Including useful information and web links we have collected.

 The web links will be stored and updated at the **Link Hub on CompleteMRCGP.co.uk**
The treasure chest symbol means there is relevant information on the Link Hub.

The ring binder
- Colour-coded RCGP Curriculum Modules.
- Easy-to-use ring binder.
- Helps you remain organised and keep the cases in order.

Helpful advice
- Tips based on our experience of the RCGP Consultation Skills exams – CSA and RCA.
- A summary of consultation models.
- Useful phrases and jargon switch.

Physical examination cards
- Stepwise guides to slick and thorough examinations.
- Realistic times suggested.

Complete MRCGP's FOCUS Consultation Model
- A consultation model created specifically for the RCA and CSA – practical, straightforward and easy to remember under stress.
- Written by three experienced GP educators – two of whom sat the CSA.

Whether your exam involves submitting recorded cases (RCA) or simulated patients (CSA), *The Complete MRCGP Casebook* provides examples of HOW to overcome the challenges and demonstrate competence throughout the marking domains for all mandatory cases and across the curriculum. For every case we provide 'Example Consultations' to demonstrate how each challenge could be achieved within 10–12 minutes as well as 'Learning Points', which summarise up-to-date guidance. All RCGP Curriculum Modules are colour coded, helping you to keep the cases in order and stay organised.

Our FOCUS Consultation Model was created specifically for the RCGP clinical skills exam, to focus your skills, provide structure and give you an easy-to-use tool to help you 'mark' your own consultations.

The authors are three experienced GP educators who have run CSA and RCA courses for many years, working in collaboration with senior RCGP examiners. We have systematically condensed our experience into this comprehensive Casebook to help you complete your GP training and become a confident and independent practitioner.

How to Use the Book

The CSA was replaced by the RCA in 2020 and a 'hybrid' exam is expected. However, the principles of what you need to evidence will remain the same:

- You will need to demonstrate that you can perform well in a range of cases across the breadth of the curriculum.
- You will need to demonstrate data gathering, clinical management and interpersonal skills.
- You must perform at the level of a UK independent GP.

We have organised a selection of core cases into 20 modules, fully aligned to the new RCGP curriculum.

We recommend that some cases are specifically performed face-to-face (symbol in the corner of the page). However, for most cases throughout the book you have the option to decide for yourself whether you practise the case as a telephone call, video call, face-to-face or home visit. If there is the potential for an examination, we have written examination findings.

You could work through the book alone; however, we recommend using the book in groups of two or three, taking the parts of: a doctor, a patient and an 'examiner'. The more frequently you practise the consultation skills that you hope to demonstrate in your exam, the more likely you are to be able to use them fluently when under pressure.

Each case has one card for the Doctor (Doctor's Notes) and another card for the Patient (Patient's Story). Once you've completed your consultation, turn your cards over to find our suggested Example Consultation and Learning Points, which cover the important facts or guidelines relevant to the case.

Where we have extracted Learning Points from NICE or other sources, always refer to the latest version of the full guidance – and please remember that this is only applicable to UK patients.

When a medication is mentioned, always refer to the BNF.

Instructions for the patient	The Presenting Complaint (PC) is the *'opening gambit'*. You should freely give the doctor anything in quotation marks. Further information should be given only if the doctor asks relevant questions.
Instructions for the doctor	We suggest using our FOCUS Model, which has been broken down into elements on each Example Consultation, as a guide. Include all these elements and you have an excellent consultation; but be flexible, so that the consultation is conversational.
Instructions for the examiner or time keeper	Mark the Giving Feedback Card. We have also provided tick boxes on each Example Consultation page. The examination clock starts following, if required, identification and consent, that is from the moment the doctor asks their first question, for example 'How can I help?'

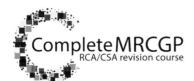

CompleteMRCGP
RCA/CSA revision course

How to Use the Book

Clinical Examinations

We provide examination findings should you choose the face-to-face option.

Constructive criticism is essential

Be honest and agree to the rules before you start! For marking, you can use:

- the RCGP marking criteria – see 'How to Demonstrate Skills: The Marking Scheme Made Easy'.
- the Generic Feedback card.
- the 'tick boxes' within the Example Consultations.

Useful information and web links will be stored and updated at the Link Hub on CompleteMRCGP.co.uk. The treasure chest symbol means there is relevant information on the Link Hub.

Symbols in the Book

Face-to-Face

See the Link Hub

RCGP Curriculum

The RCGP defines and describes the GP curriculum – the competencies and capabilities that you need to develop (and evidence!) to become an effective and safe GP. The curriculum can be found on the RCGP website, but we describe it here for convenience and to explain which areas are tested by the exam and are therefore particularly relevant to this book.

The RCGP **core statement** 'Being a general practitioner' is divided into five areas of capability and each of these is subdivided, so there are 13 specific areas of capability for general practice:

1. Knowing yourself and relating to others
   a. Fitness to practise
   b. Maintaining an ethical approach
   c. Communication and consultation
2. Applying clinical knowledge and skill
   a. Data gathering and interpretation
   b. Clinical examination and procedural skills
   c. Making decisions
   d. Clinical management
3. Managing complex and long-term care
   a. Managing medical complexity
   b. Working with colleagues and in teams
4. Working well in organisations and systems of care
   a. Improving performance, learning and teaching
   b. Organisation, management and leadership
5. Caring for the whole person and wider community
   a. Practising holistically and promoting health and safeguarding
   b. Community orientation

The RCGP website gives detailed descriptions and explanations of each of these areas and can be accessed at: https://www.rcgp.org.uk/training-exams/training/gp-curriculum-new/being-a-general-practitioner/how-the-curriculum-is-structured.aspx

As well as capabilities, six **professional modules** are listed:
   A. Consulting in general practice
   B. Equality, diversity and inclusion
   C. Evidence-based practice, research and sharing knowledge
   D. Improving quality, safety and prescribing
   E. Leadership and management
   F. Urgent and unscheduled care

Then there are 20 **clinical modules**, and these form the main content of this book, with five cases illustrating each. However, as well as assessing your clinical knowledge in these areas, the final consultation skills exam tests your ability to apply many, although not quite all, of the above capabilities. The remaining areas are tested through the AKT and the various tools of workplace-based assessment.

RCGP Capabilities

The marking scheme for the exam relates to the RCGP capabilities – see how they fit into data gathering/ technical assessment skills, clinical management and interpersonal skills. Another way to analyse your consultation is to ask yourself which capability you demonstrated.

1. Fitness to practise
Develop the attitudes and behaviours expected of a good doctor

2. Maintaining an ethical approach
Treat others fairly and with respect, acting without discrimination
Provide care with compassion and kindness

3. Communication and consultation
Establish an effective partnership with patients
Maintain a continuing relationship with patients, carers and families

4. Data gathering and interpretation
Apply a structured approach to data gathering and investigation
Interpret findings accurately to make a diagnosis

5. Clinical examination and procedural skills
Demonstrate a proficient approach to clinical examination
Demonstrate a proficient approach to the performance of procedures

6. Making a diagnosis/decision
Adopt appropriate decision-making principles
Apply a scientific and evidence-based approach

7. Clinical management
Provide general clinical care to patients of all ages and backgrounds
Adopt a structured approach to clinical management
Make appropriate use of other professionals and services
Provide urgent care when needed

8. Managing medical complexity
Enable people with long-term conditions to improve their health
Manage concurrent health problems in an individual patient
Adopt safe and effective approaches for patients with complex health needs

RCGP Capabilities

9. Working with colleagues and in teams
Work as an effective team member
Coordinate a team-based approach to the care of patients

10. Maintaining performance, learning and teaching (assessed in WPBA)

11. Organisation, management and leadership
Make effective use of information management and communication systems

12. Practising holistically and promoting health
Demonstrate the holistic mindset of a generalist medical practitioner
Support people through individual experiences of health, illness and recovery

13. Community orientation
Understand the health service and your role within it

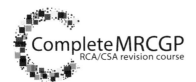

Consultation Models

You may well have been taught a framework or model for your consultations. Using a tried and tested structure can help to ensure that you remember all the key phases and don't leave anything out. The exam is marked in three different domains, and we will explore how some of the common models fit with this and which skills contribute to each domain. Although the individual models differ in their detail, most conform broadly to the following five-stage structure:

- Find out why the patient has come
- Work out what's wrong
- Explain the problem(s) to the patient
- Develop a management plan and share this with the patient
- Use time well and efficiently

Some also have a sixth stage – take care of yourself. Very important for both exam purposes and life beyond as an independent practitioner.

The exam marking domains are:

Data gathering, technical and assessment skills (find out why the patient has come and work out what's wrong)

Clinical management (make a diagnosis or state your impression, explain the problem to the patient, develop and negotiate a management plan with the patient)

Interpersonal skills (evidenced throughout the consultation from beginning to end)

Using time well and efficiently is essential because, if you run out of time before you get to the management plan, you will score no marks in that area – a recipe for failure.

Looking after yourself between each consultation is vital – otherwise one 'bad' consultation will lead to another. Some, after a difficult or dysfunctional simulated consultation, will use any time between patients to pore over the previous patient's notes. They try to work out what went wrong, rather than putting it out of their mind and spending precious moments reading and thinking about the next patient. Don't let this happen to you! Similarly, after a real consultation that may not have gone well, or has left you feeling strong emotions, it is important to regather your thoughts, 'housekeep' and focus before seeing the next patient.

Let's look at some common models and see where the different stages fit within the consultation skills exam marking structure.

Consultation Models

Pendleton (1984)

One of the first patient-centred models.

Seven tasks:

A. Data gathering

1. Find out why the patient has come, including the problem (cause, effects, history) and the patient's ideas, concerns and expectations.
2. Consider other problems.

B. Clinical management

3. Choose (with the patient) an appropriate action for each problem.
4. Achieve a shared understanding of the problems.
5. Involve the patient in the management and encourage them to accept appropriate responsibility.
6. Use time and resources appropriately.

C. Interpersonal skills

7. Establish or maintain a relationship with the patient which helps to achieve the other tasks.

Helman (1981)

Although this isn't a model of the consultation, Cecil Helman, a medical anthropologist, described six questions that any patient might have in their head when coming to see the doctor. It is well worth bearing these in mind when data gathering, particularly around ICE (ideas, concerns and expectations) and in clinical management, when you are explaining to the patient. Armed with the patient's own thoughts, fears and hopes, the answers to these questions could provide a useful framework for your explanation.

1. What has happened?
2. Why has it happened?
3. Why to me?
4. Why now?
5. What would happen if nothing was done about it?
6. What should I do about it or whom should I consult for further help?

Consultation Models

Neighbour (1987)

A five-part model 'anchored' to the fingers of the left hand, so relatively easy to remember even when you are stressed.

A. Data gathering

1. **Connecting** This stage is about rapport building (interpersonal skills) as well as gathering data. 'Connection' starts the moment the patient walks through the door. Look at the patient, what do you notice? How do they seem? What is this telling you? Tune in to the patient to get on their wavelength. Explore their story until you have enough information to summarise.

2. **Summarising** If you are unsure, or even in a consultation 'hole' where you are struggling, summarising is the best tool to get you back on track again.

B. Clinical management

3. **Handing over** This is where doctor and patient negotiate and agree a management plan and empower the patient by 'hand over' of control.

4. **Safety netting** Safety netting ensures there are safe contingency plans. Neighbour describes a really robust structure for a three-point safety net. A vague 'come back if you're no better' is unlikely to score you any marks in the RCGP consultation skills exam, so learn and use this structure:

   i.   This is what I expect to happen.

   ii. This is how you [the patient] will know if I'm wrong.

   iii. If that happens, this is what you should do.

Easy and safe!

C. Interpersonal skills

As with other models, these run as a thread from beginning to end of the consultation. Neighbour's fifth stage is 'Housekeeping'. In his book, he describes a number of quick and easy ways to deal with stress and negative feelings that have arisen during the consultation so that you can ensure you are in the best shape ready for the next patient. Well worth a read. These techniques are easy to learn and applicable to all your future consultations.

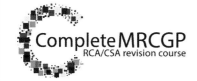

Consultation Models

Calgary Cambridge

This is a very comprehensive and evidence-based approach to the consultation – another five-stage model which includes specific detail of tools and techniques.

A. Data gathering

1. Initiating the session

    Introductions.

    Establishing rapport.

    Finding out the reason for the consultation.

2. Gathering information

    Exploring the patient's perspective using a range of verbal and non-verbal communication skills including open and closed questions, ICE, clarification, summarising, etc. Finding out 'Why now?' – the universal question of the consultation is 'Why has this patient come today with this problem?' If you can't answer this by the end of the consultation, you may well have missed something important!

B. Clinical management

3. Explanation and planning

    Finds out what the patient knows.

    Asks what the patient wants to know.

    'Chunks and checks' – information in digestible chunks.

    Careful timing of explanations – not too soon.

4. Closing the session

    Safety nets and follow-up.

C. Interpersonal skills

5. Building the relationship

    Developing rapport.

    Accepting the patient's views as legitimate.

    Using non-verbal behaviour.

    Involving the patient (e.g. thinking aloud, explicitly describing examination process and findings).

Calgary Cambridge also explores the very important feature of providing structure to the consultation by approaching it logically, using mini-summaries and keeping to time. All very important – a messy disordered consultation is inefficient.

Consultation Models

6 S for success

A newer model developed in 2013 by Alex Watson with an easy to remember alliterative '6 S' model. Story, Summarising, Sharing, Securing, Status, Sanity.

A. Data gathering

1. **Story** – connecting with the patient, being attentive, letting them tell their story, demonstrating verbally and non-verbally that you are listening to what they are saying. Find out thoughts, hopes and fears. Find the subplot if there is one.

2. **Summarising** – an opportunity to review what has been said so far, non-judgementally. The patient feels listened to and there is opportunity to clarify, add additional information and correct any misunderstandings before moving on.

B. Clinical management

3. **Sharing** – moving from listening to discussion about management, including the patient's thoughts, fears and hopes and incorporating the doctor's view. Any risks can also be discussed and shared between doctor and patient.

4. **Securing** – safety netting the consultation, securing the evidence by making notes. (Written notes are, of course, not currently assessed by the RCGP in the final clinical/consultation skills assessment exam!)

C. Interpersonal skills

5. **Status** – again, something that overarches and underpins the consultation: how we behave with others, how they perceive us and we perceive them and how this affects the consultation for good or bad. A mid-level point is the most helpful so that the clinician takes care to be warm, interested and on a level with the patient, avoiding the unhelpful extremes of arrogance/aloofness and timidity/being apologetic.

Watson's sixth stage is 'Sanity' – similar to housekeeping described by Neighbour. Making sure that you are in good shape for the next patient and for your future in general practice.

FOCUS Consultation Model

We developed the FOCUS Consultation Model to help you demonstrate the skills required for the RCGP clinical and consultation skills exam. We don't expect you to learn and remember all the elements and a formulated approach is not natural. We encourage you to find your own style – be flexible. However, the more you practise these elements, the more fluent you will become, so that you can use them with ease when you need to.

Consider how long you will allow yourself for each element. If an element is taking longer, keep bringing the patient back into the discussion, e.g. checking their understanding or reaction.

FILTER

Data gathering, starting with many open questions, then grouping together closed questions (risk assessment and red flags) to focus the history as you formulate a potential hypothesis. If appropriate, check history: past medical history (PMH), drug history (DH), family history (FH) and social history (SH) to look for relevant information which will ultimately affect diagnosis and management. Any information from the notes that you are using to help you should be clearly discussed. Examinations should be focused.

OPPORTUNITY

This is your opportunity to connect with the patient and demonstrate interpersonal skills (IPS) – remember that these are not an assessment of being polite or articulate. IPS are about making a connection, demonstrating a genuine interest in the person, and most importantly, how you tailor the rest of the consultation to meet the patient's needs based on information they have shared. Use identified **cues** to give the patient the opportunity to discuss their ICE (ideas, concerns and expectations).

Be curious, sense how they are feeling and assess the impact of their symptoms on their life.

It is intended that Filter and Opportunity can be done in any order, or often interspersed. We would encourage trying to discover the 'Opportunity' information early in the consultation.

CONTEXT

This is where you question 'What is going on here?' and is the moment for the doctor and patient to come together on the same page. Think about how the information discovered in Filter is affected by/relates to the information gathered in Opportunity. The skill includes stating your impression regarding the potential diagnosis or differential diagnoses. Another important skill is referring to ICE within your explanation and a statement of empathy reflects the challenges they are facing (problem + fears + social context).

UNITE

Share the management plan to unite doctor and patient. Discuss your recommendation as well as options: what can the patient do (demonstrating empowerment); what can I do; what can others (specialists/family) do; and finally what resources (websites, support groups, patient information leaflets) are available? Be specific regarding medicines, follow-up plans and logistics.

SAFETY

Always offer a specific safety net – what do they need to look out for? How long should they wait before returning? What should they do if they feel they are getting worse? What actions are required for both the doctor and patient?

The diagrammatic model illustrates how the model links to the RCGP mark scheme.

FOCUS Consultation Model

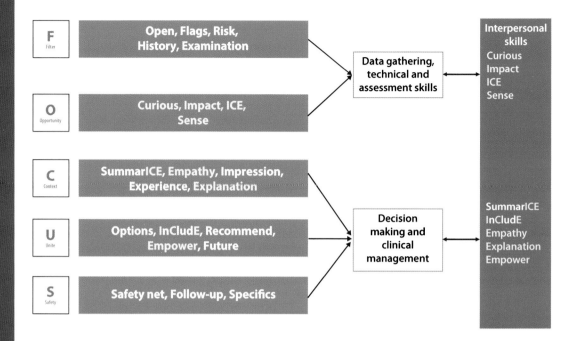

FOCUS Consultation Model

The **FOCUS Consultation Model** groups the key elements of the consultation.

FILTER

Open	Ask as many open questions as possible to collect the story.
Flags	Use focused questions. Check for red flags and whittle down differentials.
Risk	Ask about risk factors for your suspected diagnosis.
History	Take the history: past, systemic, family, medicines and social.
Examination	A focused examination to confirm or refute your hypothesis or exclude significant disease. Explain exactly what you would like to examine and gain informed consent.

OPPORTUNITY

Curious	Respond to verbal cues and explore.
	E.g. *'You mentioned your friend. What is their experience of…?'*
Impact	Find out how the problem has affected the patient: open questions about impact work really well at the beginning of the consultation. Use this information to smoothly transition to ICE. Impact questions make great open questions at the beginning of the consultation.
ICE	Explore ideas, concerns and expectations. *'This is clearly affecting you a lot day to day, have you had thoughts about what is going on?'*
Sense	Reflect what you sense (feelings or emotions) from non-verbal cues.
	E.g. *'I feel/can see that (fidgeting/breathless/distracted/in a rush)…'*

CONTEXT

SummarICE	Demonstrate that you have listened by summarising the ICE.
Empathy	Show you have put the problem into the context of their life.
	E.g. *'I can see your past experience of…can lead you to consider…'*
Impression	State your impression! Make a diagnosis if you can, or state the likely differentials.
Experience	Check their understanding or experience of what you have diagnosed. Incorporate what you have learnt from ICE.
Explanation	Provide a concise and jargon-free explanation. Tell the patient what they need to know; don't bombard them with extra unnecessary detail, however much you know.

UNITE

Options	Provide an organised list of options, Confirm their understanding and interest. A useful framework includes: *'Things that you can do…, I can do…, others can help with…'*
InCludE	Incorporate what you have learnt from asking and listening to the patient's expectations.
Recommend	As well as options, you should also help guide the patient's decision by stating your own recommendation for the way forward.
Empower	Suggest what the patient can do themselves to help the problem.
Future	Explain what you believe should or is likely to happen at the next steps.
	E.g. *'Thinking ahead…Return to the GP in…'*
	E.g. *'At the hospital you can expect to…'*

FOCUS Consultation Model

SAFETY

Safety net   Give clear instructions about what to look out for and what the patient should do in these circumstances.

Follow-up   Will you need to see the patient again? If so, when and how should they make this arrangement?

Specifics   Remember to be specific about time intervals, for example – who is booking an appointment, with whom, in what situation?

Remember to ask:

Paediatrics: gestation, delivery, postnatal, immunisations and development.

Women's health: last menstrual period, cycle, post-coital bleeding, intermenstrual bleeding, discharge, smears, parity and operations.

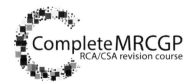

ICE, SummarICE and InCludE

Working with many hundreds of trainees preparing for their consultation assessment exams, both CSA and RCA, we have frequently noticed that ICE, if asked at all, is often then neglected or ignored in the remainder of the consultation. For good consultations and excellent marks, it is essential not just to elicit ICE, but also to use it. We suggest the following easy-to-remember technique.

1. Elicit ICE – see below for how to do this.
2. Use this information in the midpoint summary – **SummarICE**, to demonstrate that you have heard the patient.
3. Include this information when stating your impression or negotiating a plan – **InCludE**.

Elicit ICE. With good rapport and attentive listening, any or all components of ICE may emerge naturally as the patient is talking to you, particularly if you use open questions. If not, you may need to use some specific prompts:

Ideas/thoughts. What does the patient think about their symptoms? In their eyes, what might the problem be? If it's not crystal clear, ask! If the patient says 'nothing', this is unlikely to be true: it's just that the patient has not yet felt able to tell you. Ask again, rephrase the question, show that you are interested in the patient's thoughts through rapport, such as eye contact, nodding, minimal encouragers, giving the patient your whole attention and allowing space to listen. Remember, their thoughts may have come from:

- Past experience
- Others' experience – friends, work colleagues, neighbours
- The internet
- Newspaper articles, TV programmes – factual and fictional

There may be cues to follow – '*I read in the paper that...*', '*John thinks...*', '*I had this before and...*', '*A friend at work...*'

Concerns/worries. What has worried the patient enough to make an appointment with you? You could try:

'*I sense you are worried about this.*' (Pause and listen). This is a statement used as a question, so is softer and less blunt than '*What are you worrying about?*' which may lead to the answer '*nothing*' (unlikely to be true) or something that may not be directly relevant (my job/debt/the neighbours).

'*Is there anything, however unlikely, that you are particularly worried this might be?*'

If someone else has been mentioned (my friend, John, my husband/wife/daughter), make use of this and ask '*Tell me what worries your friend/John, etc. about this.*'

Remember that you cannot second-guess what the patient's worries might be – they are unique to that person. If you try and guess, you may well be wrong. Their thoughts or worries may be incorrect or implausible, but they are the patient's reality – hold on to them so that you can use them later.

Expectations. Finding out what the patient is hoping for from you will potentially save you a lot of time later, whether or not it is a practical or appropriate way forward. Try:

'*What did you have in mind that I might be able to do for you?*' '*When you booked the appointment/were sitting in the waiting room, was there anything in particular you were hoping for from today?*'

Remember not to ask this too early, otherwise it might come across as if you don't know and are asking the patient for a clue to the way ahead. Try '*I've already got some thoughts myself about what we could do but I am interested to hear what you think.*'

SummarICE (Summarise ICE). When you know you have enough information to formulate a diagnosis and a plan, including all three components of ICE, summarising is an excellent way to demonstrate to the patient that you have heard what they've said and to mark the transition from data gathering to clinical management.

Instead of summarising all the history, try summarising ICE, i.e. SummarICE. Perhaps also include impact – the way the problem is affecting the patient's life.

'You've had this cough for more than a week. You thought it might be a chest infection needing antibiotics, but at the back of your mind you are worried about cancer, given that you smoked until recently. It's been hard to sleep at night for coughing so your husband's moved into the spare room.'

'For a month or so you've had chest pain when you walk which you thought might be muscle strain from trimming the hedge, but you were also concerned about your heart and were hoping I might do a chest X-ray and heart tracing/refer you to the hospital.'

This is a more time-efficient and tailored summary than going through all the symptoms again.

InCludE (Include ICE). The midpoint summary will remind you to include the patient's ideas and concerns when stating your 'Impression':

'You thought this might be a chest infection – having listened to your symptoms and examined you, I agree/I don't think it is.'

'I don't think it's likely that chest pain when you walk is connected with muscle strain from using the hedge trimmer. The fact that it comes on when you exercise and goes when you stop might suggest pain from the heart muscle, called angina.'

'You were worried about cancer – although unlikely because you haven't lost weight or coughed up blood [red flags], I agree it is something we should exclude.'

You can either include expectations here, or a little later when negotiating the plan:

'As you've had the symptoms for a week, and I can hear signs of infection in your chest, I agree an antibiotic may well help.'

'You mentioned a chest X-ray – I don't think that would add much at this stage but if you still have symptoms in a week, we should think about one then.'

Practising the Skills within FOCUS

Recognise your strengths! Then consider which elements you find the most challenging.

Target your revision. Analyse and fine tune each microskill, a day at a time.

FILTER Be assertive and sharpen your history

Non-verbal   Use videos to analyse non-verbal communication.

Open   Concentrate on routinely asking a series of encouraging/open questions – at least three before you move to semi-closed or closed questions. Can you rephrase your questions? For example, '*When did it start?*' is a semi-closed question, but '*How did it start?*' is open and will yield much richer answers.

History   Critique your consultations. Do you ask questions which actually change your management?

Examination   Use the examination examples in Chapter 22 to practise your skills.

OPPORTUNITY

Curious   Work on reacting to those cues, e.g. repeating phrases back to patients.

ICE   We find asking ICE early is helpful and continues the use of open questions. Ensure you have found the answers to all three questions. If a patient has already provided you with the information, to demonstrate you were listening, acknowledge this and consider asking questions to explore if there's more to be found. The way the questions are phrased can make or break a consultation. E.g. 'What would you like me to do?' may be received negatively, whereas 'I'm going to be making many suggestions, but was there anything specific you were hoping for today?' enhances rapport and shared understanding.

Impact/Sense   To find out impact, you need to know something about the patient's life as well as the problem and ask or explore how the two are related. Put a Post-it Note on your desk at work to remind you to do this.

CONTEXT

Empathy and SummarICE   With every patient you see, practise summarising their ICE followed by a statement which links the ICE to their background, experience or situation.

Impression and Experience   Always ensure you state your impression/diagnosis at 5–6 minutes followed by a pause.

Explanation   Practise giving clear and concise explanations for diagnoses and your recommendations.

Practising the Skills within FOCUS

UNITE

Options   Organise your thoughts and practise using a 3-dimensional approach. Think about what you can do, what the patient can do (self-help) and where others (friends, family, referrals) could help . Using this framework will help you to produce a structured management plan for almost any presenting problem.

InCludE   *'You were worried about… and thought we should do… however what's going through my mind is… what would you like to do?'*

Recommend   Have the confidence to state *'My recommendation is…, other options are…'*

Empower   *'Things you may be interested in are… what are your thoughts?'*

Future   *'We should catch up to discuss this again, how about in…'* Have you been specific? Is it clear to the patient what steps you and they are taking regarding any agreed logistics and management?

SAFETY

Safety net   Practise excellent documentation to reinforce this. Remember, be specific. Watching back recorded consultations can help you check how clear your safety netting is. Remember the 3-point safety net – *'This is what I expect to happen…this is how you will know if I'm wrong…this is what to do then.'* The safety net should of course always be tailored to the patient and the problem. It should flow naturally from what has been discussed in the consultation and should provide reassurance and empowerment for the patient, rather than baffling or scaring them unnecessarily. It is unhelpful and inappropriate to use *'Call 999'* as a backstop at the end of a safety net for a self-limiting and relatively minor problem.

Remember that few consultations need a catch-all safety net for every eventuality, however unlikely. For example: a 30-year-old female patient phones you and describes intermittent diarrhoea and vague abdominal pain for the last year. There are no red flag symptoms at all and she has had no symptoms of any sort for several days. You are planning to see her tomorrow to examine her and suspect she might have IBS. A 'safety net' that infers she might develop an acute abdomen before you see her, and need to go immediately to hospital is inappropriate for this patient and her symptoms. It is likely to be confusing and unnecessarily increase any anxiety. A much simpler statement *'I'll see you tomorrow as we agreed. I don't imagine your symptoms will change between now and then but please phone the surgery if they do'* is all that is needed.

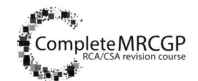

How to Demonstrate Skills: The Marking Scheme Made Easy

Data gathering is about uncovering the clinical information appropriate to the problem/s presented by the patient. This process should be efficient and logical, using appropriate open and closed questions, including finding out risk factors and red flags. Any physical examination described or undertaken should be relevant and slick, performed in a logical order and any instruments should be used fluently. This domain may include limited near-patient investigations if appropriate to the presentation, such as urinalysis.

Clinical management should reflect the differential diagnosis and be feasible and evidence based and reflect any identified risks. In a remote or telephone consultation, the management may include the description of any examination planned and how this will help with the diagnosis and management.

Interpersonal skills are the communication skills and collaboration with patients, including ethics, values and attitudes, that you demonstrate throughout the consultation. For example, in the first half, these would include finding out ICE, responding to cues and responding with interest to the patient's views. Any examination should show sensitivity for the patient's feelings and consent through clear explanations of what you hope to examine and why it is helpful.

Any plan would demonstrate that you have responded to the patient's feelings, preferences and hopes, including explaining risk effectively.

Interpersonal skills also include values and ethics – such as demonstrating equality, responding positively to problems, admitting mistakes, being open and non-judgemental.

Demonstrating IPS as a GP requires proactive and reactive communication skills. Our FOCUS model (Filter, Opportunity, Context, Unite, Safety) reminds you to take the opportunity to connect with the patient. Careful IPS should be demonstrated at every step of the consultation.

Our useful E's for interpersonal skills

Encourage	Their contribution. Not only ask ICE, but also return to it during your explanations or recommendations.
Explore	Their cues or anything you sense from the patient. Explore ICE and the impact of the issue.
Empathy	Pulling together all the patient's challenges and collectively reflecting these back to them. How we break this down to teach it… Symptoms + fears + social challenges = impact + offer your support.
Explain	(a) Provide explanations of why your questions are important, e.g. you could do this with ICE questions. (b) Share your thought process clearly, using language tailored to the individual patient.
Engage	The patient in shared management and health promotion.
Empower	Share your knowledge to empower the patient and involve them at every step in the plan. Provide them with the opportunity to (a) make an informed decision and (b) consider self-help strategies.
Elephants	E.g. issues either the patient or doctor is nervous to mention. Address them early in a sensitive way to allow time to deal with them.

This is not a finite list and you should carefully read the RCGP document – 'Generic grade descriptors' for a more comprehensive description.

Easy-to-Use Generic Feedback Card

Below are some pointers that you can look for when marking each other's cases. On the next page there is a blank grid that you could photocopy to make marking easier. Look for what the doctor has done well and what could be improved in each domain.

Data gathering:
- Was the main reason for attendance established? Were relevant red flags checked?
- Was an organised system used for gathering background information: PMH, DH, FH, SH?
- Was there an appropriate and slick examination where necessary?
- Did the doctor use information from the notes and was this made explicit and discussed?
- Were any instruments required during the examination used proficiently?

Clinical management:
- Was an appropriate working diagnosis made?
- Was the plan tailored to the patient?
- Did the doctor state their recommendation and other possibilities?
- Was an appropriate management plan discussed with the patient including appropriate tests, medication, referrals, follow-up, etc.?
- Were opportunities to tackle health promotion found?
- Did the doctor add an appropriate safety net?

Interpersonal skills:
- Were cues in the history picked up and addressed?
- Were ideas, concerns and expectations elicited?
- Did the doctor adopt a sensitive approach? Without prejudice, judgement and assumption?
- Did the doctor provide clear explanations using appropriate language?
- Did the doctor involve the patient in decisions?
- Did the doctor demonstrate active listening skills?
- Did the doctor demonstrate empathy through their communication skills?
- Did they find out how the patient's problem and individual psychosocial situation were intervolved?
- How did the doctor show that they were genuinely interested in the patient?
- Did the doctor empower the patient and how?

Possible negative descriptors for feedback and to discuss:
- The consultation appeared disorganised.
- A significant agenda, abnormal result or red flag was missed.
- Failure to examine (if appropriate).
- Poor time management.
- The focus of the consultation was on the wrong agenda/complaint.
- The doctor provided little or no opportunity to involve the patient in management decisions.
- Cues were missed.
- The consultation was low challenge.

Easy-to-Use Generic Feedback Card

Case

Data Gathering	
POSITIVE	NEGATIVE

Clinical Management	
POSITIVE	NEGATIVE

Interpersonal Skills	
POSITIVE	NEGATIVE

Structure and Time Management

For every consultation, you need to find the answer to the question: *'Why has this patient presented today with this problem?'*

How to achieve this in a 10–12-minute consultation

1. Be concise. Use as few words as possible and choose words carefully to ask concise, clear questions. Remember that open questions are most likely to reveal the detail you need.

2. The 'golden minute' is usually rich in important detail. The patient's flow can be extended by using open questions. Choose questions that guide the patient to give information that is crucial to your assessment. E.g. *'How did it start?'* Rather than *'When did it start'* which is a closed question.

3. Repeat their words, with a rising inflexion so they sound like questions. *'Chest pain? Feeling low?'*

4. Absorb the answers that follow and don't ask questions where you already know the answers.

5. Be organised – lots of open questions first, then group your closed questions (red flags).

6. Aim for the important moment of the consultation at 5–6 minutes – where you state your impression.

7. Be systematic with how you present your management plan.

8. Be assertive. See below.

9. Keep up momentum. Imagine you are on a ski slalom and quickly need to go around all the gates on the way down the hill. The gradient is the same throughout, so avoid being too slow at the start then speeding up in panic towards the end. Certainly, don't turn around and go back up the hill to cover old ground!

10. Avoid wasting time with unnecessary phrases. Every second counts in a 10–12-minute consultation. We often hear *'May I ask you some questions'* which is always followed by *'Yes of course'*. There's no need to say this unless you are signposting that you are about to ask some very personal questions.

11. Too much sympathy is neither helpful nor efficient. Interpersonal skills require an assertive not just a 'nice' doctor. Always be sensitive, however. Continue to move the consultation forward and demonstrate you are 'nice' by:

    - asking thoughtful questions *'What is it like living with <x>?'*
    - demonstrating an interest in the person *'What's this past year been like for you?'*
    - connecting through exploring cues and ICE.

This information helps you to work towards demonstrating 'proactive empathy' (you've worked for it) which silently, yet powerfully suggests to the patient 'I hear you'.

Remember our empathy equation: problem + fears + social context = an understanding and expression of how things are: e.g. *'really tough'*.

How to develop your time management skills

- Go back to basics. Write down a structure you hope to follow (allowing flexibility).
- Dissect your consultations in detail. Listen to your videos and be critical with your chosen words within questions. Could you have rephrased to ask more skillful questions which efficiently provide important answers.
- Practise going from the moment you give a diagnosis to how you present a recommended management plan and involve the patient in the decision-making process.
- Practise giving slick explanations of diagnoses to different patient groups, e.g. migraine to a lawyer, asthma to a 7-year-old who just wants to play football.

Structure and Time Management

Remember you can be assertive and yet remain patient centred. You can be assertive through having a structure, asking questions that demonstrate your curiosity and interest, reacting to the patient's needs, agenda and cues, being organised, using signposting and keeping the momentum of the consultation going. Encourage the patient's contributions, provide clear explanations to empower the patient and provide them with opportunities for informed decision making.

Signposting
Can be useful during data gathering and clinical management. It provides structure for both doctor and patient and facilitates organisation of the consultation. Signposting is especially useful if the patient has questions that require answering or there are many problems. In both situations, the GP can propose an 'agenda' based on the patient's requests and any risk the doctor may have detected.

Managing the consultation with multiple problems
Sometimes the problems may be connected or require management in parallel, e.g. a physical symptom and the psychological impact.

However, should the problems not be connected, remain organised, risk assess for each problem if appropriate, agree where to focus your remaining time, then signpost that you will move on to their second problem afterwards or if required in another consultation. In a recorded consultation, the examiner will stop listening after 12 minutes so in this situation, with unconnected problems, you should focus on one in the first 12 minutes, moving on to the second problem later or scheduling a further consultation. Prioritise which problem to deal with first, either because of the level of clinical risk or, if all problems are minor and there is no stand-out issue, then let the patient guide you to the problem they would most like help with today.

Consider how you come across to the patient (and in this case the examiner) when the patient mentions a symptom that you know requires time to safely explore. You appreciate that it is likely to require another consultation and therefore their comment instantly increases the demands of the 12-minute consultation. You may feel frustrated and under pressure, but you need to appear calm.

For example, the patient mentions another unrelated symptom (e.g. headaches) when you have only just started discussing their breathlessness… Phrases which may help: *'Tell me more about that.'* This gives you time to consider if they could be related (potentially a rare condition). Or *'We need to give each problem, the breathlessness and the headache, the time it deserves. Which do you feel we need to concentrate on today'* or *'first today?'*

Risk assess! Ask them the red flags for both problems. You can then reassure the patient and yourself why you have not explored it further today. If the patient is being vague, you may need to say, *'I need to ask you some specific questions* (red flags) *that will help me to rule out* (e.g.) *a blood clot on the lung.'* Then thank and reassure. If the patient selects the symptom which you feel is less important, e.g. tension-type headache over breast lump or haematemesis, explain your concern to the patient and ask their permission to redirect the consultation. *'Would you mind if we discuss … first as I am concerned about …?'*

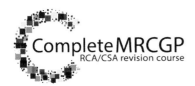

Structure and Time Management

Structuring management plans

Here is a possible sequence to the latter half of a consultation. Remember in order to also demonstrate IPS, after each point invite the patient into the consultation by pausing or asking for their thoughts.

1. **State your impression or differential diagnosis.** We refer to this as the pause or pivotal moment. You share your thoughts with the patient and allow them a moment to absorb this information. The consultation has just swung from data gathering to clinical management. Practise the moment of providing a differential diagnosis. Consider our mantra, 'Common things are common but what mustn't I miss?' You may find yourself in the following scenarios:

    i. You believe the worrying diagnosis (e.g. cancer) is low on your differential list, but still needs to be ruled out or discussed, to address the patient's fears or the potential 'elephant in the room'. Use a reassuring tone, explaining your suspected diagnosis. Use negative red flags to explain why you do not suspect cancer. Explain the importance of your recommendation of appropriate investigations to confirm your hypothesis and rule out a diagnosis of cancer.

    ii. The cancer is at the top of your differential list. You therefore combine your breaking bad news skills as you sensitively approach the seriousness of the unconfirmed problem and the need for the 2WW referral.

2. **Pause.** Give the patient space to think or talk. If required, encourage their understanding or response to this information.

3. **Explanation (and empower).** Consider incorporating the patient's ICE here so you haven't just asked it, you've woven their answers into the explanation to ensure you've addressed each health belief in turn. Ask yourself, do I agree or disagree with the patient's thoughts? Do I share the patient's worries or can I reassure? Are the patient's expectations realistic or not?

4. **Empathy** – could be useful here if not already expressed.

5. **'My recommendation is**… what are your thoughts?'

6. **Aim for five appropriate things that you offer the patient, to ensure you have provided a comprehensive management plan, which may include:**

    • **Investigations** that may be needed to include or exclude differentials. Consider resources and avoid over-investigating. It is good practice to explain which tests you believe are necessary and why, and this also tells the examiner.

    • **Medications.** Use the 5-point process – what is the drug, why you're recommending it, how to take it, potential problems and ask them how they feel about this option. Leave the issuing of the prescription until the end. Avoid spending time with your head in a BNF.

    • **Referral**. The logistics of the referral process and what to expect from the referral.

    • **General health.** If there is more than one problem, or coexisting health issues, these should also be considered in the plan. Discuss what the patient can do through health promotion, disease prevention and rehabilitation (empowerment). A practical way of helping you do this is to consider the three dimensions of self, GP and others:

        • This is what you can do….
        • This is what I, the GP can do.
        • This is what 'others' can do. Others may include other professionals, family members, exercises, resources such as educational material or leaflets.

    • **Specifics** (who/what/when/how), when describing appropriate **follow-up** and a **safety net**.

Demonstrating Interpersonal Skills

Softening and normalising

If questions are asked with a formulaic approach, this does not demonstrate the doctor's ability to tailor the questions to the information the patient has already provided. There are approaches that can soften questions and explanations and demonstrate that you are sensitive to the impact of your conclusions. We encourage you to find what feels authentic to you.

Here are some examples:

'Sometimes when people come to see me with acne, it is affecting their life in different ways. I'm wondering if this is the case for you?' (Normalising)

'What is it like living with this pain every day?'

'Some people find x helpful.'

'If I were to suggest you had x diagnosis, what are your thoughts?'

How the patient should feel when they leave the consultation

- Understood.
- With a diagnosis or, as a minimum, the most likely of a list of differentials.
- With an understanding of the plan and the specific actions required.
- Empowered – the doctor's knowledge and involved in the plan.
- Feeling positive and reassured, if not from the diagnosis, from the comfort of receiving excellent care with a feeling of trust in their doctor.

Child consultation

When possible, involve the child using language appropriate to their stage of development. Try to involve both child's and parent's perspective, including ICE, where possible. The parent may wish to lead, but keep asking and including the child.

Connection and empathy

Rapport means connection with the patient. We avoid using the words 'I understand' and instead suggest you explore and absorb all the information and reflect it back to silently show 'I hear you.'

When we teach how to demonstrate empathy, we suggest using the following equation of challenges to reflect back to the patient:

$$\text{Problem} + \text{Fears} + \text{Social context} = \text{What you sense (e.g. really tough, exhausting)}$$

Follow this with silence for a response.

Another very useful question is 'What is it like living with x?'

The good news is, the more challenging the case, the greater the opportunity to shine and overcome the challenge if you have skills to connect and empathise with the patient.

A useful approach to elicit the psychosocial context may include:

'Tell me about you … who is in your life?'

'Do you work?' Then either 'What does work involve?' or 'What do you do in a typical day?'

'What is home like at the moment?'

'Have there been challenges or changes in your life?'

'How have you been feeling with all this going on?'

Demonstrating Interpersonal Skills

Avoiding assumptions

Avoid leading questions and make no assumptions. Trainees may fall into this trap when they believe a patient has told them their concern. We recommend ensuring you acknowledge the concern you have heard and then ask explicitly about further thoughts, fears and hopes. If medication is potentially linked to the problem, don't assume compliance – ask about medication taken and doses.

Detecting and responding to verbal cues

A doctor on the phone has to work harder with their senses. Without visual cues, the doctor's ears need to be listening out for hesitations, changes and emotions within the voice. Remember we encourage you to make a statement about what you 'Sense' (see FOCUS model).

Although we would encourage you to submit some cases which are face-to-face, as we believe it is easier to connect with your patient in person, there is no statistical difference between candidates' scores received for the different formats – face-to-face, video or telephone consultations.

Verbal cues are often expressions that are unique to the person, e.g. a description of a feeling (subjective rather than fact). A person may also be mentioned. Be curious, repeat the word they have chosen to find out why. Use your senses to also detect the non-verbal cues. Imagine you are opening a hyperlink to another page of information. Cues will be obvious to an examiner, but will require you to be receptive, remembering that you are in the 'hot seat' with the combined challenge of receiving, processing and formatting information. Do not fear that you may go down 'the wrong track', you will soon discover if your hunch was wrong. Cues are clues to help us treat both the problem and the person.

Avoid 'parking' cues. We often hear doctors say 'We'll come back to that' or state afterwards that they did hear the cue but feared going down the wrong path if they explored further. In a simulated case, an actor would normally 'shut you down' rather than fabricate an answer, if you were on the wrong track. In your consultation room, however, we appreciate that anything can happen when patients are trying to be helpful. Remember, though, that if you hear a potential cue, the examiner will have heard it too! If you don't explore it, firstly, you may miss important information but also you are not demonstrating to the examiner that you have heard the cue. Always remember that cues are clues – for example leading you to important psychosocial factors which are affecting the patient.

Try asking or repeating a word the patient has used, but in the style of asking a question – perhaps using a rising inflexion in your voice. In a recorded consultation, you may then discover vital information. Should the patient take you down the garden path with a problem that you conclude is not relevant, don't submit the case. But do ensure that you submit some cases which demonstrate your cue-spotting skills.

Explanations of grey areas

There are many grey areas in general practice! Holding the responsibility of potential risk is the greatest challenge. Diagnoses and management plans don't always fit into boxes or guidelines. Use present AND absent red flags to help direct your management or possible referral. It is usually helpful to verbalise the dilemma: if you explain clearly why the symptom or your management suggestion is atypical, the standard guidance and what details have led to your uncertainty. Both the patient and the examiner will then understand your thought process.

The doctor should present their rationale using evidence-based medicine and provide a recommendation to empower the patient and enable an informed decision. Consider if you can tailor your recommendation to the important features of the history. Be organised with your explanations and ensure you are clear. Remember that patients shouldn't be expected to advise the doctor and some patients do not want the emotional burden of making a decision. A doctor should never share responsibility solely to make themselves feel better or lighten the weight of responsibility.

Examinations

For the RCA, clinical examination is no longer a mandatory requirement. Despite this, there will of course be occasions when it is clinically appropriate to examine the patient in a face-to face consultation, or describe a planned examination in a remote consultation.

Examination advice for the RCA

- Do not stop or edit the tape – it must be a continuous recording.
- Ensure that any examination or description of a planned examination is solely to enhance patient care and for the benefit of the patient, not the examiner. Don't over-describe. The patient needs to know what you will examine and why and how it will help, but they don't need endless details.
- You may well LOSE marks in IPS and CM if the examiner thinks your description of a proposed examination was unnecessary or inappropriate, perhaps confusing the patient or increasing anxiety.
- In a face-to-face consultation, if you do physically examine a patient, be sure you are doing so solely for the patient's benefit and that the examination is not in any way 'staged' for the examiner. The RCGP rightly takes a very dim view of this – there may be serious sanctions such as referral to your Responsible Officer (RO).
- If the patient has sent you a photograph, describe what you see using plain English.
- At all times, ensure that your descriptions are free of acronyms and jargon.

Performing an examination is generally part of data gathering and usually occurs before you state your diagnosis. In a remote consultation, however, you may well share your impression of the diagnosis **before** discussing an examination, explaining why the examination is important to confirm your diagnosis.

Before any examination, obtain informed consent:

- Explain what you would like to examine and the details (take your pulse, listen to your chest).
- Offer a chaperone if appropriate.
- Explain how it will be helpful to establish a diagnosis, e.g. what it may rule in or out.
- Confirm their consent.

During the examination talk the patient through the examination (see our final chapter for examples of how to do this). Take the patient to the examination couch unless it is more helpful for them to be sitting in a chair (e.g. thyroid examination). Examine behind the curtain for recorded consultations if removing clothing, or if the examination requires exposure in the 'swimsuit area', i.e. swim shorts for males ≥2 years, bikini area for females ≥2 years and nappy area for an under 2-year-old. Remember that you will score no marks for the consultation if there is any exposure of this kind.

After the examination sit the patient down and present your findings sensitively. In their eyes you may be breaking bad news. Explain what this means – did you confirm your diagnosis?

How to describe a proposed examination during a telephone consultation when you plan to bring the patient in for an examination

One approach, checking the patient's response at each step:

- Explain what you would like to examine and why.
- Discuss your differential diagnosis.
- Explain how the examination may confirm your impression or rule in/out different hypotheses.
- If at this point the patient clearly wants to know more: 'If the examination findings support the diagnosis of x, my recommendation at this point would be… Other options may be… If, however, the examination supports the diagnosis of y, my suggestions would be…'
- 'A heads up about other suggestions I have, for you to be considering before I see you…'

Patients Returning for Test Results

In this book, there are some cases focused on patients returning for test results, which is a normal part of everyday general practice. The pitfall here is that your data gathering may be curtailed or even non-existent, scoring no marks in this domain. Be careful to ensure that you take an appropriate and comprehensive history from the patient and that you have collected the information yourself rather than summarising what a colleague may have already discussed. This ensures that you give yourself the opportunity to score good marks. For recorded consultation assessments, you may find it easier to demonstrate data-gathering skills in new presentations rather than follow-up consultations. Although follow-ups can be done well, there are potential pitfalls and you may have to critique your data gathering with additional care.

When a patient consults for a test result, remember the following:

- If you are choosing this consultation as part of recorded assessment, ensure you actually elicit new information in the consultation. Summarising what you know so far does not demonstrate data gathering skills.
- Put the investigation into context – why was the test performed and what is the patient expecting?
- There is a balance between keeping the patient waiting for the result but ensuring you have enough information to help you put the result in to appropriate context. You may need to collect some information, provide the results, but then remember to return to complete your data gathering.
- The result may be the 'elephant' in the room. Any result could be perceived by the patient as 'bad news', so ensure you leave enough time to manage their feelings and expectations.
- If the patient tries to move the consultation ahead before you are ready, pressing you for the result, acknowledge their anxiety or question (e.g. blood test or diagnosis of CKD3) straight away and give them the answer. However, do not be pressured into immediately discussing management options and go back to the beginning to take the history. It is difficult to score marks for data gathering if you gather no data!

E.g. *'I can see you are keen for your results. The tests show your blood sugar is raised. I'm sure you are keen to know what that means and where we go from here but, to put this result into the context of you, I need to find out more about you and go through your medical history in more detail first please.'*

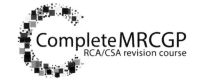

Vulnerable Patients

For vulnerable and elderly patients, the following questions may be helpful when speaking to them (e.g. teenager or a person with a learning disability):

- **Home**. Relationship with family. Any stress within the home? Are they a carer? Do they have any responsibilities (e.g. work to financially support the family)?
- **School**. Exams, stress with workload, relationships with friends and bullying?
- **Mental health**. Low self-esteem, mood, anxiety, self-harm or suicidal thoughts? Social habits. Alcohol, drugs and smoking?
- **Physical health**. Eating, exercise habits and weight changes?
- **Sexual health**. Are they sexually active? Who with? Discuss pregnancy and STI risk.
- **Vulnerability and abuse**. Which adults do they have time alone with? Use of social media? Does anyone upset them, hurt them, make them feel uncomfortable or encourage them to have sex?

And when consulting with an elderly patient:

- **ADL.** Shopping, meals, cleaning, washing.
- **Medications**. Compliance, polypharmacy and risks (e.g. anticholinergic burden). Is a dosette needed?
- **Memory and mood.**
- **Risk**. Leaving hob on/locking doors/wandering/falls/driving.
- **Isolation/loneliness**. When do they feel vulnerable?
- **Weight**. Are clothes loose? Are they eating?
- **Continence and bowels.**
- **Risk factors for AKI.**

COVID-19

The submission to publishers of *The Complete MRCGP Casebook* was during the rollout of the coronavirus vaccination programme in 2021. At the time of writing, we therefore do not know what the future holds regarding the incidence of coronavirus cases and the impact that coronavirus variants may have. We hope the majority of patients presenting with a cough will have been vaccinated and by the time the book reaches your eyes the incidence of this disease will have fallen. We have therefore decided not to include coronavirus in our list of differential diagnoses, e.g. for a cough. However, we urge you to do so if appropriate and also advise the patient of the correct management, should the ongoing situation require this consideration.

Phrasing Your Questions

Top Tips – when a case feels like it's going wrong or you have a brain freeze

There are ways to pull it back. Can you summarise ICE or is there information you need?

'What's been on your mind?' is a good rescue question, especially if the patient has an unusual opening gambit.

'What's most important to you today?' Or ask the patient if they have any questions.

'I'm going to be making suggestions but was there anything you were particularly hoping for.'

Can you empathise to reconnect with the patient?

Be honest. *'I feel I am not being as helpful as I could be. I'm sorry. Can we take a step back to… and go from there so I can do a better job?'*

FILTER

Clarify understanding… *'Can you describe what you mean by wheeze/palpitations?'*

Instead of the vague *'Tell me more'* which will waste time because the patient will ask you what you want to know, try… *'Tell me the story of (your headaches) from the beginning.'*

If they've had the symptom for months… *'What prompted you to come now?'*

Checking past history and investigations, etc.… *'As we haven't met before, would you mind telling me…'*

OPPORTUNITY

ICE, ICE, ICE. It is vital that these questions come across naturally and do not sound robotic, so consider what information you need. To understand a patient and, more importantly, for the patient to feel understood, the GP needs to explore their health belief; this means their thought process, what is on their mind, their fear, where this has come from, their experience of a 'similar' problem or what they have read, who they have spoken to and why they have presented now. Be curious! Being aware of what is going through the patient's mind will lead you towards what they may be assuming you will do.

If you miss any (or all!) of this, the patient may feel you have missed something crucial and they may be right.

Try variations on the following:

'Is there anything else that you have been wondering?'

'Have you had any thoughts about what might be causing your symptoms?'

'Is there anything else that has been on your mind?'

'Do you have any thoughts about what you would like us to do?'

'What is important to you when considering what needs to be done today?'

CONTEXT

Summarise ICE… this is a powerful way to show you understand the patient.

'Am I on the right track?' or *'Have I understood you correctly so far?'*

ICE and empathy help address health beliefs in the context of the individual.

Incorporate their thoughts and experience together with their background (social history) to help you empathise.

'I can see that because your father had… you are worried this could be… and because you are under a lot of pressure at the moment with… I can see you have been frightened for what this could mean and had fears of… but I think what is going on here is….'

Phrasing Your Questions

The result

The patient feels listened to and understood.

The doctor understands the patient's health beliefs and can educate.

You can only genuinely empathise when you have explored the person's experience.

Another example…

'*You wonder if it could be … I see why you would think that, especially when you have experience of/have gone through/your mother has gone through… However, my impression is… which may have been caused by…*'

You could use the positive and negative red flags to help you here, explaining why you have reached that conclusion. Check experience (understanding): '*What do you know about…?*' Then educate: '*… is… and the course of the problem is often…*'

UNITE

An inappropriate request… '*Have you thought about any problems with that?*'

'*Let's think through this together.*'

Acknowledge their expectation before giving options. '*I understand you were hoping for… My suggestion of options for where we go from here include …*'

Remember you are the doctor… '*My recommendation would be…*'

But include the patient in the management plan, especially if there are a couple of appropriate options…

'*What do you believe is best for you?*' or '*What is your preference?*'

Structure your management plan within your mind. What can the patient do (e.g. lifestyle factors), what can I do (e.g. medications, referrals), what can others do (e.g. primary care team, charities, friends/family, specialists).

If you give a patient an information leaflet, you must explain its contents.

SAFETY

Remember to be specific: '*If you find your child is not able to keep down fluids, they are at risk of becoming dehydrated, so please contact us at the surgery. If the surgery is closed, dial 111 to speak to an on-call GP.*' '*If you find you require more than 10 puffs of your inhaler over four hours, please call the surgery. However, if you require 10 puffs at the same time, please call 999.*'

The motivational interview

Fantastic for health promotion cases…

'*How is your general health do you think?*'

'*What could be improved?*'

'*Do you want… to change?*'

'*Do you feel confident you can change…?*'

'*How could you improve…?*'

'*What challenges might you encounter with this?*'

'*How could you overcome these obstacles?*'

'*What steps do you think you may take?*'

'*In what time frame should this change happen?*'

'*When do you want to meet again to discuss this?*'

Jargon Switch

Consider the patient in front of you. You may need to change your language.

You may decide to tell your revision partner to tap their pen on the table whenever you use jargon.

For example…

'2-week wait'	An urgent referral where you should be seen by the hospital doctor within 2 weeks
'Abdomen'	Tummy
'Acute'	New symptom
'Benign'	Harmless
'Cervix'	The neck of the womb
'Chronic'	Symptoms you have had a long time
'Cyst'	Fluid-filled lump that is usually harmless
'DNA'	The genetic information passed down from our parents
'ECG'	Test where we put stickers on the chest to see a tracing of the heart, which we call an ECG
'Fracture'	Broken bone
'Inflammation'	Swelling/redness
'Observations'	Heart rate and blood pressure
'Over the counter'	From the pharmacy
'Positive/negative'	Test result. Avoid using this term and explain exactly what the test shows. Patients may believe positive means good, negative means bad which may not actually be the case! 'Clear' can often be used to describe a normal result, e.g. your chest X-ray was clear, your urine sample was clear.
'Ultrasound'	Jelly scan called an ultrasound
'Vital signs'	Heart rate and blood pressure

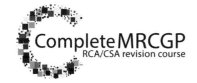
CompleteMRCGP
RCA/CSA revision course

Resitting the Exam

What may have gone wrong…

Poor choice of recorded cases – lack of complexity. With a straightforward case, you do not give yourself the opportunity to demonstrate that you have the clinical skills needed for independent UK practice and so, no matter how well you perform the case, you will not gain top marks and may not even 'pass' that case.

Too slow – you do not reach the management plan. Practise your time management. You may be spending too long on data gathering (for fear of missing something) but to the detriment of the rest of your case. Go back to basics, e.g. lots of well chosen open questions that help you obtain lots of information quickly, then group the red flags.

The doctor talks more than the patient. Consider the many opportunities within the FOCUS model to **engage** and involve your patient before giving information.

Missing the subtleties of the consultation and hence the reason for the patient's attendance.

The patient leaves not knowing their diagnosis. Even if you are unsure, you should reassure yourself and the patient with the important negatives, e.g. why it is not a sinister/serious diagnosis. Or share what you need to do to rule out the sinister/serious and how you will get more information (tests, referral, and colleague advice) to make the diagnosis.

You do not produce a safe management plan. Ask yourself if this is because you have not considered the sinister/serious causes of their symptoms.

Poor organisation. Disorganised consultations don't give a good impression to the examiner or patient.

Try to stick to your consultation model structure and don't jump between the story, the examination and information giving.

Still not sure? Think about the basics – whose needs aren't being met?

PATIENT NEEDS
- Wants to feel understood.
- Wants to share everything they have noticed.
    - To offload anxiety and hand over responsibility.
    - Just in case it may be relevant.
- Wants to know what is wrong.
- Wants reassurance.
- Wants to get better.

DOCTOR AGENDA
- To know the facts that will change the management.
- Wants clear information so they can make the diagnosis and plan… within 10–12 minutes.
- Wants to fix the problem.
- Wants the patient to be satisfied with the plan.

Nuts and Bolts for RCA

The RCGP produces an excellent online handbook for candidates and, if you are submitting recordings, you should read this carefully, more than once, as it is a live document and does change relatively frequently. At the time of writing:

- You need to submit 13 cases online.
- These can be face-to-face, video, audio or any combination of these.
- Six population groups/clinical areas MUST be covered:
  - Child ≤16 years
  - Maternal or reproductive health problem
  - Older adult ≥65 years
  - An acute problem that requires investigation or treatment
  - A chronic problem
  - A mental health problem
- There must be a minimum of two examinations or explanations of examinations.
- Other than this, cases can be drawn from any areas of the curriculum but no more than two consultations from any one area.
- The cases are marked individually by 13 different examiners and may be double marked. This reduces any possible risk of bias or 'halo/horns' effect.
- Scoring – there are nine marks per case and a maximum achievable score of 117 if single marked and 234 if double marked.
- The pass mark is determined by the scores of borderline candidates, so is not a fixed number, but is likely to be around 143–144, if double marked.

Preparing for the RCA

You can submit cases that have been recorded up to 182 days before the results date, so it makes sense to start early. This will also make sure that you are familiar with your recording equipment so you don't find that a wonderful consultation cannot be submitted because of avoidable technical problems. You may also find you have some that can be saved for submission, and this will ease any pressure to find cases in the run up to the final date.

Note that you cannot 'double dip': a case that has been used for a CBD, COT or other workplace-based assessment, cannot also be submitted for the RCA.

Be organised and have a system so you can easily identify, over time, which are your stronger cases for submission. Consider using a grid, across the curriculum and including all mandatory cases where you perhaps colour code or self-score titles of recordings. Then, when it comes to deciding which cases to submit, you can identify your preferred recordings more easily.

Consent and confidentiality

It is essential to have appropriate consent from the patient – this needs to be requested beforehand and checked afterwards. Patients are of course free to withdraw their consent. Some platforms such as FourteenFish automatically build in consent, therefore you don't need to verbally repeat it. Whichever recording method you use, it is your responsibility to check that this is in place for every patient consultation and upload evidence of this with your workbook.

Should another person appear, seen or heard, within a recording, they must have also given consent.

Case Selection and Demonstrating Skills of Managing Complexity

Case selection

Whether submitting recorded consultations or being given simulated cases within the exam, you need to demonstrate competence across the curriculum and especially within the mandatory population groups/clinical areas.

If you are submitting recorded consultations, we recommend that first presentations provide a greater opportunity to demonstrate your data gathering. See also our advice within the section 'Patients returning for test results'.

Choosing the right cases to demonstrate your skills is critical. The list of mandatory cases does change periodically so keep checking the RCGP website. When recording you will have a range of consultations which fit into these criteria, so which should you choose? How do you maximise the marks you can score? The answer to this is pitching the complexity level just right. It is possible to perform a good GP consultation which you, your trainer and the patient are happy with, but scores poorly in the assessment. You can also make life very difficult for yourself by tackling very complex cases. Too simple and you are restricting the available marks you can score. Too complex and you will struggle to complete in 12 minutes. Look for 'Goldilocks' cases – where the complexity level is just right.

Balance the combination of clinical challenge and complicating factors to provide you with the best chance of demonstrating competent skills within the given time.

Remember, the examiner can only mark what they see/hear and so you need to demonstrate your skills. You have lots of skills you can showcase: risk management, breaking bad news, negotiation, shared management, the list goes on. How do you demonstrate these?

Patients who are new to you or present with a new problem may well give you the opportunity for higher marks. Your data gathering will be broader and deeper if, from the outset, you are unfamiliar with the patient or the problem. Follow-up cases are generally less suitable, although they can be used if you consider carefully how to do this. To score well in data gathering, you must elicit NEW information. Summarising the history back to the patient is not sufficient – either in follow-up cases or in those you may have triaged earlier.

Similarly, in a case in which the patient has perhaps been on a long and complex journey with their problem already, simply discussing and following a pre-existing plan, e.g. from a consultant, is not likely to gain you marks for management. Think about 'What have I added to this case?' 'Has the patient been moved forward in their journey by your consultation?'

This is an exam to demonstrate the competent skills of an independent GP. Therefore, if the same outcome could have been achieved by the nurse minor illness clinic or practice pharmacist, don't submit it.

Look at the mark scheme to see how you can achieve the third mark, e.g. for data gathering and clinical management, your clinical approach should be focused and justifiable. For interpersonal skills, there should be a demonstration of sensitivity and empowering the patient.

How to identify suitably complex cases

First of all, consider the following areas of challenge:

- **Diagnostics** – is the diagnosis difficult to make? Is the condition inherently difficult to manage or are there lots of differentials which need to be ruled out?
- **Situation** – is the problem having a significant impact? Do the patient's personal circumstances provide a challenge or do limitations in services available provide a complication?
- **Patient** – do they have unrealistic expectations, significant worries or concerns or communication difficulties?

- **Management** – are standard guidelines or protocols unsuitable for this patient? Do the patient's individual comorbidities or polypharmacy restrict your options?

From the above you can see each provides some form of challenge, and each of these could be considered as a 'layer' or a 'dilemma' to add into the consultation. For example, a headache case may be very straightforward, but if the patient has significant worries about a brain tumour, perhaps due to prior experience, and is requesting a CT scan, this will make the case more complex. It is likely the doctor will need to be expert in discussing risk, reassurance (without inappropriate reassurance), negotiation and shared management to manage this case well. The patient's ICE may have provided extra levels of complexity to the case. Similarly, you may have a case where there is a mixture of positive and negative red flags. Your gut instinct may be that the condition is likely to be benign, but there is some nagging doubt to be addressed – or, in other words, a dilemma. How you discuss your thought process with the patient, and how you manage this risk and uncertainty, will demonstrate lots of skills.

There doesn't need to be a lot of complexity in the cases. Take the example of a UTI, something we all see very often. A young, fit, female patient with classic symptoms is unlikely to pose much of a challenge. However, an older patient with CKD, perhaps who has also become a little confused, does have complexity. You must be aware that the patient's prior conditions alter the medication you will provide and there may even be a safeguarding element to consider if the patient lives alone or a carer is struggling to cope. As long as you voice this to the patient, i.e. 'as your kidneys no longer work as well as they used to, I would recommend we choose a slightly different antibiotic from usual…' you can demonstrate that you are taking prior information into account and managing the patient safely and appropriately.

When analysing your case's potential for submission, consider if it demonstrates your ability to manage complexity. Ask yourself what makes it a suitable case. The following are examples to give you inspiration. However, there are many more potential complexities which may present to a GP.

Diagnostics
- Red flags/risk factors – were there elements of risk or red flags which muddied the picture? Have I discussed risk and/or uncertainty with the patient and explained my thought process well?

Situation
- Impact – is the problem having a significant impact on the patient and have I helped manage this in my plan?

Patient
- Was the patient vulnerable and did I consider this in my plan?
- ICE – did the patient have a false health belief, significant concerns or unrealistic expectations which I have addressed?
- Were there compliance issues which I addressed?

Management
- Did the patient's past medical history affect/restrict the options? Have I explained any deviation from standard care to the patient? Did I explain the difficulty conflicting problems pose to the patient?, e.g. heart failure and CKD.
- Did the patient's drug list pose difficulty regarding interactions? Did I voice this in my explanation/management?

If you can answer Yes to any of the above points you are likely to have a case with a suitable level of complexity and you will have had the opportunity to demonstrate GP skills.

The RCA Mark Scheme

Make sure you are familiar with the RCGP sheet 'Generic Grade Descriptors' (https://www.rcgp.org.uk/training-exams/mrcgp-exam-overview/mrcgp-recorded-consultation-assessment.aspx#marking).

Data Gathering, Technical and Assessment Skills	Clinical Management Skills	Interpersonal Skills
1a Takes a focused history to allow for a safe assessment to take place	2a Appears to make a safe and appropriate working diagnosis(es)	3a Encourages the patient's contribution, identifying and responding to cues appropriate to the consultation
1b Elicits and develops relevant new information	2b Offers appropriate and safe management options for the presenting problem	3b Explores where appropriate, patient's agenda, health beliefs and preferences
1c Rules in/out serious or significant disease	2c Where possible, makes evidence-based decisions re prescribing, referral and coordinating care with other healthcare professionals	3c Offers the opportunity to be involved in significant management decisions reaching a shared understanding
1d Considers and/or generates any appropriate diagnostic hypotheses	2d Makes appropriate use of time and resources whilst attending to risks	3d When undertaken, explains and conducts examinations with sensitivity and obtains valid consent
1e Explores where appropriate the impact and psychosocial context of the presenting problem	2e Provides realistic safety netting and follow-up instructions appropriate to the nature of the consultation	3e Provides explanations that are relevant, necessary and understandable to the patient
1f Plans, explains and where possible, performs appropriate physical/mental examinations and tests		
1g Appears to recognise the issues or priorities in the consultation		

When you look at the mark scheme, it becomes much clearer why you cannot gain high marks for simple consultations. The straightforward medication check is unlikely to gain any marks in:

1c – Rules in/out serious or significant disease.

2a – Candidate appears to make a safe and appropriate working diagnosis.

2e - Provides realistic safety netting and follow-up instructions appropriate to the nature of the consultation.

3d – When undertaken, explains and conducts examinations with sensitivity and obtains valid consent.

3e – Provides explanations that are relevant and understandable to the patient.

So, the maximum possible score for a very easy consultation may be as low as 3.

Real patients don't behave like simulated patients...

When preparing for assessment through simulated surgeries, a common issue that trainees raise is that actors don't behave like real patients – and the converse is true as well. For example, all simulated cases that form part of a consultation skills exam have an important or significant psychosocial aspect and, if you seem interested and ask, the simulator will generally readily tell you what you need. This is not always the case with real patients – and they may misinterpret or not understand questions that you ask. For example, typical questions that would normally successfully elicit ICE from a simulated patient.

'What thoughts have you had about [these symptoms]?'

'Has anything worried you about [x]?'

'Did you have anything in your mind that you were hoping I might be able to do for you?'

If these are asked in context and with rapport, any simulated patient will tell you exactly what you need to know. Many 'real' patients will respond in the same way, but some may be puzzled that you are asking or simply say *'None/nothing.'* You may need to ask again, or differently, or work hard to demonstrate that you are interested and that you care about what they say.

Real patients may also talk more, not knowing that there is a 12-minute deadline, so you may need to use skills to move them on if they are being repetitious or not answering your questions:

'John – can I just check I've got this right so far?'

'So, to recap –...'

Using a patient's name to interrupt and punctuate can be a useful way to get them to pause and listen. You can read more about this in *The Naked Consultation*, Chapter 4 – 'Building Rapport' which describes some techniques to manage a chatterbox patient.

Analysing your cases

Self-analysis of cases is essential to sort the wood from the trees – the cases that you will save, and those that you will delete. Try using the mark scheme critically. Ask your trainer to do this with you a few times to see if your own benchmark is in the right place. Remember how the mark scheme works:

0 = Unsafe, or nothing a lay person with no training couldn't do (e.g. being nice to a patient)

1 = Some skills displayed but inadequate, does not follow accepted practice, does not listen to the patient

2 = Safe but not fluent

To score a 3:

- Performance must be competent and safe AND
- There must be complexity (no 3s for easy cases)
- Data gathering and clinical management must be fluent and efficient
- You must show that you have picked up cues
- Interpersonal skills must demonstrate patient empowerment.

It is common for trainees to be overgenerous with their own ratings – be critical!

Making it easier to collect good recordings

- During the consultation, listen carefully and leave typing until the end. This takes time and the sound can be distracting. Jot a few notes by hand as reminders.
- If the patient has been triaged so you know in advance what the problem is, look up the NICE guideline or the relevant section of the BNF so you are aware of your options – BUT be very careful to then tailor any advice to the individual patient rather than giving them a mini-lecture. The examiners want to hear you put guidelines into context.
- Always remember that any description of a proposed examination should be solely for the benefit of the patient, not the examiner. An elaborate description will do little to improve the patient's understanding

of their problem and may well make them more anxious. This is likely to mean you lose marks in IPS and/or CM.

- If it's a face-to-face consultation, a good examination of something that can be done on camera (e.g. testing for carpal tunnel syndrome) will gain marks. If clothing needs to be removed (in the nappy area for children age <2, trunks area for male patients age ≥2, bikini area for female patients age ≥2), you must examine off-camera and should then make a running commentary about what you are doing. Then sit down and provide a clear explanation of your findings.
- If the patient has two problems, see if you can complete 1 in the first 12 minutes rather than trying to merge them both.

Helping your trainer to help you

It's your assessment, not your trainer's, but they can help you to perform at your best. Some discussion areas might be:

- Patient selection. Perhaps you can pick from others' triage lists?
- Timing – useful to have gaps between the 12-minute consultation slots when you are collecting your recordings.
- Ask your trainer to look through and analyse some recordings with you – BUT only those which last no longer than 12 minutes and where you think you may have scored more than 6 marks. Do not overload them or ask which you should submit.

Enough is enough!

For those who are perfectionists, it may be tempting to reject cases that are good enough, but not perfect, in order to gain a very high mark indeed. This can be time consuming and stressful. You need to pass safely, but there are no 'Distinctions' awarded for particularly high marks in the RCGP consultation assessment exams. When you have 13 cases that you are sure will each gain more than 6 marks, we suggest that you stop!

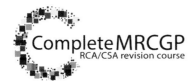
CompleteMRCGP
RCA/CSA revision course

Abbreviations

#	fracture
°C	degrees centigrade
♀	female
♂	male
1/12	1 month
20/40	20 weeks' gestation
2WW	2-week wait
3/7	3 days
αFP	α fetoprotein
2°	secondary
μg	micrograms
A&E	accident and emergency department
AA	Alcoholics Anonymous
AAA	abdominal aortic aneurysm
AAI	adrenaline autoinjector
ABC	airway, breathing, circulation
ABPI	ankle brachial pressure index
ACE	angiotensin converting enzyme
ACEI	ACE inhibitors
ACL	anterior cruciate ligament
ACR	albumin creatinine ratio
ACS	acute coronary syndrome
ACTH	adrenocorticotropic hormone
ADHD	attention deficit hyperactivity disorder
ADL	activities of daily living
AF	atrial fibrillation
AKA	also known as
AKI	acute kidney injury (acute renal failure)
AKT	applied knowledge test
ALP	alkaline phosphatase
ALT	alanine aminotransferase
AMD	age-related macular degeneration
AMS	acute mountain sickness
AMTS	abbreviated mental test score
ANA	antinuclear body
APC	adenomatous polyposis coli
APQ	alcohol problems questionnaire
APTT	activated partial thromboplastin time
ARB	angiotensin receptor blocker
AREDS2	Vitamin C 500 mg, Vitamin E 400 IU, lutein 10 mg, zeaxanthin 2 mg, zinc 25 mg and copper (cupric acid 2 mg)
AS	ankylosing spondylitis
ASD	atrial septal defect
AST	aspartate transaminase
AUDIT	alcohol use disorders identification test
AUTI	atypical urinary tract infection
AV	arteriovenous

AVSD	atrioventricular septal defect
β-blockers	beta-blockers
β-hCG	beta-human chorionic gonadotropin
B12	vitamin B12
BC	bone conduction
BCC	basal-cell carcinoma
BCG	bacillus Calmette-Guérin
BD	twice daily
BDD	bone dysmorphic disorder
BM	blood sugar level
BMD	bone mineral density
BMI	body mass index
BNF	British National Formulary
BNP	B-type natriuretic peptide
BP	blood pressure
BPH	benign prostatic hypertrophy
bpm	beats per minute
BPO	benzoyl peroxide
BPPV	benign paroxysmal positional vertigo
BRCA	breast cancer
BV	bacterial vaginosis
Ca^{2+}	calcium
CA125	cancer antigen 125
CAMHS	child and adolescent mental health services
CAPRIE	clopidogrel versus aspirin in patients at risk of ischaemic events
CBD	case-based discussion
CBT	cognitive behavioural therapy
CCB	calcium-channel blocker
CCB	coercive controlling behaviour
CCG	clinical commissioning group
CEA	carcinoembryonic antigen
CF	cystic fibrosis
CFTR	CF transmembrane conductance regulator
CHA_2DS_2-VASc	clinical prediction calculator for estimating risk of stroke in patients with AF
CHC	combined hormonal contraception
CI	contraindication(s)
CIDP	chronic inflammatory demyelinating polyneuropathy
CK	creatinine kinase
CKD	chronic kidney disease
CKS	Clinical Knowledge Summaries (NICE)
CMV	cytomegalovirus
CN	cranial nerve

CNS	central nervous system
COC/COCP	combined oral contraceptive pill
COPD	chronic obstructive pulmonary disease
COT	consultation observation tool
CPAP	continuous positive airway pressure
CPPS	chronic pelvic pain syndrome
CRB-65	confusion, respiratory rate, BP, age – assessment tool for community-acquired pneumonia
CRC	Clinical Research Council
CRP	C-reactive protein
CSA	clinical skills assessment
CT	computed tomography
CT CAP	CT chest abdomen and pelvis
CT KUB	CT kidney ureters and bladder
Cu-IUD	copper coil
CURB	confusion, urea, respiratory rate, blood pressure
CV	cardiovascular
CVA	cerebrovascular accident (stroke)
CVD	cardiovascular disease
CXR	chest X-ray
DAAT	Drug and Alcohol Action Team
DBP	diastolic blood pressure
DC	direct current
DEET	*N,N*-diethyl-meta-toluamide
DEXA	dual energy X-ray absorptiometry
DH	drug history
DHEAS	dehydroepiandrosterone sulfate
DKA	diabetic ketoacidosis
DLA	Disability Living Allowance
DM	diabetes mellitus
DMPA	depot-medroxyprogesterone acetate
DNA	did not attend (i.e., missed appointment)
DNACPR	do not attempt cardiopulmonary resuscitation
DOAC	direct oral anticoagulant
DPP4	dipeptidyl peptidase 4
DRE	digital rectal exam
DSM-IV	Diagnostic and Statistical Manual of Mental Disorders, 4th Edition
DUB	dysfunctional uterine bleeding
DV	domestic violence
DVLA	Driver and Vehicle Licensing Agency
DVT	deep vein thrombosis
EBV	Epstein–Barr virus
ECG	electrocardiography
ECHO	echocardiogram
ECP	emergency contraceptive pill

ED	erectile dysfunction
EEG	electroencephalography
eGFR	estimated glomerular filtration rate
eGFRcysC	glomerular filtration rate (eGFR) by standardised cystatin C
ELISA	enzyme-linked immunosorbent assay
ELSCS	emergency lower segment caesarean section
ENT	ear, nose and throat
ESR	erythrocyte sedimentation rate
ETP	essential thrombocytopenia
F	female
F2F	face-to-face
FAP	familial adenomatous polyposis
FBC	full blood count
FBG	fasting blood glucose
FEV1	forced expiratory volume in 1 second
FH	family history
FIT	faecal immunochemical testing
FOB	faecal occult blood
FOCUS	Filter, Opportunity, Context, Unite, Safety
FODMAPs	fermentable oligosaccharides, disaccharides, monosaccharides and polyols
FRAX	fracture risk assessment tool
FSH	follicle stimulating hormone
FSRH	Faculty of Sexual and Reproductive Healthcare
fT4	free thyroxine
FVC	forced vital capacity
g	grams
GAD	general anxiety disorder
GAD-2	general anxiety disorder 2-item
GCS	Glasgow Coma Scale
GCSE	general certificate of secondary education
GF	glandular fever
GFR	glomerular filtration rate
GGT	gamma-glutamyl transferase
GI	gastrointestinal
GI	glycaemic index
GLP	glucagon-like peptide
GMC	General Medical Council
GnRH	gonadotropin-releasing hormone
GOLD	Global Obstructive Lung Disease
GORD	gastro-oesophageal reflux disease
GP	general practitioner
GQ	gender-queer
GTN	glyceryl trinitrate
GUM	genitourinary medicine

HACE	high altitude cerebral oedema		IVF	in vitro fertilisation
HAPE	high altitude pulmonary oedema			
HAS-BLED	score for major bleeding risk		JVP	jugular venous pressure
HbA1c	glycated haemoglobin			
HbeAg/Ab	hepatitis B e antigen/antibody		K	potassium
HBsAg	hepatitis B surface antigen			
HBV DNA	hepatitis B virus deoxyribonucleic acid		LA	local anaesthetic
HCA	healthcare assistant		LABA	long-acting beta agonist
Hct	haematocrit		LAMA	long-acting muscarinic antagonist
HCU	homocystinuria		LARC	long-acting reversible contraception
HCV RNA	hepatitis C virus ribonucleic acid		LD	learning disability
HF	heart failure		LDH	lactate dehydrogenase
Hib	*Haemophilus influenzae* type B (vaccine)		LFT	liver function test
			LH	luteinising hormone
HIV	human immunodeficiency virus		LIF	left iliac fossa
HLA B27	human leukocyte antigen		LMP	last menstrual period
HMB	heavy menstrual bleeding		LMWH	low molecular weight heparin
HOCM	hypertrophic obstructive cardiomyopathy		LNG-IUS	levonorgestrel-releasing intrauterine system
HONK	hyperosmolar non-ketotic acidosis		LOC	loss of consciousness
HPV	human papillomavirus		LRTI	lower respiratory tract infection
HR	heart rate		LTOT	long-term oxygen therapy
HRT	hormone replacement therapy		LUTS	lower urinary tract symptoms
HS	heart sounds		LV	left ventricular
HSP	Henoch–Schönlein purpura			
HTN	hypertension		M	male
			m	metre
IBD	inflammatory bowel disease		M/R	modified release
IBS	inflammatory bowel syndrome		MASI	Melasma Area and Severity Index
ICD-10	International Classification of Diseases 10th Revision		MCADD	medium chain acyl-CoA dehydrogenase deficiency
ICE	ideas, concerns and expectations		MCS	multiple chemical sensitivity
ICP	intracranial pressure		MCUG	micturating cystourethrogram
ICS	inhaled corticosteroids		MDT	multidisciplinary team
ID	intellectual disability		MenC	meningitis C (vaccine)
Ig	immunoglobulin		mg	milligrams
IgG	immunoglobulin G		MI	myocardial infarction
IgM	immunoglobulin M		mL	millilitres
IHD	ischaemic heart disease		MMR	measles, mumps and rubella
IM	intramuscular		MRC	Medical Research Council
IMB	intermenstrual bleeding		MRI	magnetic resonance imaging
IMP	progesterone-only implant		MS	multiple sclerosis
INR	international normalised ratio		MSK	musculoskeletal
IPS	interpersonal skills		MSU	mid-stream urine
IPSS	International Prostate Symptom Score		MUSE	medicated urethral system for erections
IQ	intelligence quotient			
ISMN	isosorbide mononitrate			
IT	information technology		N&V	nausea and vomiting
ITU	intensive treatment unit		Na	sodium
IUD	intrauterine device (copper coil)		NAD	no abnormality detected
IUS	intrauterine system (e.g. Mirena)		NHS	National Health Service
IV	intravenous		NICE	National Institute for Health and Care Excellence
IVDU	intravenous drug use			

NIPT	non-invasive prenatal testing		PR	per rectum (rectal examination)
NKDA	no known drug allergies		PRN	as required
NOGG	National Osteoporosis Guideline Group		PSA	prostate specific antigen
			PSC	primary sclerosing cholangitis
NOK	next of kin		PSV	public service vehicle licence
NSAID	non-steroidal anti-inflammatory drug		PT	prothrombin time
NVD	normal vaginal delivery		PTH	parathyroid hormone
NYHA	New York Heart Association		PUD	peptic ulcer disease
			PV	per vaginam (vaginal examination)
OA	osteoarthritis		PVD	peripheral vascular disease
OCP	oral contraceptive pill			
OD	once daily		QDS	four times daily
O/E	on examination		QIP	quality improvement project
Ofsted	office for standards in children's education, children's services and skills		QOL	quality of life
			QRISK2	algorithm for cardiovascular disease
OGTT	oral glucose tolerance test			
OM	once in the morning		RACPC	rapid-access chest pain clinic
ON	once at night		RCA	recorded consultation assessment
OOH	out-of-hours GP		RCGP	Royal College of General Practitioners
OTC	over the counter		RCO	Royal College of Ophthalmologists
ORBIT-AF	Outcomes Registry for Better Informed Treatment of Atrial Fibrillation		RFs	risk factors
			RLQ	right lower quadrant
			RNIB	Royal National Institute of Blind People
OSA	obstructive sleep apnoea		ROM	range of movement
OSAHS	obstructive sleep apnoea/hypopnoea syndrome		RR	respiratory rate
			RUTI	recurrent urinary tract infection
OSAS	obstructive sleep apnoea syndrome		RUQ	right upper quadrant
			Rx	treatment
PA	personal assistant			
PC	presenting complaint		s/c	subcutaneous
PCB	post-coital bleeding		SABA	short acting beta agonist
PCDS	Primary Care Dermatology Society		SI	sexual intercourse
PCKD	polycystic kidney disease		SADQ	severity of alcohol dependence questionnaire
PCN	primary care network			
PCOS	polycystic ovary syndrome		Sats	oxygen saturation
PCR	protein creatinine ratio		SBP	systolic blood pressure
PCV	pneumococcal conjugate vaccine		SCC	squamous cell carcinoma
PE	pulmonary embolus		SD	standard deviation
PEF	peak expiratory flow		SGLT	sodium-glucose linked transporter
PEFR	peak expiratory flow rate		SH	social history
PERLA	pupils equal and react to light and accommodation		SHBG	sex hormone binding globulin
			SIGN	Scottish Intercollegiate Guidelines Network
PF	plantar fasciitis			
PID	pelvic inflammatory disease		SLE	systemic lupus erythematosus
PIL	patient information leaflet		SLR	straight leg raise
PIP	Personal Independence Payment		SMART	self-management and recovery training
PMB	post-menopausal bleeding			
PMH	past medical history		SNHL	sensorineural hearing loss
PN	practice nurse		SNRI	serotonin–norepinephrine reuptake inhibitors
PND	paroxysmal nocturnal dyspnoea			
POP	progesterone-only contraception pill		SOB	shortness of breath
POI	primary ovarian insufficiency		SOL	space occupying lesion
PPI	proton pump inhibitors			

SPC	summary of product characteristics	U&E	urea and electrolytes and eGFR
SSRI	selective serotonin reuptake inhibitor	UC	ulcerative colitis
STI	sexually transmitted infection	UKMEC	UK medical eligibility criteria for contraceptive use
SUFE	subluxation of the upper femoral epiphysis	UMN	upper motor neurone
SVT	supraventricular tachycardia	UO	urinary output
		UPA	ulipristal acetate
T1DM	type 1 diabetes/diabetics	UPSI	unprotected sexual intercourse
T2DM	type 2 diabetes/diabetics	URTI	upper respiratory tract infection
T4	thyroxine level	USS	ultrasound scan
TAH	total abdominal hysterectomy	UTI	urinary tract infection
TB	tuberculosis	UV	ultraviolet
TCA	tricyclic antidepressant		
TCI	to come in	VA	visual acuity
TDS	three times daily	VC	vital capacity
TENS	transcutaneous electrical nerve stimulation	vs	versus
		VTE	venous thromboembolism
TFT	thyroid function test	VZV	varicella-zoster virus
TIA	transient ischaemic attack		
TIBC	total iron binding capacity	WPBA	workplace-based assessment
TSH	thyroid stimulating hormone	WCC	white cell count
TURP	transurethral resection of the prostate	WHO	World Health Organization
TV	*Trichomonas vaginalis*		
TVUSS	transvaginal ultrasound		

Disclaimer

The information or guidance contained in this book is intended for use by medical professionals (specifically General Practitioners or General Practitioner Trainees) only and is provided strictly as a supplement to the reader's own judgement, their knowledge of the patient's medical history, relevant manufacturers' instructions and the appropriate best practice guidelines. The guidance we refer to within this book is specifically for General Practitioners based in the UK, and international readers should refer to local guidance and advice. Because of the rapid advances in medical science, any information or advice on dosages, procedures or diagnoses should be independently verified. The reader should take into account that the information within this book is only part of any guidance mentioned and is strongly urged to consult the full text of up-to-date guidance. The text is not to replace specialist advice. The reader is strongly urged to consult the relevant national drug formulary and the drug companies' and device or material manufacturers' printed instructions, and their websites, before administering or utilising any of the drugs, devices or materials mentioned in this book. This book does not indicate whether a particular treatment is appropriate or suitable for a particular individual. Ultimately, it is the sole responsibility of the medical professional to make his or her own professional judgements, so as to advise and treat patients appropriately. We do not accept any liability or responsibility for any form of loss or any decision made by the reader.

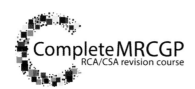
CompleteMRCGP
RCA/CSA revision course

CHAPTER 2 OVERVIEW

Allergy and Immunology

	Cases in this chapter	Within the RCGP 2020 curriculum: Allergy and Immunology	Learning points in this chapter include:
1	Angioedema	'.... understand how to take an allergy-focused clinical history and understand the differentiation of different types by appropriate testing and referral' 'Recognising and recording of food and drug sensitivities' 'Managing emergencies but supervising the ongoing management of risk factors and prescribing' 'Prescribing issues (e.g. adrenaline devices)'	Rapid assessment of potentially acutely ill patient Negotiation with parent Resuscitation Council UK guidelines
2	Venom Allergy	'Anaphylaxis' 'Venom allergy: referral and emergency management; the role of immunotherapy' 'Patient safety measures (e.g. systems to document allergies in the patient record; Medic Alert bracelet)'	Immunotherapy for venom allergy – Pharmalgen (dried bee sting powder used for desensitisation)
3	Asthma Diagnosis	'Atopy – asthma, eczema and hay fever' 'The UK has one of the highest prevalences of asthma, rhinitis and eczema. Allergy-related conditions may present in a significant number of consultations. The GP has the lead role in identifying underlying allergic symptoms that can be difficult to distinguish from the range of normality or other illness' 'Risk factors including lifestyle, socioeconomic and cultural factors' 'Diagnostic features and differential diagnosis'	Asthma diagnosis – adult and child
4	Varicella in Pregnancy	'Management of specific situations such as chickenpox in pregnancy'	Varicella in pregnancy – Risks to mother Risks to fetus Assessing 'significant exposure'
5	Occupational Allergy	'Contact allergies such as hair dye…'	Management of allergic contact dermatitis
Extra Notes	Allergy and immunology in everyday practice		Taking an allergy-focused history Management of allergy/immune conditions Common and important conditions – allergy Common and important conditions – immune disorders

CHAPTER 2 REFERENCES

Angioedema
1. NHS inform. https://www.nhsinform.scot/illnesses-and-conditions/skin-hair-and-nails/angioedema. Sep 2020.

Venom Allergy
1. NICE CKS. https://cks.nice.org.uk/insect-bites-and-stings#!scenario:1. Sep 2020.
2. Golden D.B., Moffitt J., Nicklas R.A. et al. Stinging insect hypersensitivity: a practice parameter update 2011. *J Allergy Clin Immunol* 2011; 127: 852–4.e1.
3. Eich-Wanger C., Muller U.R. Bee sting allergy in bee keepers. *Clin Exp Allergy* 1998; 28: 1292–8.
4. https://www.nice.org.uk/guidance/qs119/chapter/Quality-statement-3-Specialist-assessment-for-venom-immunotherapy. Mar 2016.
5. NICE guidance TA246. Pharmalgen for the treatment of bee and wasp venom allergy. https://www.nice.org.uk/guidance/ta246. Aug 2017.

Asthma Diagnosis
1. Pellegrino R., Viegi G., Brusasco V. et al. Interpretive strategies for lung function tests. *Eur Respir J* 2005; 26: 948–68.
2. SIGN158 British guideline on the management of asthma. Jul 2019. https://www.sign.ac.uk/media/1773/sign158-updated.pdf.
3. NICE CKS. Asthma. https://cks.nice.org.uk/asthma. May 2021.
4. NICE Guideline NG80. Asthma: diagnosis, monitoring and chronic asthma management. Mar 2021.

Varicella in Pregnancy
1. NICE CKS. Chickenpox. https://cks.nice.org.uk/chickenpox#!management. Aug 2018.
2. Royal College of Obstetricians and Gynaecologists Green Top Guideline No. 13. https://www.rcog.org.uk/en/guidelines-research-services/guidelines/gtg13/. May 2015.

Occupational Allergy
1. NICE CKS. Dermatitis – contact. https://cks.nice.org.uk/dermatitis-contact. Jul 2018.

Information taken from NICE guidelines with kind permission. Please note the guidelines change frequently and you should ALWAYS check for the latest updated guidance. Remember that NICE guidance is only applicable to patients in the UK.

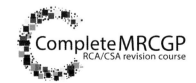

Allergy and Immunology

Doctor's Notes

Emergency walk-in patient

Patient	Joshua Middleton	11 years	M
PMH	Eczema		
Medications	Oilatum		
	Hydrocortisone		
Allergies	No information		
Consultations	Medication review. Eczema controlled. 1 year ago.		
Investigations	No information		
Household	David Middleton	46 years	M
	Angela Middleton	43 years	F
	Samantha Middleton	13 years	F

Open ☐	Hello Joshua, I'm Dr Blount. What happened? Is there anywhere else in your body that doesn't feel right? Angela, is there anything else you have noticed?
Flags ☐	Joshua, does your breathing feel different? Does it feel swollen in your mouth?
Risk ☐	Has this happened before?
O/E ☐	Because this has happened so quickly, I would like to first have a closer look at you Joshua; at the rash and swelling… now your temperature in your ear… now this will squeeze your arm… now please put your finger in this gadget… may I look in your mouth please and listen to your chest? I can see the swelling around your eyes and the rash. You are okay Joshua, but let's give you some medicine to get rid of this rash.
History ☐	What time did this happen? When did the swelling around the eyes start? Has it got worse since you left the football pitch or stayed the same? How is your eczema? Angela, does Joshua have any other medical conditions? What medicines or creams is Joshua using? Any known allergies? Who is at home? Any pets?
ICE ☐	Joshua, what do you think has caused this? Do you know why this might have happened? What did you think I may say today? What about you Angela: what has gone through your mind?
Impression ☐	Joshua, you have had an allergic reaction, most likely to the peanuts. The diagnosis is angioedema, which means swelling from the allergic reaction.
InCLudE ☐	It is frightening to hear about other people's reactions; however, Joshua is doing fine and we will keep you safe Joshua. It's helpful to know you have had training with EpiPens and we can inform the allergy team who prescribe first EpiPens. What are your thoughts Angela?
Experience☐	Have you heard of the word allergy Joshua? What do you know about it?
Explanation ☐	That's right Joshua. An allergy means your body doesn't like something. If you have an allergy you can have a rash or it can make your breathing difficult if you eat or touch the thing it doesn't like. Your friend cannot eat eggs. Lots of people have allergies. I would like you to see the allergy doctor at the hospital who will likely do tests to confirm the peanut allergy and may suggest other things you should avoid. For now, please avoid eating and touching all nuts until we know what is safe.
Empathy ☐	The reaction on your face and skin must have been very frightening and it must be worrying you that it has not gone back to normal.
Options ☐	Because Joshua's breathing has been normal, the swelling has not got worse since leaving the pitch and his body measurements are normal, I do not believe Joshua has had an anaphylactic reaction. Therefore, we could give Joshua an antihistamine and steroid tablets to take the swelling and rash down. I would expect these to work over the next few hours to a couple of days. The other option would be to go into hospital for a drip. I mention this option because, although I think it is unlikely, there is always a chance the swelling could get worse and affect the breathing.
Recommend ☐	My suggestion, if you feel comfortable with this, is starting the tablets now, staying in the surgery for the next hour to make sure the swelling does not get worse, then if all is okay go home and complete the course of tablets, but with the plan that if anything gets worse or you are worried, then go to hospital. Or do you want to go there now?
Safety net ☐	Okay, let's give you tablets. If in the meantime you feel unwell or different, or your tongue or breathing feels funny, please let me know. If, when you get home, any of these symptoms happen, call 999. If in the future you ever notice this happen again, call 999 straight away because it can happen quickly and affect your breathing.
Future ☐	We will refer Joshua to an allergy specialist. EpiPens are prescribed initially by the specialist if they feel it is necessary. Because Joshua has not had an anaphylactic reaction, they may say it is not necessary. I appreciate allergies can get worse the next time a reaction happens; however, we should be guided by their expertise because EpiPens can be dangerous. I will let them know in my referral letter that you have training to use EpiPens. What are your thoughts about the plan? Is there anything you'd like to ask or clarify?
Specifics ☐	So I'll make that referral today and if you haven't received an appointment in the next month then please let me know. Let's take you through to the treatment room and I'll keep popping in between patients to see you. If you are worried, just call for help.

Doctor's notes		Emergency walk-in patient.
		Joshua Middleton, 11 years. PMH: eczema. Medications: Oilatum and hydrocortisone.
History	**Mum**	*'Joshua was eating peanuts and he immediately came out in a rash.'*
		This has never happened before. Joshua is well and his eczema is controlled with emollients alone. He has no other allergies.
		There is no family history.
	Joshua	You were playing football and felt well.
		Afterwards your friend gave you some peanuts. This was one hour ago now.
		You can't remember if you've had peanuts before.
		Within a minute you had come out in a rash and your eyes had started to swell.
		Since then, there has been no change.
		Your lips are slightly swollen but there is no tongue swelling and your breathing feels normal.
Social	**Joshua**	You are in the first year of secondary school.
		You live with your parents and older sister.
ICE	**Mum**	You would like Joshua to have some medicine straight away.
		You've heard of a child who died from a peanut reaction and this thought frightens you.
		You would like to go home with an Epi-Pen but are happy to follow the doctor's advice.
		You are a district nurse and have had Epi-Pen training.
	Joshua	You feel scared and would like the swelling and rash to go away.
		You don't know what this is.
		Your friend has an allergy to eggs which means he can't have them.
Examination		Sats 98%. RR 18. HR 90 bpm regular. Temperature 36.8 °C. BP 106/60.
		Widespread urticarial rash. Chest clear. Mouth and tongue normal. Mild lip swelling and mild swelling of the eyelids.

Doctors are aware that anaphylaxis requires intramuscular adrenaline. However, the misuse of intramuscular adrenaline can be dangerous. When faced with a patient with swollen eyes and lips and a generalised urticarial rash, anaphylaxis is at the top of the differential diagnosis list.

Angioedema

Angioedema is a sign of a possible frightening medical emergency. Therefore, the above case of an acute IgE-mediated reaction in the haemodynamically stable patient without respiratory compromise (which is not an uncommon scenario) may be approached differently by different GPs. GPs are likely to ask themselves:

Do I need to call an ambulance?

Do I need to give intramuscular adrenaline?

Should I give hydrocortisone and chlorphenamine (IM or slow IV) or oral treatment?

Anaphylaxis is a life-threatening risk to airway, breathing and circulation. Adrenaline is required if there are signs of risk to life.

The NHS website tells us angioedema 'sometimes occurs in combination with anaphylaxis ...', which reminds us that they are two separate diagnoses.

Although many cases of angioedema get better without treatment after a few days, medication is often used.[1]

For cases of allergic and idiopathic angioedema, antihistamines and oral steroids can be used to relieve the swelling.[1]

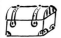

Anaphylaxis

See the **Link Hub at CompleteMRCGP.co.uk** for a useful link to anaphylaxis guidance from the Resuscitation Council (UK).

Consider keeping a printout of this in your doctor's bag for reference in real-life emergencies.

Egg allergy is a contraindication to IM influenza/MMR/yellow fever/rabies vaccines.

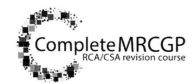

CompleteMRCGP
RCA/CSA revision course

Allergy and Immunology – 1

Doctor's Notes

Patient	Marian Harker	58 years	F
PMH	None. Recently registered with little in the medical records.		
Medications	No current medications		
Allergies	No information		
Consultations	Recent attendance at A&E with insect sting. No GP consultations for >5 years.		
Investigations	None		
Household	Jennifer Harker	59 years	F

Open☐	I'm really sorry to hear that. Please can you tell me more about what happened.
History ☐	Can you describe how the stings looked and felt? And what happened at the hospital?
Flags ☐	Did your throat or mouth swell? Any difficulty breathing or swallowing? Did you feel dizzy or pass out? Did you feel nauseous or vomit?
Sense ☐	I sense this was a very frightening experience for you. What went through your mind?
ICE ☐	You asked for a referral for desensitisation. Was there anything else you hoped for today?
Curious ☐	What's brought you to this area? What was your previous work? Who is at home with you? What does your partner think? You seem to have had few contacts with health professionals in the past – have you had any screening checks, for example BP checks or tests for diabetes or cardiovascular disease?
Impact ☐	How has this affected how you feel about your health? And about your move to the country?
Risk ☐	Have you or any close family member had severe reactions to stings or bites in the past?
Impression ☐	It sounds as if you had a significant reaction to the stings, although not a life-threatening reaction, which we call anaphylaxis.
Experience ☐	Have you known or heard of anyone who has had a really serious reaction to bee stings?
Explanation☐	Everyone gets stung from time to time but for most people it is a painful nuisance that soon gets better. Because you had a significant reaction, you were right to go to A&E.
InCludE ☐	If there were 100 people like you, between 5 and 10 of them might have a more severe reaction, called anaphylaxis, on a future occasion, although 90–95 would not.
Recommend ☐	So I agree that we should refer you to an allergy specialist and I will do this today. I would also recommend an Alert bracelet and I will add an alert to your records.
Options ☐	I will contact the specialist to find out if they advise that we should prescribe an adrenaline injector pen for you to carry with you whilst waiting for the appointment. If so, we will prescribe this and our PN will teach you how to use it. At the hospital they may do some blood tests to find out how susceptible you are to a future bad reaction. Especially because you are so worried about stings, they may suggest desensitisation with a series of injections of a weak bee venom called Pharmalgen. There's an initial course of injections and then maintenance injections for up to 3 years. It is usually very effective and would keep you safe from reacting to bee stings so badly in the future. How do you feel about this?
Empathy☐	It can be difficult adjusting to a new way of life – leaving a job that you loved, moving away from city life and sometimes the countryside can feel isolating. Getting stung by the bees and the long trip to hospital must have felt very different from living and working in London.
Empower ☐	There are many local social groups and activities and I am sure there would be some that would interest you. They would offer opportunities for you to get more involved in the local area and make some contacts and friends. Some groups would no doubt be really pleased to make use of your financial experience and expertise. There are details of local groups on our notice board in the waiting room.
Future ☐	I would also like to arrange some routine blood tests to check for diabetes and heart disease as well as kidney function. How do you feel about doing this? We could meet again in a week or two to see how you are feeling and go through the results together. Is there anything that you'd like to ask?
Specifics ☐	I'll make the referral today and I'll contact you if the allergy team advise an adrenaline pen. Please make an appointment for a blood test, then to see me a week later. Also contact our secretary if you have not received your appointment letter within the next month.
Safety net ☐	For the moment, I would suggest leaving the beekeeping to your partner. If you do get stung, it is more likely than not that you will have the same sort of reaction as last time which is unpleasant but not serious but, if your throat or mouth swell, you feel dizzy or vomit, then call 999.

Doctor's notes	Marian Harker, 58 years. No PMH. No medication. Recent attendance at A&E with insect stings.
How to act	Anxious.
PC	*'I was stung by a swarm of bees last week – my arms were so swollen. Do you think I can be referred for desensitisation?'*
History	A week ago, you and your partner were checking the hives on your smallholding when the bees started to swarm. This was very frightening. They got inside your protective clothing and you were stung a few times. You were scared but not SOB and your throat and mouth did not swell. You felt a bit queasy but did not vomit. Over the next 24–48 hours, the stings on your arms swelled up to 10 cm across, and were red, swollen and itchy. Your arms were so bad your partner drove you to A&E. This was a 20-mile drive away and you were very anxious on the journey there. At the hospital, they gave you antihistamines and advised you to see your GP to ask if you needed to be referred to an allergy clinic. You were occasionally stung by bees as a child but did not have a bad reaction. No one you know, or in your family, has had anaphylaxis or a severe reaction to stings.
Social	You were made redundant from your job as a banker in the City a few months ago but received a good pay-off and have recently moved with your partner to a smallholding in the countryside where you keep chickens, goats and bees. You were unsure about this move, but your partner was persuasive. You have a good relationship with her. You have always been nervous about bees, but your partner had kept them in the past and was keen that you both get involved in the good life. But – *'I think it was a mistake moving here'* – you feel isolated and lonely. You miss your old way of life. The last straw was that A&E was so far away, when you used to have a large teaching hospital down the road, although you never needed it. Your health has always been excellent and you have rarely consulted doctors in the past. You have ignored invitations for well person screening checks. But now – *'I feel so far away from hospital help if I need it.'*
ICE	You are anxious about getting stung again and have read in the newspaper about people dying from bee stings. *'Am I going to die?'* You would like to stop beekeeping but your partner is keen to carry on and wonders if desensitisation would help. You have never smoked and drink minimal alcohol.
Examination	Nil to find.

Most insect stings result in minor local reactions, lasting a few hours to several days but some people will develop large local skin reactions, or potentially life-threatening systemic reactions including anaphylaxis.

If systemic reaction is suspected or stings are on the face or mucous membranes, risking airway obstruction or compromised vision, arrange immediate admission. Treat angioedema or anaphylaxis whilst awaiting emergency transfer.[1]

Consider referral to allergy specialist if large local reaction or previous systemic reaction.

Whilst patients are waiting to be referred to an allergy specialist:

1. Seek interim advice, e.g. about self-administered adrenaline pens.

2. Provide information about medical bracelets.

3. Discuss avoidance methods.

Explain what to expect at their appointment, e.g.

1. Skin or antibody testing.

2. Consideration of venom immunotherapy.

If at 24–48 hours after a bite or sting the area of erythema or oedema has developed to be >10 cm, discuss with an allergy specialist because there is an increased chance of systemic reaction.[2]

Tell patients that an AAI is not a substitute for emergency medical care – if patients have used it, they should seek emergency medical attention.[2]

Beekeepers are strongly exposed to honeybee stings and therefore at an increased risk to develop IgE-mediated allergy to bee venom. Venom immunotherapy is effective and well tolerated and the majority of allergic beekeepers can continue beekeeping successfully under the protection of venom immunotherapy.[3]

Specialist Pharmalgen venom immunotherapy is an option for IgE-mediated bee and wasp venom reactions if severe or high risk.[4,5]

General

Many consultations have an opportunity for general health promotion. This 58-year-old woman is new to the practice and does not appear to have had screening for cardiovascular disease or diabetes. She has made a significant career move from a high-flying job in the City to a rural area where she knows few people. This may lead to an adjustment reaction, including anxiety.

Doctor's Notes

Patient	Peter Atkins	12 years	M
PMH	Eczema		
	Hay fever		
	Viral-induced wheeze		
Medications	Current medication:	Oilatum cream PRN	
	Previous medication:	Salbutamol	
		Spacer	
		Loratadine	
Allergies	No information		
Consultations	3 months ago. Mild eczema – emollients encouraged.		
Investigations	No information		
Household	Rachel Atkins	40 years	F
	Alexander Atkins	40 years	M

Open ☐	How can I help today? Tell me more about this cough, Peter. Have you had any problems with your breathing? Are you well at the moment or are you poorly?
Flags ☐	Have you had a cold? Any phlegm? Does it hurt anywhere? Has Peter had a fever? When with your friends, do you run around like they do or do you need to stop more?
Risk ☐	I see Peter has hay fever and eczema. Has any family member had asthma at all?
History ☐	Any other medical history? Any complications when Peter was born? Or any other medical problems afterwards? And the medicines that he takes at the moment? Any allergies?
Curious ☐	Peter was previously given an inhaler; how often does he use it? When did he last use it?
ICE ☐	Why was Peter given the inhalers? Peter, why do you think you have a cough? You could be right Peter; why do you think that? Tell me more about your friend, Peter. Has John ever struggled with his breathing? Are you worried about your breathing too? And Mum, what do you think is causing this cough? Are you worried about anything in particular? And, today, what did you hope we would do at this stage?
Sense ☐	I can see you are both concerned.
O/E ☐	I would like to examine your chest, Peter, if you can lift up your shirt. Now I will check your pulse and oxygen level with this gadget. Have you seen this blowing tube (peak flow meter) before? I will demonstrate. Can you try?
Summary ☐	So, Peter, you have been coughing for months but otherwise feel fine. You are worried you could have asthma like John and would like an inhaler. Mum, you have had many doctors tell you this is viral wheeze not asthma and therefore thought his cough must be an infection because he has not been wheezy. Is that correct?
Impression ☐	Viral wheeze is very common as a young child but you are older now, Peter, and you feel your breathing isn't as good as your friends' so it sounds like this is asthma. Coughing can be the only symptom but, Peter, you think you have been wheezy at times too. Asthma is also more likely if you suffer with hay fever or eczema.
Experience ☐	Do you know what asthma is, Peter? What about you, Mum?
Explanation ☐	Asthma is where the air tubes in your lungs become narrow so there is less space for the air.
Empathy ☐	I appreciate this may worry you, Peter, after you have seen John go to hospital.
InCludE ☐	We can use inhalers to prevent breathing from getting worse. This may be why John has his inhalers before playing. If you do have asthma, it may be different to John's asthma.
Options ☐	Firstly, to confirm the diagnosis our nurse can do some special blowing tests. May I give you a new blue inhaler, called salbutamol, and a spacer to use it with? You simply put the spacer in your mouth and spray the inhaler into the other end. Take five normal breaths for each puff. It's likely you will need a brown preventer inhaler too, but ideally we should do the tests before starting this so the results are more accurate. What do you think? Use the blue inhaler whenever you feel wheezy, breathless or cough a lot. If this is happening frequently, call me and we can discuss starting the brown inhaler straightaway.
Empower ☐	I'll write the details down in your asthma plan. Peter, can you keep a diary of each time you need your blue inhaler? Any questions so far?
Future ☐	Please see me again in 2 weeks so we can discuss your blowing tests and potentially start the brown inhaler. At this point, I can update your asthma action plan so it tells you what to do if your asthma gets worse.
Safety net ☐	If you ever struggle with your breathing and need more than 10 puffs of your inhaler at once, then this is when an ambulance should be called, but I don't expect that to happen before we meet again. In the past you may have given Peter ibuprofen Mum? We advise only paracetamol for anyone with asthma and speaking to a doctor if required, because ibuprofen can make asthma worse.
Specifics ☐	Please can you arrange to see the nurse as soon as you can, keep your diary and arrange to see me a week later? So, can you tell me, Peter, when you should ask for help? Yes, and if at any time your breathing gets worse, you should see a doctor. That's a lot of information that I've given you today. I'll write down instructions and leave it with the nurse to give you. Any questions?

Doctor's notes		Peter Atkins, 12 years. PMH: eczema, hay fever and viral-induced wheeze.
		Medications: Oilatum cream. Past medication: salbutamol with spacer, loratadine.
How to act		Peter is quiet and requires encouragement from the doctor to speak.
		Mum speaks first if the question is not directed to Peter.
PC		*'Doctor, Peter keeps coughing every night and it has been going on for months.'*
History	**Mum**	Peter has had a dry cough for months, especially at night and it keeps you awake.
		He is not breathless and has no sputum or fever. He has not complained of pain.
		He is well and you have not heard him wheeze.
		Peter has had no other symptoms for months.
		Peter has not used his (very) old inhaler for months, since winter.
		He was born around his due date and was always well. Immunisations are up to date.
		No FH. Eczema is mild and controlled with Oilatum.
History	**Peter**	You are *'fine'*. When you play football, you feel wheezy and out of breath.
		Your friends can run around for longer. You have had no pain, no fever and no sputum.
		You do not have an itchy nose at present. You recall that you used to use an inhaler.
Social		No pets. Only child. Parents both smoke *'but not in the house'*.
ICE	**Mum**	You know that Peter has *'viral wheeze'* after multiple doctors have said so.
		You are not worried but have brought him here today for antibiotics.
		Peter has not told you about his friend John or his worries about asthma.
	Peter	If asked, you think the diagnosis is *'asthma'*.
		Mention *'John has asthma too'*.
		John is your friend and, if asked about John, tell the doctor that once John *'went to hospital because he couldn't play football'*. He was using his inhaler a lot that day and was sat on the football pitch with it.
		You think you need the inhaler like John. You don't want to have to go to hospital too. If asked what you understand about asthma, say *'John uses his inhaler before he plays football.'*
Examination		Height 140 cm. Peak flow 270 L/min. Chest clear and no wheeze. HS normal. Sats 98%. RR 17. HR 80 bpm regular. Apyrexial.

Symptoms　　　Wheeze, cough, difficulty breathing and chest tightness. Especially at night or in the morning. Variability in symptoms.

Triggers　　　　Exertion, weather, emotion, pets and hay fever. Screen for occupational asthma. Minus features which lower the probability: only with a cold, no interval symptoms, moist cough, dizziness, light-headedness, no wheeze. Also in adults: smoking history, cardiac disease, voice change.

Atopy　　　　　PMH or FH of hay fever, eczema or asthma.

Medications　　Symptoms with aspirin, NSAID or beta-blockers.

Examination　　May be normal or findings may include expiratory polyphonic wheeze reduced air entry low saturations and reduced peak flow levels.

Investigations　Spirometry and fractional exhaled nitric oxide testing are first-line tests.

　　　　　　　　If ongoing uncertainty, peak expiratory flow variability testing for 2–4 weeks.

　　　　　　　　Specialist tests may include bronchial challenge test with histamine or methacholine

　　　　　　　　For older children and adults, history alone should not provide a diagnosis.

Supporting the diagnosis

Symptoms.
- Positive FeNO level (positive levels according to age). Check prior to initiation of inhaled corticosteroids when possible (FeNO suppressed by IHCS).
- Obstructive spirometry (FEV1/FVC <0.7) and positive bronchodilator reversibility (increase from FEV1 baseline of >12% (child) and in adults also 200 mL volume increase).
- Positive peak flow variability (>20%).

Criteria and algorithms for diagnosis according to age are available at NICE.

Also, for treatment see the SIGN asthma management guidance[2] and Chapter 19 – Respiratory Health.

Initiating treatment

Use clinical judgement to start treatment at the appropriate step according to symptom severity.

If two or fewer episodes wheeze a week, PRN salbutamol and 'Consider monitored initiation of treatment with very-low-dose to low-dose ICS'.[2]

If three or more episodes of wheeze a week or waking at night with symptoms, or symptoms not controlled with SABA, consider moving to the next step on the SIGN pharmacological management ladder.[2]

Refer if diagnosis is uncertain, suspected occupational asthma, asthma is uncontrolled and following poor response to treatment.

Making a diagnosis in a child <5 years

Under 5s　　　　Will be based on symptoms, judgement and observation following treatment.

Once >5 years　Repeat tests every 6–12 months until a diagnosis is confirmed.

Education　　　Provide a written asthma self-management plan, training regarding use of inhalers and information about how to seek help. Provide regular monitoring according to symptoms and control.

Allergy　　　　Consider allergy screening. Skin prick testing or IgE tests may be helpful.

Doctor's Notes

Patient	Jennifer Adeyemi	27 years	F
PMH	No information		
Medications	No current medications		
Allergies	No information		
Consultations	Nil		
Investigations	No information		
Household	Amire Adeyemi	29 years	M

Open ☐	How can I help? That must be worrying for you. What has led you to worry about chickenpox?
Experience ☐	Have you come across chickenpox in pregnancy before?
ICE ☐	What has been going through your mind about getting chickenpox whilst pregnant? Were you hoping I would do anything particular today?
Risk/history ☐	When were you spending time with your niece? Would you say you were in close contact with her for more than 15 minutes? When did she become unwell? Do you know if you have had chickenpox before? How are you feeling? Have you felt unwell? How has your pregnancy been going so far? Is this your first baby?
Sense ☐	I sense you are very worried about miscarriage. Is this something you have experienced before? Or did you have difficulty conceiving?
Impact ☐	How have these worries been affecting you?
Curious ☐	How are things at home? Who do you live with? Are you working at the moment?
SummarICE ☐	So you are 16 weeks' pregnant with your first baby and have been exposed to chickenpox after babysitting your niece. You struggled to conceive so are frightened about any complications, in particular you are worrying about miscarriage or the baby being born with deformities. You don't think you have had chickenpox before but aren't certain. You hoped I could arrange a test and possibly a scan to check the baby is okay.
Empathy ☐	I can tell this baby is very precious so this must be very worrying for you.
Explanation ☐	Chickenpox in pregnancy can cause problems, particularly if the mother hasn't had it before. The chickenpox may make the mother more poorly with complications like pneumonia and rarely the baby can be affected. However, because you have come in so quickly, there are things we can do to try to prevent you getting chickenpox and therefore prevent your baby being affected.
Include ICE ☐	Reassuringly, even in babies which are affected by the chickenpox virus, very few develop problems like deformity and there doesn't appear to be an increased risk of miscarriage.
Recommend ☐	Usually the first step would be to check the mother's immunity to chickenpox – we do this with a simple blood test. If it comes back that you are immune (which means your body has fought chickenpox before and is ready to act) then we don't need to worry – it is unlikely you will develop chickenpox again. If you aren't immune, we would refer you to the hospital to have a special injection which protects you. This should help prevent the infection developing. How does this sound? As long as you don't develop any symptoms, you shouldn't need any extra scans.
Future ☐	You will get your detailed scan as normal in 4 weeks. If you did develop a rash or symptoms you would need to let us know straight away. We would then need to discuss giving you a medication to help treat the virus with a specialist. The rash usually develops about 2 weeks after exposure so although this seems a while to wait to see if you have caught it, it does give us time to act.
Empower ☐	To help protect yourself, it would be a good idea to avoid seeing your niece until all her spots have scabbed over. This usually takes about 5 days. It's important to avoid anyone with shingles too, which is caused by the same virus.
Specifics ☐	So I will ask our nurse to squeeze you in for the blood test this morning. The lab should send us the result in the next 48 hours. I will call you then to explain the next step. Is there anything that I can clarify or explain in more detail for you?
Safety net ☐	In the meantime, if you feel unwell with a fever, flu-like symptoms or develop a rash, please get in touch straight away.

Doctor's notes	Jennifer Adeyemi, 27 years.
How to act	Anxious.
PC	*'I'm worried I may have caught chickenpox from my niece. I'm 16 weeks' pregnant.'*
History	You are 16 weeks' pregnant. Two days ago, you were babysitting your 2-year-old niece. You spent the whole day together and were playing together on the floor a lot. Your sister-in-law has called this morning to say your niece has come out in a chickenpox rash. You don't know if you have had chickenpox or not, but are aware it can be harmful to babies. You want to know what to do – will the baby be okay? You are anxious about the pregnancy because you struggled to conceive. You are worried the baby may be deformed if affected by chickenpox or that it may even cause a miscarriage. So far you have had an uneventful pregnancy – all seemed well at the dating scan. You feel well at present and haven't noticed any symptoms.
Social	You moved to the UK from Nigeria when you were 18. You came to the UK to study History and English Literature. You met your now husband at a Nigerian Students Society dinner at university. You are very happy and have a good relationship with your husband. You got married 5 years ago. You were keen to start a family straight away but have struggled to conceive so your current (first) pregnancy is very precious to you. Your husband grew up in the UK and has a lot of family around. They are supportive. You do not smoke or drink. You are currently not working. Since your research role at the university came to an end you have been a housewife. Your husband works in pharmaceuticals and so has a little medical knowledge. He encouraged you to come and get checked out.
ICE	Ideas: you have probably caught chickenpox from your niece.
	Concerns: your baby may be harmed or you may have a miscarriage. You worry your child may have deformities; you don't know how you would cope with a disabled child.
	Expectations: you hope the doctor can do a test and maybe even arrange a scan to check the baby is okay. You would like to know how quickly the rash will come out if you have caught chickenpox.

Varicella in pregnancy[1]

Varicella in pregnancy can be serious with consequences to both mother and baby. In Europe, most women have been exposed to chickenpox and so are less likely to be seronegative, whereas women from the tropics and subtropics have a higher chance of being seronegative. A clear history of previous chickenpox infection is reassuring. If there is doubt, a blood test for VZV IgG can be done to check immunity.

Risk to mother:

- Severe infection resulting in increased risk of pneumonia, hepatitis, encephalitis and even death.

Risk to fetus:

- Scarring of skin, eye and limb deformity, neurological problems, e.g. intellectual disability, microcephaly.
- Even in infected fetuses, the risk of fetal varicella syndrome is small, although it has been reported to occur in gestations from 3 to 28 weeks.
- Post-exposure prophylaxis in seronegative women is protective to the fetus.
- There is no apparent link to miscarriage in the first trimester.

What is significant exposure? Take into account *type of varicella rash (e.g. exposed lesions), timing of exposure (e.g. between 48 hours prior to onset of rash to crusting of lesions)* and *closeness (e.g. in the same room for 15 minutes).*[1]

Management[2]

- Clear history of previous infection or proven immunity on testing – reassure.
- No previous history of chickenpox or doubt – check VZV IgG (if result available within 48 hours).
- If seronegative or unable to get result within 48 hours discuss with specialist about immunoglobulin prophylaxis.
- If seropositive – can reassure.
- If chickenpox develops, discuss treatment with a specialist.

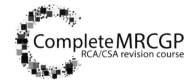

Doctor's Notes

Patient	Lacey Archer	21 years	F
PMH	No information		
Medications	No current medications		
Allergies	No information		
Consultations	Nil		
Investigations	No information		
Household	No information		

Open ☐	How can I help? I'm sorry you are having problems. What difficulties are you having with your hands? You mentioned a placement – where is this?
Sense ☐	I sense you seem worried about the rash; how has it been affecting you?
ICE ☐	Have you had any thoughts about the cause of the rash? What worries have you had about it? Have you had any thoughts about what I may be able to do to help?
History ☐	When did you first notice the rash? What does your role at the salon involve? How quickly does the rash come on? Does it itch? Is it sore? Have you noticed a rash anywhere else? Have you noticed any blisters? Has the skin been oozing at all?
Risk ☐	Do you or any family members have a history of skin problems? Do you suffer with asthma or hay fever? Do any family members have asthma or allergies?
Experience ☐	Have you come across anyone else with similar problems, perhaps at the salon?
Curious ☐	Have you spoken to your college about the problem? Or anyone at the salon? Why not?
Summary ☐	You have recently started a hairdressing placement in a salon and found your hands becoming itchy and sore a day after you have been there. You wonder if it is from washing up the hair dye pots and worry it may be work-related because you love hairdressing and don't want to have to give it up. You hoped I could give you a cream to make it better.
Empathy ☐	It must be worrying to feel your skin may force you to give up your passion.
Impression ☐	Looking at the picture I can see areas of dryness and redness on your hands and it appears you have a condition called contact dermatitis.
Experience ☐	Have you come across this term?
Explanation ☐	This is a condition in which the skin becomes sore due to touching a chemical. This can sometimes be caused by the chemical causing irritation directly or sometimes the body can be allergic to the chemical. Because your rash has been coming on a day or two later and it is very itchy, I think you may have the allergy type. This would also fit with your personal and family history of allergy. Allergy to hair dye is quite common, so you may be right that this is the cause.
Options ☐	It is treatable, but avoiding the chemical is really important.
Empower ☐	Can you think of a way that you could avoid touching the dye? Could you wear gloves? Could you speak to your tutor or mentor? Hair dye allergy is common so I suspect they will have come across it before.
Recommend ☐	Other things that can help are moisturising creams called emollients. It's important to put these on frequently to prevent the skin drying out. You can also use the creams instead of soap when washing because soap can also make the rash worse. Because the rash is quite angry, I would also suggest applying some steroid cream, called Eumovate, every night for a week. Steroid creams should be used in moderation because they can cause skin thinning and be absorbed into the body over time but, when required, steroid creams are helpful. What are your thoughts? Do you remember your sister using emollients and steroids for her eczema? You need to put two fingertips worth of steroid on each hand at night. Allow this to soak in, then apply the emollient on top – this is called Doublebase. Unfortunately, it can take many weeks for this rash to settle, but it will get better with time.
Future ☐	It would be great if we could speak again in about 4 weeks to see how the rash is settling. Could you send another photo then for us to look at together? Perhaps you could speak with your tutor in the meantime to explain about your allergy?
Specifics ☐	So I'm going to prescribe you the deep moisturising and a steroid cream – I'll send this through to the pharmacy for you to collect. Please can you book a convenient follow-up appointment with me. Any questions?
Safety net ☐	If the rash doesn't improve with the week's course of steroid or at any time you notice it become more painful, red or weepy, please come and see us straight away because it may be infected. Also, should the rash spread, please come to see us.

Patient's Story

Occupational Allergy

Doctor's notes	Lacey Archer, 21 years. No other information.
How to act	Concerned.
PC	*'It's my hands – I'm really struggling with this rash since I started my placement.'*
History	You are a 21-year-old hairdressing student who has just started her first placement in a salon. To help out, you have been washing out hair dye bowls for the qualified hairdressers but have noticed irritation to your hands. At first you thought it was due to washing your hands so often, and perhaps because of the cold weather, but now you aren't so sure. The rash tends to appear a day or two after you have been touching hair dye so you didn't make the link straight away. Usually, the following day you notice a strong itch, then the skin becomes red and can crack. This can happen at weekends and on college days when you aren't in the salon. You have tried E45, which soothes the skin a little, but it's getting worse. You haven't tried wearing gloves at work because no one else does and you were embarrassed to ask. You have started wearing gloves when you go out, more to hide your hands because the skin is no longer recovering before you go back to the salon.
	Your mum has asthma and your sister had terrible eczema as a child, but this has improved as she has grown up. You do get bad hay fever in summer but manage this with over-the-counter medication. You haven't suffered with your skin before.
Social	You have just moved into your own flat with a fellow hairdressing student. You are happy at home and happy with your course. You have done really well in the theory parts of the course.
ICE	You are starting to wonder if the chemicals you touch at work are causing the symptoms because when you went on holiday for 2 weeks your hands seemed better. But because the symptoms tend to appear a day or two later you weren't sure if this could be related. You are worried that if you can't do what other hairdressers do you will have to quit your course. This makes you upset because you love what you do. You hope the doctor can give you a cream which will help.
Examination findings	See photograph.

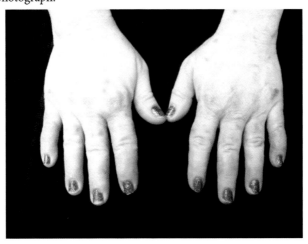

Reproduced from *Clinical Handbook of Contact Dermatitis* (2015), CRC Press. With thanks to Michael P. Sheehan, Monica Huynh, Michael Chung, Matthew Zirwas and Steven R. Feldman.

Allergic contact dermatitis[1]

Allergic contact dermatitis is a type IV (delayed) hypersensitivity reaction which can occur on repeated exposure to an allergen. Common allergens include hair dye, cosmetics, nail varnish, metals such as nickel and cobalt (often found in jewellery), plants, rubber and cement. Therefore, occupations such as floristry, hairdressing, catering and those handling metal have a higher incidence.

There is an overlap in presentation, and often causation, with irritant contact dermatitis. This is caused by direct irritation rather than an allergy. It can be difficult to distinguish between the two and the conditions may coexist.

With allergic contact dermatitis there is often a delay of more than 24 hours before the symptoms appear. Itching is more predominant than in irritant contact dermatitis. You may get symptoms in areas of the body not directly exposed to the allergen.

Management[1]

Removal of the allergen is key. It may take 8–12 weeks of allergen avoidance before the dermatitis settles. Frequent and liberal use of emollients is required, and topical steroid may be needed – the strength requires depends on the severity of the rash. Sometimes antibiotics are required if there is superadded infection.

When removal of the allergen is not possible, advise use of gloves, although these should be removed frequently to prevent sweating. Hands should be washed with soap substitute because water alone or with soap can exacerbate the rash.

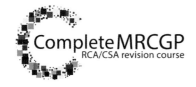

Allergic conditions are becoming more common so may present in many consultations. Anaphylaxis is life threatening. Learn how to manage it in primary care. Also:

Taking an allergy-focused history

- When and how did symptoms start?
- Symptoms – oral, e.g. tongue swelling/tingling lips?
- Triggers?
- Getting worse on each exposure?
- Family history of allergy/atopy.
- Patient health belief.

Management of allergy immune conditions

- Investigation, e.g. patch test, skin prick, blood tests, challenge testing.
- Acute management – doses of adrenaline for different ages.
- Ongoing management – adrenaline devices, shared management plans (e.g. with school).
- Alert bracelets.
- Appropriate documentation of allergies in GP notes.

Common and important conditions to be aware of: allergy

- Anaphylaxis including doses of adrenaline.
- Autoimmune conditions in primary care.
- Drug allergies and their mechanisms.
- Food allergies including milk allergy.
- Occupational allergies (latex, hair dye, metals, plants).
- Pollen food syndrome.
- Types of allergic reaction – immediate, delayed, possible mechanisms.
- Venom allergy.

Common and important conditions to be aware of: immune disorders

- Immune deficiency states, e.g. HIV, chemotherapy, inherited.
- Antibiotic use and immunisation of people with immune deficiency.
- Interpreting antibody results, e.g. chickenpox in pregnancy, rubella, hepatitis B and C.
- Immunisation schedule for children.
- Immunisations for occupational medicine, e.g. health workers.
- Needlestick injuries – risks of hepatitis B and C and management.
- Kaposi's sarcoma.
- Transplant medicine (heart, lung, liver, kidney, cornea).
- Indications for and consequences of transplantation, e.g. immunosuppression.

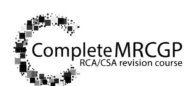

Cardiovascular Health

	Cases in this chapter	Within the RCGP 2020 curriculum: Cardiovascular Health	Learning points in this chapter include:
1	Chest Pain of Recent Onset	'Risk factors for coronary heart disease' 'Manage cardiovascular emergencies in primary care'	Differential diagnosis of chest pain NICE Guideline CG95. Recent-onset chest pain of cardiac origin: assessment and diagnosis. November 2016
2	Heart Failure	'Monitor and manage the care of patients with long-term cardiovascular conditions such as...chronic heart failure'	NICE Guideline CG187. Heart failure: diagnosis and management. October 2014 NICE Guideline NG106. Chronic heart failure in adults: diagnosis and management September 2018
3	Atrial Fibrillation	'Monitor and manage the care of patients with long-term cardiovascular conditions such as.... atrial fibrillation'	NICE CKS https://cks.nice.org.uk/atrial-fibrillation May 2021
4	Hypertension	'Consider involving the patient in self-monitoring and self-management' 'Advise your patients appropriately regarding lifestyle interventions'	NICE Guideline NG136. Hypertension in adults: diagnosis and management. August 2019
5	Angina	'Demonstrate an understanding of the importance of risk factors, including chronic kidney disease, in the diagnosis and management of cardiovascular problems'	NICE Guideline CG126. Stable angina: management. August 2016
Extra Notes	Managing the Stroke Risk in Atrial Fibrillation		CHA_2DS_2VASc ORBIT-AF DOACs
	Hypertension		Referral to cardiology White coat HTN Resistant HTN

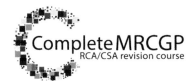

CHAPTER 3 REFERENCES

Chest Pain of Recent Onset
1. NICE Guideline CG95. Recent-onset chest pain of cardiac origin: assessment and diagnosis. Nov 2016.

Heart Failure
1. NICE Guideline NG106. Chronic heart failure in adults: management. Sep 2018.
2. NICE Guideline CG187. Acute heart failure – diagnosis and management. Oct 2014.
3. Heart.org. Classes of Heart Failure. https://www.heart.org/en/health-topics/heart-failure/what-is-heart-failure/classes-of-heart-failure. Oct 2020.

Atrial Fibrillation
1. http://patient.info/doctor/atrial-fibrillation-pro. May 2021.
2. NICE Guideline NG196. Atrial fibrillation: diagnosis and management. Jun 2021. Patient decision aid.
3. NICE CKS. Atrial Fibrillation. http://cks.nice.org.uk/atrial-fibrillation#!scenario. May 2021.

Hypertension
1. He F.J., Li J., MacGregor G. Effect of longer term modest salt reduction on blood pressure. Cochrane systematic review and meta-analysis of randomised trials. *BMJ* 2013; 346: f1325.
2. NICE Guideline NG136. Hypertension in adults: diagnosis and management. Aug 2019.
3. Whelton P.K., Carey R.M., Aronow W.S. et al. ACC/AHA/AAPA/ABC/ACPM/AGS/APhA/ASH/ASPC/NMA/PCNA Guideline for the Prevention, Detection, Evaluation, and Management of High Blood Pressure in Adults: Executive Summary: A Report of the American College of Cardiology/American Heart Association Task Force on Clinical Practice Guidelines. Circulation 2018; 138: e426–e483.
4. NICE Guideline NG28. Type 2 diabetes in adults: management. Dec 2020.
5. https://www.nice.org.uk/guidance/ng17/chapter/1-recommendations. Dec 2020.
6. NICE Guideline CG82. Chronic kidney disease in adults: assessment and management. Jan 2015.

Angina
1. NICE Guideline CG126. Stable angina: management. Aug 2016.
2. http://patient.info/doctor/stable-angina-pro. Accessed 4 August 2021.
3. NICE Guideline CG94. Unstable angina and NSTEMI: early management. Nov 2013.
4. Bosch J., Lonn E., Pogue J. et al. Long-term effects of ramipril on cardiovascular events and on diabetes: results of the HOPE study extension. *Circulation* 2005; 112: 1339–46.

Managing the Stroke Risk in Atrial Fibrillation
1. NICE Guideline NG196. Atrial fibrillation: diagnosis and management. Jun 2021.
2. https://www.practical-haemostasis.com. Risk assessment algorithms: atrial fibrillation and the risk of bleeding.
3. NICE CKS. Atrial Fibrillation. http://cks.nice.org.uk/atrial-fibrillation#!scenario. May 2021.

Useful Resource
https://www.mdcalc.com/orbit-bleeding-risk-score-atrial-fibrillation for an online tool to calculate the ORBIT-AF score.

Hypertension
1. NICE Guideline NG136. Hypertension in adults: diagnosis and management. Aug 2019.
2. Beckett N., Peters R., Fletcher A.E. et al. Treatment of hypertension in patients 80 years of age or older. *N Engl J Med* 2008; 358: 1887-98.

Information taken from NICE guidelines with kind permission. Please note the guidelines change frequently and you should ALWAYS check for the latest updated guidance. Remember that NICE guidance is only applicable to patients in the UK.

Doctor's Notes

Patient	Mary Jones	45 years	F
PMH	New patient questionnaire: smoker, BMI 40.2, three children. No further information.		
Medications	No information		
Allergies	No information		
Consultations	No information		
Investigations	No information		
Household	No household members registered		

Open ☐	Please tell me more about the pain, from when you first noticed it until now. How did it start? Please describe the pain to me? And tell me about any other symptoms.
Flags ☐	What are you doing when the pain comes on? Do you feel sick, sweaty or short of breath? Have you injured your neck? Any headache? Any weakness or tingling in the arms?
Risk ☐	Do you suffer with raised BP or cholesterol? Has a family member under the age of 65 had a problem with their heart? Do you smoke?
History ☐	Do you have any other medical conditions? Or take any medications?
ICE ☐	What do you think might be going on? I'll be explaining my recommendations today. Apart from prescribing co-codamol, was there anything else that you were hoping I would do today? What has been on your mind about this pain? Any other worries?
Impact ☐	Has this pain stopped you from doing anything?
Sense ☐	I'm sorry that I have kept you waiting. I can see that you are in a rush; however, I am concerned about your pain.
O/E ☐	May I examine your BP in both arms, pulse and heart rate, take your temperature and listen to your heart please?
Summary ☐	So you've had this pain a few times, initially when quite active, but this time it started whilst you were resting. It has now been present for 30 minutes in your chest and neck and you feel nauseous and sweaty.
Impression ☐	I am concerned that this pain is from your heart (pause); this could be a heart attack.
Explanation ☐	A heart attack is where a vessel to the heart becomes blocked and the lack of blood flow causes the pain.
InCludE ☐	I see why you thought it was a neck problem. However, pain from your heart is commonly felt in the neck.
Empathy ☐	I appreciate this is very frightening and completely unexpected.
Recommend ☐	I'd like to take you through to our treatment room where we can do a heart tracing called an ECG. I'm going to ask the receptionist to call an ambulance. I appreciate this sounds frightening, although if the pain is coming from your heart it is treatable. But we must not delay this treatment. I'd like to give you an aspirin tablet to help with the blood flow.
Empower ☐	I appreciate you need to go to your son. However, I must tell you what is at risk here. You need to go to the hospital now otherwise your life could be in danger.
Options ☐	I'm sorry. Do you have anyone our receptionist can call? Your husband? We will keep a close eye on you and have you seen by hospital staff straight away.
Future ☐	At the hospital I expect they will do a blood test and they may take you to have a procedure which looks at the vessels to the heart. Do you have any questions? Sometimes when people are new to an area, they can feel isolated. I'd really like to catch up with you and see how you are.
Specifics ☐	When you are discharged from the hospital, please make an appointment to see me so that we can discuss what has happened, make sure your medication is up to date and answer any questions you might have.
Safety net ☐	I expect the hospital doctors will treat your heart to prevent this from happening again. However, if you ever notice similar symptoms again – feeling breathless or in pain – then call 999.

Doctor's notes	Mary Jones, 45 years. New patient. BMI 40.2. Smoker. Three children.
How to act	You are in a rush. Tell the doctor this as he/she is running late.
	You want to reassure the doctor it's just a pulled neck.
PC	*'Doctor, I've got a pain in my neck.'*
History	The pain in the upper left chest and neck has now been present for 30 minutes. You had not rushed here and this time it started 5 minutes after you arrived at the surgery.
	It feels like something is pressing. You feel nauseous, sweaty and slightly SOB. You can't think of anything that takes it away. It just comes and goes but you think movement makes it worse because whenever you are doing something it comes on.
	You also had the same pain 2 days ago when you were in the garden, but it went away after 5–10 minutes when you rested.
	You have had this pain a few times in the past 2 weeks.
	For example, when running upstairs or watching television.
	Your old GP gave you co-codamol for back pain so you would like this for your neck.
	Your father died when you were a child due to his heart.
Social	Mother of three. You have moved areas as your husband has been relocated. You have not found a job and used to work in a local tea room. Your husband works in the building supplies industry. You smoke 10 a day. You drink alcohol rarely.
ICE	You believe you have pulled your neck. You have not made any connection with the heart.
	You would like a prescription for co-codamol and you will return another time if the doctor suggests anything else.
	You can't go to hospital now. You have to go and watch your son in a school play.
	You would just like the codeine. However, when the doctor explains the seriousness of the problem, you become upset and agree.
Examination	HS normal. HR 124 bpm regular. Sats 97%. RR 18. BP 130/80 in both arms.
	Temperature 36.5 °C.
	No neck or cervical spine tenderness and full range of movement.

Beware: cardiac pain at radiation sites + nausea/vomiting/sweating especially in women/elderly/diabetics.

Do they need to go to hospital today?

Yes, if history of ACS within 72 hours[1], or if the patient shows signs of acute decompensation or other complications, or if clinical judgement concludes a troponin level is required.

Otherwise refer to RACPC.

Do I need to call for an ambulance?

Yes, if current chest pain and consider in all possible ACS.

Always refer to full guidance.

Differential diagnosis

ACS:	Pain >10 minutes or increasing frequency or onset with less activity or at rest.
Dissection:	Sudden tearing pain radiating to the back between the scapulas.
Pericarditis:	Sharp, relieved by sitting forward ± radiation, fever, cough and arthralgia.
Acute heart failure:	Orthopnoea and breathlessness.
Arrhythmias:	Associated with palpitations and syncope.
PE:	SOB, tachycardia, hypoxia, ± haemoptysis ± leg swelling± risk factors for VTE.
Pneumothorax:	Risk factors include injury, tall male and COPD.
Pneumonia:	SOB, fever, purulent sputum, cough ± pleuritic pain. Check the CRB65 score.
GORD/PUD:	Belching, reflux and sharp/burning pain ± melaena.
MSK causes:	From Tietze's, costochondritis or rib fracture. Recent activity, tender.
Anxiety:	Tight chest, tingling in fingers, feeling of needing to breathe.
Referred thoracic pain:	Back pain with possible back pain red flags.
When to give oxygen?	Sats <94% and not at risk of carbon dioxide retention (aim for 94–98%).
	Sats <88% and with COPD history (aim for 88–92%).

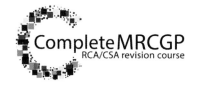

CompleteMRCGP
RCA/CSA revision course

Cardiovascular Health – 1

Doctor's Notes

Patient	Brendon Phillips 74 years M
PMH	Irritable bowel syndrome
	Barrett's oesophagus
	Severe mitral valve regurgitation
	Heart failure
	Essential hypertension
Medications	Bisoprolol 1.25 mg
	Ramipril 2. 5 mg
	Furosemide 40 mg
Allergies	NKDA
Consultations	6 months ago for ankle oedema: GP prescribed 40 mg furosemide OD.
Investigations	1 year ago:
	Echo: ejection fraction 55%, severe mitral valve regurgitation.
	ECG: sinus rhythm 70 bpm.
	Bloods: FBC, U&E, LFT, TFT, HbA1c, lipids – all normal.
	Chest X-ray: mild pulmonary congestion, cardiomegaly.
Household	No household members registered

Open ☐	What have you noticed about your breathing? When does this affect you? How is your breathing with exercise? At night? Anything else you have noticed? How quickly has it changed?
Flags ☐	Any chest pain? Do you feel your heart beating in an unusual way? Coughing? Phlegm or blood? Whistling in your chest? Swelling or pain in your ankles/legs? Weight loss? Fever or sweats? How many pillows do you sleep with? Do you suddenly feel breathless at night?
Risk ☐	Any heart or breathing problems or blood clots in the family? Have you smoked? Or drank much alcohol? Have you travelled or been off your feet recently? Any exposure to asbestos or animals?
History ☐	Tell me about your medical history? How do you take your medicines? How do you spend your days. Is anyone else at home? Do you enjoy anything?
Impact ☐	How is this affecting you? What other changes have you had to make? How is your mood?
Sense ☐	I sense you feel quite concerned about this change in health.
ICE ☐	What do you think is causing the problem? Is there anything you have been worried about? I'll be making many suggestions, but did you have any particular help in mind?
Curious ☐	When you say damaged, what have other doctors explained? What have you read?
O/E ☐	I would like to bring you in to examine you: your hands, BP, pulse, oxygen level, breathing rate, temperature, listen to your heart and lungs, the veins in your neck, feel your tummy and look at your legs. Would that be okay? Are you free to come in at 3 p.m? I'll talk through what I think is going on so you can be considering your options before we meet.
Summary ☐	To summarise, you were prescribed medication for your heart a year ago, but over the past 4 months your breathing has worsened causing worry about your heart.
Impression ☐	We know you have a leaky valve that affects your heart. Your BP is slightly raised and this may be putting additional strain on the heart. I believe it is your heart that is causing your breathlessness and swollen ankles. What are your thoughts?
Explanation ☐	The mitral valve is in the left side of the heart, which receives blood from the lungs and pumps blood to the body. Your valve doesn't close fully, causing blood to leak backwards. The term heart failure has a frightening name but is a common condition where the heart doesn't pump efficiently. Fluid often gathers in legs and lungs. Do you have any questions?
Empathy ☐	Connecting what you have read and heard from your mother, and with a diagnosis which sounds scary and not being able to walk your dog, it sounds like this has been tough? (Pause)
InCludE ☐	You're right; rheumatic fever may have caused it. Being told your heart is not right will give you a feeling of doom and fear. Let's talk options to improve your heart.
Recommend ☐	Firstly, up-to-date blood tests would be helpful, e.g. to check anaemia isn't contributing to breathlessness, and your kidneys are coping with the water tablet, and I'd like to increase your ramipril to 5 mg as this can help both the BP and the heart. However, we will need a further kidney blood test 2 weeks later to check your kidneys are happy. How does this sound? Also, an up-to-date ECG can check the heart rhythm is okay. Is that also possible? Then I would like to put all this information together and ask the cardiologist to see you. I would expect them to make further changes to medications and talk to you about surgical options. How would you feel about seeing the cardiologist?
Specifics ☐	So, today you are coming in to see me at 3 p.m. When you get here, please ask reception to book you in for a blood test and ECG, followed by a call with me to discuss those results. I will then write to cardiology.
Safety net ☐	I do not expect this to happen but, if you ever suddenly feel very breathless or get chest pain, you need to call 999. If your symptoms change or worsen whilst you are waiting to speak to me again, seek help through us or 111. Do you have any questions?
Include ICE ☐	Together we can make this problem much better for you and you'll have some options to choose from, so stay positive if you can. I'll see you at 3 p.m.

Patient's Story

Doctor's notes Brendon Phillips, 74 years. PMH: IBS, Barrett's oesophagus, severe mitral valve regurgitation, heart failure, essential hypertension. Medications: bisoprolol 1.25 mg, ramipril 2.5 mg, furosemide 40 mg.

How to act Concerned for your health.

PC *'My breathing is not very good doctor.'*

History You used to enjoy hiking but, 18 months ago, you noticed you could not manage the same strenuous walks. You had tests and the doctor had said you needed medication to help with the flow through your heart. In the past 4 months, you have gradually noticed that normal life is more difficult, due to your breathing getting worse around the home, for example after climbing the stairs you feel tired and breathless at the top and you generally feel more tired. You have given up walking the dog around the block and your neighbour helps with this. You have noticed a return of the ankle swelling. Your legs are not swollen and you have no chest pain. No palpitations.

You have noticed it is easier to sleep with three pillows but have had no PND recently.

You have noticed that you are wheezy sometimes when walking.

You have had no cough or weight loss and have been well with no temperature.

You have no RFs for CVD or VTE.

You have never smoked or had any exposure to asbestos or animals/birds.

No recent travel. No drenching sweats.

You were born in India where your parents worked until you were 14 years old, then your family moved back to the UK.

Social You retired 3 years ago from your job as a surveyor.

Divorced 10 years ago and have since lived alone.

You have a good network of friends who share your interests. You go to play bowls and can still do this. You enjoy listening to sport and reading the newspaper. You have fun at the pub quiz in a village where you know everyone. So, if not thinking about your health, you're content with life. You rarely see your children as they are busy in London.

ICE You have also done some reading since the ultrasonographer last year mentioned your valve is affected. You ask *'Is my heart damaged?'* You remember your mother telling you that you had rheumatic fever as a child and you have read that this can affect the valves.

The prospect of a problem with the heart has given you a sense of doom that you can't explain. You are not sure what the GP may suggest today.

Examination Pansystolic murmur heard at the apex. Chest: bi-basal crackles in lower zones. HR 72 bpm regular. RR 15. Sats 96%. Apyrexial. BP 158/94. No hepatomegaly. Ankle oedema to lower calf. JVP 4 cm. No palpable thyroid. No lymphadenopathy. No clubbing.

Refer to full NICE Guideline NG106. Chronic heart failure in adults: management. September 2018.

History	Dyspnoea, exercise tolerance for NYHA class, PND. Alcohol, nutrition and mood.
	Bloods FBC (anaemia), U&E and LFTs (baseline/reliability of BNP)
	TFTs (secondary cause), lipids and glucose (secondary prevention).
	BNP if no previous MI.
Other tests	Urinalysis (protein). ECG (ischaemia/LV hypertrophy). CXR (HF and malignancy).
	Consider spirometry if diagnosis uncertain.
Echo	Systolic and diastolic function and valve disease.
BNP	BNP <100 pg/mL = NT-proBNP <400 pg/mL – low clinical suspicion of HF.[2]
	BNP >400 pg/mL = NT-proBNP >2000 pg/mL – raised clinical suspicion of HF.[2]
	Beware of factors that may influence the BNP level including medications, comorbidity (e.g. renal, liver, diabetes), acute illness, obesity and age.
2-week echo	if previous MI + suspected HF or BNP >400 pg/mL.[1]
6-week echo	for initial diagnosis and BNP between 100 and 400 pg/mL.
	If valve disease present, follow cardiology advice.
Refer back	if NYHA class IV, not responding to treatment[2] and admit if can't be managed at home.
Health advice	Smoking, alcohol, salt, cardiac rehabilitation, flu and pneumococcal vaccine.[1]
	Weight – report if 2 kg ↑ in 2 days. Consider referral to a rehabilitation programme.[1]

Medication for left ventricular systolic dysfunction[2,3]

For each medication check licensing (for indication), contraindications and interactions.

Diuretics – titrate up or down according to congestion symptoms.[1]

ACEI – titrate to maximum tolerated dose. If intolerant consider an ARB.

Measure creatinine, U&E (e.g. 2 weeks) after each dose increment.[1]

Caution includes valve disease – await cardiology advice.

β-blockers – increase slowly and check HR and BP after each increment.

Consider even if elderly, diabetic, COPD, PVD and ED.

Switch previous β-blockers to one licensed for HF.[1]

ARB – if intolerant of ACEI and monitor creatinine/U&E.[1]

Hydralazine with nitrate – seek specialist advice. An option if intolerant of ACEI/ARB.[1]

Spironolactone, e.g. if NYHA class III–IV.

Following an MI – initiated within 3–14 days preferably after ACE.[1]

Monitor creatinine/U&E – for hyperkalaemia and ↓renal function.[1]

Digoxin – if worsening HF despite 1st and 2nd line Rx and seek specialist advice.

Aspirin 75 mg if indicated for vascular disease.

CCBs – Amlodipine may be considered if coexistent HTN or angina.[1]

HFPEF	Heart failure with preserved ejection fracture (e.g. due to diastolic dysfunction).
	Diagnosis symptomatic, ↑ BNP (other causes excluded) and normal ejection fraction on echo.
	Symptomatic Rx diuretics for congestion. Treat comorbidities and seek advice.

Doctor's Notes

Patient	Elizabeth Alderton	65 years	F
PMH	Hypertension		
Medications	Amlodipine 5 mg		
Allergies	No information		
Consultations	The nurse has added Elizabeth to your list after a routine ECG for HTN.		
Investigations	BP today 128/72. Recent blood tests normal (U&E, glucose, cholesterol).		
Household	Patrick Alderton	67 years	M

Impression ☐	Thank you for waiting. I can see you are keen for your results so may I suggest that we discuss them briefly, then go into detail about your health. Is that okay? Your ECG has shown an irregular heart beat. (Pause). This is called atrial fibrillation or AF for short and it is very common.
Experience ☐	Have you come across atrial fibrillation?
Explanation ☐	Your BP may have been a trigger. Atrial fibrillation can cause problems if we don't control it. But that's what I'd like to help you with to keep you healthy and safe.
Sense ☐	I can see this is unexpected and you're keen to know what needs to be done. But, in order to make the right decisions for you, can we start at the beginning; so we can make a plan tailored to you?
Open ☐	Please take me back to any events that led you to having this ECG. Had you experienced any symptoms that you now wonder may be related?
Flags ☐	Have you had any pain, dizziness or breathlessness? Faints, visual changes? Episodes where your arms or leg felt weak?
History ☐	Does amlodipine suit you? Any other tablets? Ibuprofen? Tell me more about you.
Risk ☐	How much alcohol and caffeine do you drink? Any recent illness, fever, cough or weight loss?
O/E ☐	Please may I examine your heart and lungs and take your BP?
Summary ☐	So, to summarise, a routine ECG for HTN has detected AF. You had no symptoms.
Explanation ☐	Within the heart, an electrical current makes your heart muscles pump. In AF the electrical current is disorganised. The electrical pulse starts at the top of the heart in the atria. When this happens in an uncoordinated way, the atria twitch, or fibrillate as we call it, hence the name AF. Any questions? The heart can beat fast and ineffectively, so medication is given to prevent this. The risk of AF is that clots can form and then cause problems, e.g. strokes. We can prevent this by using medication to thin the blood.
Options ☐	So the treatment for AF is in two stages. Firstly, a tablet to slow down the heart rate if needed. Your resting rate is normal, but we need to monitor it. If it goes fast we will need to slow it down. Secondly, we need to discuss whether to make your blood less likely to clot.
Recommend ☐	As high BP also increases stroke risk, I recommend a tablet to reduce clotting. Have you come across drugs such as warfarin or apixaban?
Curious ☐	Warfarin was used until recently for AF. What was your uncle's experience of warfarin?
Options ☐	Aspirin is no longer recommended as it does not work well; the stroke risk remains high. All blood thinners increase the risk of bleeding from the stomach, brain or nose. However, apart from your BP, which is controlled, you are well and may feel the benefits of preventing a stroke outweigh the risks. A newer type of drug is now recommended as first choice - apixaban. It's important to take it daily but no blood tests are required. This is a lot of information. What are your thoughts? I can print out a patient decision aid leaflet produced by NICE to help you decide if you like.
Future ☐	So shall we try apixaban? It is taken twice a day. If you experience any persistent nausea with this tablet, let me know. A great way to monitor your heart is if you have a watch that does this and we could look at results together when you've been exerting yourself. Or we can arrange a 24-hour ECG monitor? Do you have a preference? If we find we need to slow the heart, we could consider swapping your amlodipine to diltiazem, a cousin tablet of amlodipine, which slows the heart rate and reduces BP. Or we could start a β-blocker, alongside the amlodipine which is already working well for you.
Specifics ☐	So please can you arrange a call with me in a couple of weeks' time, after you've had a chance to exercise and monitor your heart rate with your watch. Please keep the readings for me. If you notice HRs over 100 frequently please call sooner.
Empower ☐	Other things that you can do include decreasing caffeine and alcohol intake.
Safety net ☐	The apixaban is very protective, however if you ever notice your vision changes or arms or legs feel different or weak, you must call an ambulance as these may be signs of a stroke. If you ever feel lightheaded, breathless or have chest pain, this may be due to AF, so please seek help straightaway.

Doctor's notes	Elizabeth Alderton, 65 years. PMH: hypertension. Medication: amlodipine 5 mg.
	BP today 128/72 and a routine ECG.
How to act	Very pleasant.
PC	*'I had an ECG with the nurse and he said I had to wait to see you. Is something wrong?'*
History	After a series of home BP readings you were recently diagnosed with HTN.
	You were told to get an ECG but you have been on holiday.
	You feel very well and are very active.
	You have had no symptoms.
	Your father suffered with high BP but you have no other FH.
	You feel well on amlodipine 5 mg.
Social	You are a librarian. You live with your husband and you have two dogs.
	You walk the dogs daily and enjoy swimming.
	You have never smoked and you drink 14 units of alcohol a week.
	You enjoy coffee.
	You often go on holiday.
ICE	After being informed you have AF you are keen to know the plan.
	'What does that mean … is it dangerous?' Then *'So what needs to happen?'*
	You have never heard of atrial fibrillation.
	If the doctor talks about anticoagulants, say: *'My uncle was on warfarin. You need blood tests. Can't I take aspirin?'*
	Your uncle had lots of nose bleeds after which his nose would need packing.
	You will not take warfarin under any circumstances due to the blood tests.
	You hate needles and have another holiday planned.
	Once aware of the risks/benefits of a DOAC, this is your preferred option.
Examination	HS normal. HR 80 bpm irregular. Chest clear. BP 120/70. Please see ECG in Extra Notes

Cause[1]	Idiopathic.
	Heart: hypertension, ischaemia, valve disease and other cardiac conditions.
	Metabolic: hyperthyroid or diabetes.
	Acute changes: Infection or electrolyte imbalance.
	Respiratory: PE or lung cancer.
	Drug/food: alcohol, caffeine, salbutamol or thyroxine.
	Correct any underlying cause then manage the heart rate or rhythm.
Symptoms	Asymptomatic, SOB, palpitations, syncope, dizziness, chest pain, stroke, TIA.
Complications	Stroke, TIA, heart failure, cardiomyopathy or ischaemia.
Investigations[2]	ECG, if an irregular pulse is detected,[2] to make the diagnosis and for possible signs of old ischaemia.

If paroxysmal AF (PAF) is suspected and an ECG has not captured AF:

- 24-hour ambulatory ECG monitor if asymptomatic or episodes <24 hours apart.[2]

Ambulatory ECG monitor, event recorder or other ECG technology if episodes >24 hours apart.[2]

Check FBC, TSH and electrolytes for reversible causes.

U&E and LFT are needed for the bleeding risk assessment and medication choice.

CXR if a lung cause suspected.

24-hour tape if daily palpitations or event recorder if infrequent palpitations.

Echocardiogram If concern of underlying structural disease (murmur) or functional heart disease – which influences medication.[3]

AF can be managed in primary care but see reasons for referral in Extra Notes*

Rate control[2]	Beta-blocker (bisoprolol) if not contraindicated.
	Do not prescribe amiodarone for long-term rate control or sotalol in primary care.
OR	Rate-limiting calcium-channel blocker (diltiazem) if not contraindicated.
	If still not effective may add digoxin to either of above.
OR	Digoxin monotherapy for non-paroxysmal AF if they are sedentary or other medications rejected due to comorbidities or preference.

If still poor rate control and symptomatic consider combination therapy with any two of following: a beta-blocker, diltiazem, digoxin.

See Extra Notes at the end of this chapter for CHA_2DS_2-VASc and ORBIT bleeding risk score, DOACs and reasons to refer to cardiology.

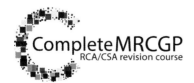

Doctor's Notes

Patient	Richard Turner	57 years	M
PMH	No medical history		
Medications	No current medications		
Allergies	No known drug allergies		
Consultations	BP 162/102 at a check with the nurse		
Investigations	Average ambulatory BP reading 151/96		
Household	Gillian Turner	56 years	F

Open ☐	What led you to have this tested? Do you know your readings?
ICE ☐	When you saw the 151/96 figure what went through your mind? Is this a worry for you? What did you think I was going to say?
History ☐	Do you have any medical conditions?
Risk ☐	Has a family member had a heart problem, high BP or a stroke?
Sense ☐	So this has come out of the blue? How do you feel about being told your BP is raised?
Flags ☐	When talking about BP, I usually check you haven't suffered with any headaches? Or any chest or calf pains? Does your heart ever feel like it is beating too fast?
Curious ☐	You mentioned your wife was helping you test it and she wanted you to have a check; what does she think? Why do you think she is worried?
SummarICE ☐	So to summarise, you've been very well and therefore you were surprised when your BP was high. You were hoping that I'd say we'll keep an eye on it but your wife wants you to take tablets, especially with her father's experience. Is that right?
Empathy ☐	I can see you take this seriously and your wife is concerned as her father had high BP.
Impression ☐	Your diagnosis is Stage 2 hypertension, which is the medical word for high BP. It is Stage 2 because the top number is >150 and the bottom >95.
Experience ☐	What do you understand about why we treat high BP?
Explanation ☐	High BP can increase your risk of a stroke, angina or a heart attack, which is why it is important to control it. It can also harm your kidneys and eyes. Stage 2 hypertension is not dangerous; however, it does suggest that we should be treating the BP with tablets as well as lifestyle advice.
Recommend ☐	Whether to start treatment is your decision. My recommendation would be to start a tablet called amlodipine 5 mg each morning. This helps to relax the blood vessels to decrease the pressure. Like any tablet there may be side effects, such as the possibility of ankle swelling, tummy upset or headaches, in which case we could consider a different tablet. How do you feel about taking the tablet? I also suggest you see your optician and inform them that you are now receiving BP medication. Rarely, eyesight can be affected. However, if they see small changes from the effects of BP this is useful for us all to be aware of so do let me know if this is the case please.
Empower ☐	Things you can do to help include exercising more, reducing alcohol and restricting salt in your diet. A 6 g reduction in salt each day reduces your BP number by 10.[1] Do you feel these suggestions will be possible?
Future ☐	Thinking ahead, we need to do some routine tests with the nurse to check your general health including an ECG, which is a heart tracing, a urine test and blood tests including cholesterol and to check your kidneys. Is this okay?
Specifics ☐	So to summarise, you will start a morning tablet, make an appointment with the nurse for a heart tracing, blood test and urine test, then see me in 1 month. Please also see an optician. If you're having a problem with the tablet or have any concerns, please let me know.

Doctor's notes.	Richard Turner, 57 years. PMH: none. Medications: none.
	Last consultation: BP 162/102 right arm and 160/102 left arm (practice nurse). Average ambulatory BP reading 151/96.
How to act	Interested in your health.
PC	*'I've telephoned to find out what I need to do about my blood pressure.'*
History	You feel well. No PMH or FH.
	You were at a friend's house for dinner and they had purchased a BP machine, so you checked yours.
	'My wife wanted me to go to the nurse to check it again.'
	The nurse found that your BP was raised and gave you a machine to check it at home.
	You discussed the average BP, 151/96, with the nurse and have been told to phone the doctor.
Social	Very healthy. You enjoy squash and consider yourself to be a healthy eater.
	You drink very little alcohol and have never smoked.
	You work as a gardener so are active during the day.
	You enjoy your work, and do not find it stressful.
	You have a good relationship with your wife.
ICE	You thought 151/96 was high but thought you'd be told to keep an eye on it. You are worried the doctor will want to start a tablet. You are not keen as this will make you feel old, but it won't otherwise impact on your life.
	You thought you had no CV risk factors, so you were quite shocked.
	You understand that it was your father-in-law's BP that led to his stroke.
	You are happy to take the tablet, once its importance has been explained.
	You are also interested in other ways to decrease your BP.
	Do not tell the doctor your wife is worried unless the doctor asks.
	You have mentioned your wife twice already. It is your wife who is worried.
	Her father was always talking about his BP before his stroke.
	She would like you to take tablets.

Refer to full NICE Guideline NG136. Hypertension in adults: diagnosis and management. August 2019.

Investigations[2]	Bloods: Lipids (for QRISK) and HbA1c (comorbidity), U&E, eGFR (baseline for Rx), FBC (anaemia) and TFT (cause).[3] ECG (ventricular hypertrophy, arrhythmia), ACR (microalbuminuria/CKD) and fundi (retinopathy).
Diagnosis[2]	Check BP in both arms, if difference >15 mmHg persists use the arm with ↑readings.
	Ambulatory monitoring (best): 2 measurements/hour during waking hours.
	Home BP monitoring twice/day (2 readings 1 minute apart) for 4–7 days.
	Discard 1st day's reading and average remaining.
Stage 1 HTN	Clinic BP ≥140/90 and home BP ≥135/85. Treat if* (see below).
Stage 2 HTN	Clinic BP ≥160/100 and home BP ≥150/95. Start treatment.
Stage 3/severe HTN	Clinic SBP ≥180 or DBP ≥110. Treat immediately.
Accelerated HTN	Papilloedema or retinal haemorrhage. Admission.
	Suspected phaeochromocytoma. Admission.
Aims of clinic	BP:
	<140/90 if <80 years or <150/90 if >80 years with treated HTN.[2]
	<140/80 if type 2 DM or <135/85 if type 1 DM.[4,5]
	<130/80 if DM and either CKD or retinopathy or cerebrovascular disease.[4,6]
Treating hypertension[2]	(Check you have stopped the OCP!)
	A = ACE inhibitor. B = β-blocker. C = calcium-channel blocker. D = thiazide-like diuretic
	If <55 years start with ACEI. If required A + C + D.
	If >55 years or people of Black ethnicity and of African/Caribbean descent start with CCB. If required C + A + D.
	NB Always check adherence before adding new drug.
	* Adult <80 years with persistent stage 1 hypertension AND ≥1 of:
	target organ damage
	established cardiovascular disease
	renal disease
	estimated 10-year risk CVD ≥10%
	Use clinical judgement if frailty or multimorbidity.[2]
Secondary causes of HTN	Primary hyperaldosteronism, phaeochromocytoma, CKD and sleep apnoea.
	Ask about UTIs as a child. Investigations: urinary normetadrenalines, USS kidneys + referral to exclude fibromuscular dysplasia of the renal artery.

See Extra Notes at the end of this chapter for white coat hypertension and resistant hypertension.

Doctor's Notes

Patient	Hibiki Hayashi	75 years	M
PMH	Hypertension		
Medications	Ramipril 5 mg		
	Bendroflumethiazide 2.5 mg		
Allergies	NKDA		
Consultations			
Investigations	Last BP 132/78 (1 month ago)		
Household	No household members registered		

Open ☐	Tell me about this pain, perhaps from when it first began.
History ☐	How frequently does it happen? Have you noticed anything that brings it on? What takes it away? Do you have any other symptoms with the pain?
Flags ☐	Have you had a pain that has lasted more than 10 minutes? Do you have pain when you are sitting or lying down? Is this pain becoming more frequent?
Impact ☐	Has it stopped you from doing anything?
ICE ☐	When you have had this pain, what has gone through your mind? What do you think is causing the pain? What did you think I might say we should do about this pain?
Risk ☐	Apart from HTN, do you have any other medical problems? Has anyone in your family had heart problems or a stroke? Do you smoke? Do you get any pain in the lower legs when you are walking?
Sense ☐	You seem very quiet…are you very worried?
Curious ☐	I'm sorry to hear you lost Maho and Hisae. That must have been devastating. You sound very low just now. Sometimes when people feel so low, they don't want to be alive. Do you feel like this? Have you had thoughts about ending your life?
SummarICE ☐	So you have also been feeling lonely and, since Maho died, you have had chest pains which you thought may be a heart attack. You thought I might say you need an operation, but you don't want this. Is that right?
O/E ☐	May I have a listen to your heart, feel your pulse and take your BP?
Empathy ☐	The past 2 years have been life changing for you.
Impression ☐	Mr Hayashi, I think you may be suffering with angina. It is unlikely that you have had a heart attack. If pain goes away when you stop, this is called angina. Angina and depression are very common together, as angina can affect a person's daily life.
Experience ☐	Have you come across angina? Do you know anyone with it?
Explanation ☐	Angina is where the blood flow to the heart is not as good as it could be due to furring of the vessels – a bit like clogged drains. A heart attack is different; this is when the pipe becomes completely blocked.
Recommend ☐	I can make some recommendations to help your symptoms and protect your heart.
Options ☐	I would like to give you a spray to use once under the tongue if you have pain. It widens the vessels to your heart. If the pain is still there after 5 minutes, take a second spray. If you feel unwell, or the pain is present 5 minutes later, call an ambulance. You may notice a headache and, if dizziness occurs, sit for a few minutes. Please also use this spray before exercise. Are you happy to try it? Please repeat back to me how and when you would use it. Are you happy to take aspirin to thin your blood to help the blood flow through the vessels? Have you had tummy ulcers, because aspirin can make stomach problems worse? We should also start bisoprolol, every morning, to slow the heart and prevent pain when you are walking. If it makes you feel tired or lightheaded let me know. May I prescribe all three medications? I would like to send you to our chest pain clinic where you will be seen within a couple of weeks to confirm the diagnosis. Any concerns from what I have said? I will write it all down for you as there is a lot to remember.
InCLudE ☐	Yes, you can drive, unless angina happens during driving, in which case stop driving until the angina is controlled.
Empower ☐	You've mentioned getting another dog to go for walks and for company. When your angina is under control, this would be an excellent idea to help both your mood and heart.
Future ☐	Have you ever wondered about stopping smoking? We can help you with this. Have a think about whether you might be interested in talking to someone about your loss and if information on community groups would be of interest.
Specifics ☐	I will book you in for a heart tracing and blood tests to check your cholesterol and sugar, then I'll make you a double appointment with me next week so we can talk about your results, your angina and have a longer talk about your mood. Is that okay?
Safety net ☐	If the pain becomes more frequent or occurs at a shorter distance let a GP know immediately. If pain occurs at rest or has been present for 10 minutes, call 999.

Doctor's notes	Hibiki Hayashi, 70 years. PMH: hypertension.
	Medications: ramipril 5 mg, bendroflumethiazide 2.5 mg. NKDA. Last BP 132/78.
How to act	You are subdued.
PC	*'Doctor, I keep getting these chest pains.'*
History	It started 3 months ago when you were walking to get the paper.
	Since then, it has happened a few times a week, usually after about 500 metres, particularly if you are in a hurry.
	The pain makes you stop. The pain is then gone after about 2 minutes.
	You have not had pain before this distance and no rest pain.
	The pain is in the centre of your chest and feels very heavy.
	There is no radiation. There are no associated cardiac symptoms.
	You have not felt the pain after eating, only when walking.
	No claudication pain.
	You take two tablets for BP. You have no FH.
Social	You live in a bungalow. You have not had pain when at home.
	You lost your wife, Hisae, 2 years ago. Since then, your dog, Maho, kept you going.
	You used to walk Maho 2 miles a day but she died 4 months ago.
	You feel very lonely and low and have stopped going to get the paper.
	You don't go out any more and don't see anybody. Your son lives 2 hours away.
	You think about getting another dog. You smoke 20/day. You do not drink alcohol.
	You moved from Japan to the UK 40 years ago.
ICE	You are not worried. You think you have probably had a heart attack.
	You don't want to die and have had no thoughts about ending your life, but you do sometimes think it would be nice to be with Hisae and Maho.
	You expect the doctor will tell you that you need an operation. You don't want this.
	You believe angina is a small heart attack.
Ask the doctor	*'Am I allowed to drive?'*
Examination	HR 66 bpm regular. BP 130/70. HS normal.

Refer to full NICE Guideline CG126. Stable angina: management. August 2016.

Investigations	ECG.
	Consider CXR if lung cancer/infection possible.
	FBC for anaemia.
Referral	To confirm diagnosis – rapid-access chest pain clinic.
	Re-refer if symptomatic despite medical therapy.

Classification

Stable angina

May be **typical** (3/3) or **atypical** (2/3) of:

- Constricting pain
- Precipitated by exertion
- Relieved by rest.[1,2]

Unstable angina

Deterioration or angina at rest. Requires immediate admission.[3]

Medications in angina

GTN before exercise and during angina (unless taken Viagra).

β-blocker or CCB.

CCB   Diltiazem is rate limiting.

However, if HF or needing to combine a CCB with either a β-blocker or ivabradine, CCB should be amlodipine, nifedipine or felodipine.

Others: Nitrate (ISMN), nicorandil.

Ivabradine, ranolazine – specialist only prescribed.

Secondary prevention drugs

Aspirin 75 mg OD. Continue clopidogrel if on this for another reason.

Statin.

ACEI if DM or other conditions, in line with NICE.[4]

Cardiac syndrome X

Consider in ongoing symptoms and normal angiography. Continue antianginal if effective. No evidence of benefit with secondary prevention treatment.

It is possible to have a complex case in a simulated surgery, as well as in real life, when you may need to manage multiple problems. In this example we suggest completing a risk assessment for depression, then focusing on the chest pain and finally signposting the need to manage the depression at a later date.

 See the Link Hub at CompleteMRCGP.co.uk or a helpful guide to DVLA guidance for medical conditions

Discuss the risks and benefits of anticoagulation with patients with AF to facilitate informed decision-making. For most people, the benefits outweigh the risks of bleeding but, for those with an increased risk of bleeding, careful monitoring is needed and the benefits may not always outweigh the risks.[1]

Remember to consider modifiable risk factors for bleeding including:[1]

- Uncontrolled hypertension.
- Poor control of INR in patients already taking vitamin K antagonists (such as warfarin).
- Concurrent medication, e.g. antiplatelets, SSRIs and NSAIDs.
- Harmful alcohol use.
- Reversible causes of anaemia.

CHA_2DS_2VASc score[1]

Consider anticoagulation for ♂ with a score of ≥1 or ♀ with a score of ≥2, after taking into account the risk of bleeding using the ORBIT toolkit.

In people aged <65 with AF and very low risk of stroke, i.e. no risk factors apart from their sex (♂ with a score of 0, or ♀ with a score of 1) – do not offer anticoagulation for stroke prevention.

'Do not withhold anticoagulation solely because of a person's age or their risk of falls.'[1]

ORBIT-AF[2]

NICE recommends using the ORBIT-AF tool to assess the risk of bleeding when considering starting anti-coagulation or when reviewing people already taking anticoagulants, as evidence shows that it has a higher accuracy than other tools when predicting absolute bleeding risk.[1]

The ORBIT-AF score takes account of five different criteria, maximum score 7:

Criterion	Score
Older age ≥ 75	1
Reduced Hb	
♂Hb < 130 g/dL	
♀Hb < 120 g/dL	
Or Hct	2
♂<40%	
♀<30%	
Or history of anaemia	
Bleeding history	2
Insufficient renal function	
(eGFR <60 mg/dL)	1
Treatment with antiplatelets	1

Score 0-2	**Low bleed risk**
Score 3	**Medium bleed risk**
Score 4-7	**High bleed risk**

DOACs[1]

Offer treatment with a DOAC to patients with AF and a CHA2DS2VASc ≥2.

Consider treatment with a DOAC for patients with AF and a CHA2DS2VASc of 1.

Choice of DOAC: NICE recommends apixaban, dabigatran, edoxaban and rivaroxaban 'when used in line with the criteria specified in the relevant NICE technology appraisal guidance'.[1]

If DOAC is contraindicated, not tolerated or not suitable, offer a vitamin K antagonist, e.g. warfarin.

If already taking a vitamin K antagonist and stable, consider continuing with this and reviewing at the next routine appointment.

*Consider referral to cardiology:[1]

'Refer people promptly at any stage if treatment fails to control the symptoms of atrial fibrillation and more specialised management is needed. This should be within 4 weeks after the failed treatment or after recurrence of atrial fibrillation after cardioversion.'

New onset AF with heart failure or secondary to reversible causes.

For possible amiodarone or catheter ablation if heart failure present.

For cardioversion following 3 weeks' anticoagulation unless there is good evidence to suggest this is a new AF within <48 hours.

Amiodarone may be prescribed (by specialist) prior to DC cardioversion.

Lone AF and in the young.

Left atrial appendage occlusion may be considered by specialists if anticoagulation is CI or not tolerated or there is a high bleed risk.

Acute admission to the medics[3]

Unwell/unstable e.g. tachycardic, hypotensive, LOC, chest pain, increasing SOB, dizziness.

Use clinical judgement.

In all cases discuss the following stroke and bleeding risk assessments with the patient: CHA_2DS_2-VASc stroke risk score for AF, PAF, atrial flutter or if risk of recurrence following cardioversion or ablation.

If possible, use the ORBIT bleeding risk score to assess bleeding risk because 'evidence shows that it has a higher accuracy'.[1]

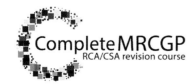

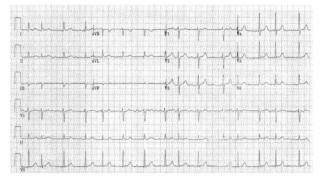

Reproduced from *Handbook of Cardiac Electrophysiology,* Second Edition (2020), CRC Press. With thanks to Rong Bai, Mohamed Salim, Luigi Di Biase, Robert Schweikert and Walid Saliba.

White coat HTN	>20/10 mmHg between home and clinic. Monitor only home readings.
	Confirm with ABPM and then treat average as per usual guidance.[1]
Resistant HTN	HTN persists despite three drugs:

- Confirm clinic BP using ambulatory or home BP readings.
- Assess for postural hypertension.
- Discuss adherence.

4th line. If K ≤4.5 mmol/L and eGFR >60 mL/min/1.73 m^2 consider spironolactone. Repeat eGFR/U&E in 1/12 and as needed thereafter.

Caution ↓eGFR = ↑ risk of hyperkalaemia.[1]

If K >4.5 mmol/L then consider an alpha-blocker or beta-blocker.

If oedema, HF or risk of HF, offer thiazide diuretic.[1]

If diabetic, caution with B and D and consider A first for microalbuminuria.

'People of black African or African–Caribbean family origin, consider an ARB in preference to an ACEI.'[1]

If >80 years, consider starting with D. If required D + A (HYVET study).[2]

We suggest U&E at baseline and 2 weeks after initiating/increasing ACEI or ARB or spironolactone.

Refer if BP remains uncontrolled on four agents[1] or earlier if concerned.

NB: Also, be aware of sodium content in drugs (e.g. effervescent).

CHAPTER 4 OVERVIEW

Dermatology

	Cases in this chapter	Within the RCGP 2020 curriculum: Dermatology	Learning points in this chapter include:
1	Skin Lesion	'Diagnose, treat and advise on common skin conditions efficiently' 'The effect of an ageing population and increased exposure to sun damage in an older population' 'Recognition of alarm or red flag features'	Skin lesions – advice from the Primary Care Dermatology Society Solar keratosis
2	Acne	'Acne vulgaris, including indications and side effects of isotretinoin'	When to refer Treatment
3	Melasma	'Hyperpigmentation'	When to refer Treatment
4	Eczema	'Dermatological disorders in childhood… atopic eczema' 'Common and important conditions – eczema: infantile, childhood, atopic' 'Prescribe appropriately and safely'	Cause Management Red flags Fingertip units
5	Psoriasis	'Recognise the importance of the psychosocial impact of skin problems' 'Appreciate the complexity of care that is needed with some skin problems' 'Examination of the rest of the skin, nails, scalp, hair and systems such as joints when appropriate'	Triggers Associations Limb/trunk treatment Scalp psoriasis treatment

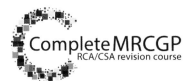

CompleteMRCGP
RCA/CSA revision course

CHAPTER 4 REFERENCES

Skin Lesion

1. http://www.dermnetnz.org/lesions/lichenoid-keratosis.html. Mar 2016.
2. www.pcds.org.uk
3. http://www.pcds.org.uk/ee/images/uploads/general/skin-cancer-detection-patient-advice-07-2012.pdf
4. http://www.dermnetnz.org/lesions/solar-keratoses.html. Dec 2015.

Acne

1. https://www.pcds.org.uk/clinical-guidance/acne-vulgaris. Aug 2021.
2. http://www.pcds.org.uk/ee/images/uploads/general/Acne_Treatment_2015-web.pdf

Useful Resource

https://patient.info/skin-conditions/acne-leaflet. Jul 2021.

Melasma

1. http://www.dermnetnz.org/colour/melasma.html. Oct 2020.
2. http://www.britishskinfoundation.org.uk/SkinInformation/AtoZofSkindisease/Melasma.aspx
3. Pandya A., Hynan L., Bhore R. et al. Reliability assessment and validation of the Melasma Area and Severity Index (MASI) and a new modified MASI scoring method. *J Am Acad Dermatol* 2011; 64: 78–83.

Eczema

1. http://www.pcds.org.uk/clinical-guidance/atopic-eczema. Aug 2021.

Psoriasis

1. http://www.pcds.org.uk/clinical-guidance/psoriasis-an-overview. Jul 2021.
2. NICE Guideline CG153. Psoriasis: assessment and management. Sep 2017.

Information taken from NICE guidelines with kind permission. Please note the guidelines change frequently and you should ALWAYS check for the latest updated guidance. Remember that NICE guidance is only applicable to patients in the UK.

Dermatology

Doctor's Notes

Patient	Paul Robson	65 years	M
PMH	No medical history known		
Medications	No current medications		
Allergies	No information		
Consultations	No recent consultations		
Investigations	No investigations		
Household	No household members registered		

Example Consultation

Open ☐	Tell me about the skin changes from the beginning please. Anything else that you noticed?
ICE ☐	What has worried you about this? What do you think it is? An SCC – tell me what you understand by this. You mentioned your daughter. What does she think? Is there anything else you hoped we would discuss today?
Sense ☐	Thank you for sending a photograph – that is very helpful. I can hear you are worried about this.
Curious ☐	Is your daughter medical? Did you have any other ideas between you?
History ☐	Tell me about you. Your general health? Any other problems to report whilst we have the opportunity today? Do you work? Have you ever smoked? How much alcohol do you drink? Is anyone else at home? Tell me about your lifestyle or hobbies.
Risk ☐	Have you had much sun exposure? Sunburn?
Flags ☐	Has the lesion changed? Over what time period? Have you noticed changes in size, colour? shape, thickness? Has it bled?
O/E ☐	Let me have a good look at the photograph. Thank you.
SummarICE ☐	To summarise, you have noticed for a few years that the skin on parts of your scalp and face is discoloured but then, over the past month, the patch on your right temple became darker and thicker. Then your daughter, who is a GP, believes it changed again over a week and she thinks it may be an SCC because it has changed quickly. You would like to be referred promptly for a biopsy and hope that I can give you my opinion as well as explain what is likely to happen at the hospital appointment. Is that correct?
Impression ☐	I agree there is sun damage to the face and scalp, which we call solar keratosis. We try to keep this under control with creams…
InCludE ☐	….as it has the potential to become cancerous and change to the SCC which your daughter talked about. But I agree it is not typical, because of the pigment. Therefore, we also need to rule out a melanoma.
Explanation ☐	Sometimes we can only be sure what we are dealing with by taking a biopsy of the skin and looking at it under a microscope.
Recommend ☐	This is certainly necessary if a lesion changes quickly. How do you feel about that?
Options ☐	At the hospital, it is likely that they will first have a look at your skin and may or may not do a biopsy on the same day. They may also talk to you about creams for the sun-damaged skin. They will write to me with their findings and advice if any treatment is required.
Empathy ☐	I appreciate it is a worry when anyone points out something which is potentially a cancer. You said you were on holiday at the time – I hope you still managed to have a good time!
Empower ☐	You have come promptly – well done – and I hope this can be dealt with quickly. Do wear a hat and factor 50 sun cream when outside. Now you're someone we don't see very often, so I was wondering if we could arrange some general health checks?
Specifics ☐	I would like to refer you on the suspected cancer pathway, which means you should be seen within 2 weeks. If this doesn't happen, I need to know straight away please. Can you also make a follow-up appointment with me 2 weeks after your clinic appointment unless the specialists at the hospital advise this is not necessary? If I receive a letter meanwhile, and action is required, I will call you.
Safety net ☐	If you ever notice any other skin changes or you are not sure, see your GP straight away.

Patient's Story

Doctor's notes Paul Robson, 65 years. No medical history or medications.

How to act Pleasant. You have written down what you need and hope to be an efficient patient. You show the doctor the photograph or examination description with your opening statement.

PC *'I am concerned about the sun damage on my face.'*

History You have had this skin damage on your right temple for about 3 years and there are other parts of the head which look similar but are not as dark and not as noticeable.

If asked about a change, over the past month it has become darker and possibly thicker. It has not changed in size.

You have no other medical problems. You are very well in yourself.

Social You are a retired physics lecturer. You have never smoked.

You drink a glass of wine most nights.

You live with your wife and keep very active playing golf.

You have had lots of sun exposure and have been burnt several times. You enjoy spending time outside both in the garden and playing golf and try to go on a couple of sunny holidays a year. You don't always wear sun cream in the UK.

ICE You think it is fine. You are not worried and wish to be pragmatic.

'Well, my daughter noticed it whilst we were on a family holiday.'

If asked, your daughter is a GP.

If asked what she thinks, explain: *'My daughter thinks it may be the beginning of an SCC because it's scaly and she thinks it has changed from the week before, but she says she isn't sure because it is pigmented.'*

If asked what your daughter thinks about management: *'She said I should have a biopsy.'*

You hope the GP will give you his/her opinion, refer you to a dermatologist and tell you what is likely to happen at the hospital.

However, you are aware how busy GPs are and are satisfied with a referral.

If the GP does not refer you, follow his/her advice.

You are not interested in a general health check at the moment. You will, however, talk to your daughter about it.

Examination Description of the lesion for the doctor: on the patient's right temple there is a 1 cm pigmented lesion with a scale and irregular outline. The base is thickened. There is no ulceration or induration. Central hyperpigmentation which is raised and surrounded by flat irregular slightly pigmented areas. There is no rolled edge or central telangiectasia. Pigmented areas over the scalp. There are no other lesions of concern on the body.

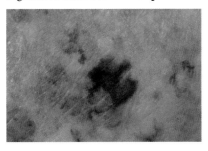

Reproduced from *An Atlas of Dermoscopy* (2013), CRC Press. With thanks to Steven Q. Wang, Harold S. Rabinovitz, Margaret C. Oliviero and Ashfaq A. Marghoob.

The biopsy returned as a lichenoid keratosis. DermNet NZ provides an excellent educational resource[1] including pictures and descriptions of common and not so common lesions.

Skin Lesions–Advice from the Primary Care Dermatology Society

 Primary Care Dermatology Society (PCDS) website is recommended reading.
See the **Link Hub at CompleteMRCGP.co.uk** for a useful patient advice leaflet for skin lesions and useful diagnostic tables from PCDS.[2]

PCDS encourages looking at the body (not the individual lesion alone) for 'pattern comparison' and spot 'the ugly duckling'.[2]

A change in a lesion or the following features (A–G) should raise concern.[3]

Asymmetry	In shape or colour
Border	Uneven, notched or irregular
Colour	Either several colours within one lesion, or a different colour to other moles.
Dimensions	Change and size
Elevated	
Firm	
Growth	

Solar (actinic) keratosis

Features	Sun-exposed sites.
	May be flat or thickened, with scale or a wart/horn surface, tender or asymptomatic and the colour can vary from skin coloured, red or pigmented.[4]
At risk of	Developing into a cancer (e.g. SCC and BCC) or cutaneous horn or actinic cheilitis.[4]
Treatment	Aimed at removing the affected cells so the epidermis can regenerate.[4]
Minor surgery	Options include cryotherapy with liquid nitrogen; shave, curettage and electrocautery of hypertrophic tissue or horns, or excision.[4]
Field Rx's	'Creams are used to treat areas of sun damage and flat actinic keratosis.'[4]
	'Pre-treatment with keratolytics (such as urea cream, salicylic acid ointment or topical retinoid), and thorough skin cleansing improves response rates.'[4]
	E.g. diclofenac gel, 5-fluorouracil, imiquimod, photodynamic therapy and ingenol mebutate gel[4] – see DermNet NZ for further advice.
	'Tender, thickened, ulcerated or enlarging actinic keratoses should be treated aggressively.
	Asymptomatic flat keratoses may not require active treatment but should be kept under observation.'

Doctor's Notes

Patient	Adelaide Bukoski	28 years	F
PMH	No medical history known		
Medications	No current medications		
Allergies	No information		
Consultations	No recent consultations		
Investigations	No investigations		
Household	No household members registered		

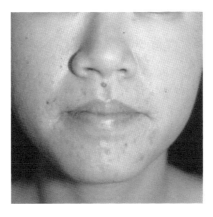

Reproduced from *Acne and Its Therapy* (2007), CRC Press. With thanks to Guy F. Webster and Anthony V. Rawlings.

Open ☐	Please tell me about your skin. Anything else you've noticed? Please tell me why a referral to an endocrinologist is important to you? Why specifically an endocrinologist? Thank you.
History ☐	Tell me about any other medical problems you have had. And in the family? What have you tried for your skin? Do you take any medicines? Do you smoke? What is your facial washing regime?
ICE ☐	What do you believe is causing the spots? What do you hope an endocrinologist will do? Is there another reason why you think there is a problem with your hormones? What concerns you most about your skin? Were you hoping I would start treatment today?
Risk ☐	Do you use hormonal contraception like the pill? Do you know your current weight?
Flags ☐	Have you noticed any hair on your face? Is your weight stable? Are your periods regular? Have you noticed that the spots increase around your period?
Impact ☐	How does your skin affect you and your self-esteem?
O/E ☐	Thank you for sending a photograph, let me have a good look at it. I can see that there are a few black and white heads on the face and back and some papules. Thankfully there is no scarring, pustules, nodules or cysts. There is no evidence of excess facial hair.
SummarICE ☐	To summarise, you believe that your spots are being caused by a hormonal problem and would like a referral to a skin specialist and blood tests to check your hormone levels.
Impression ☐	I believe you have acne, which affects 12% of women over 25.
Experience ☐	What do you know about acne? Do you know why it happens?
Explanation ☐	Pores, tiny holes in the skin, become blocked due to the skin thickening at the surface or dead skin pores can become blocked and oil can collect in the pores. Bacteria get into the oil and cause painful red spots.
InCLudE ☐	Sometimes hormonal imbalances can cause excess oils, e.g. PCOS or excess male hormones. Every woman has male hormones, but some women have more. You have no other symptoms of these hormone problems but we can do blood tests to check the hormones on your list. LH, FSH and testosterone levels will help us rule out a hormonal cause for your acne. What are your thoughts?
Options ☐	As cream alone hasn't worked, we could try a combination of a cream called Epiduo with an antibiotic tablet, called lymecycline, taken every day. The Epiduo contains two treatments which kill the germs, unblock the pores and reduce the inflammation. Lymecycline is an antibiotic which kills the skin bacteria and will help treat the pustules. Like all tablets, side effects are possible; the cream can irritate the skin and the tablets can cause nausea or headaches, but usually people feel fine. Even if you did have PCOS or a raised male hormone level, treatment options are similar, including a hormone pill used for acne. There is another treatment, called isotretinoin, which is only prescribed by skin specialists because it has risks, e.g. to the liver. We could refer you to the skin specialists should your skin not improve with the treatment I have suggested. I can give you information on all these treatments to read.
Sense ☐	Is your priority finding out if there is a hormone problem? I can see you are unhappy.
Curious ☐	What would your GP in Poland do? What do you believe the GPs role is for you?
Empathy ☐	I can imagine it is frustrating that my suggestions are different from your other doctor. I hear how important this is for you. Changes in your skin can affect how you feel and your confidence, especially in a new relationship.
Options ☐	Because acne is so common, GPs know a lot about it and we don't need to refer everyone to a skin specialist. We could start treatment today. Would you like me to prescribe you something appropriate?
Empower ☐	At first, try the cream every other day to reduce any irritation. Wear clothes like cotton, which can breathe, to avoid your back from getting sweaty. Clean your face and back twice a day. Cleaning too much may cause excess oil to be produced.
Specifics ☐	Shall we meet again in 3 months? The treatment prevents new spots forming so it may be 8 weeks before you notice a big improvement.
Safety net ☐	If you notice scarring or increased inflammation, please return earlier. You must stop this treatment before falling pregnant.

Doctor's notes	Adelaide Bukoski, 28 years. New patient.
How to act	Demanding.
PC	*'I would like to see an endocrinologist for my spots.'*
History	You moved to the UK from Poland 6 months ago.
	In Poland you were given a cream for your spots, but this was not effective.
	You do not know what the cream was called.
	You are otherwise well. You have never taken any regular medication.
	You had a copper coil inserted 2 weeks ago.
	You have regular periods and no symptoms of PCOS.
	The acne is on your face and back. You have tried eating a healthy diet.
	You wash your face four times a day and have spent lots of money on cleansing products.
Social	You work in a cafe. You drink minimal alcohol and have never smoked. You have a new partner.
ICE	You believe there is a problem with your hormones.
	You would like to see a specialist as you want to know why you have spots at your age.
	You presume the GP is not able to solve the problem and demand to see an expert.
	Before you left, your GP in Poland wrote down a list of blood tests which you could have.
	'LH, FSH, oestrogen, progesterone, testosterone.' You would like these checking.
	If the doctor does not refer, you become angry as you want to find the cause.
	You have just started a new relationship. The spots on your back are especially bad and you feel embarrassed and self-conscious about this.
Examination	A few open and closed comedones on the face and back and some papules. No scarring, pustules, nodules or cysts. No hirsutism.
	Height 162 cm. Weight 58 kg. BMI 22.
	You leave dissatisfied unless you are referred to an endocrinologist. You accept the suggested treatment but walk out looking unhappy with the doctor.

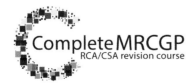

CompleteMRCGP
RCA/CSA revision course

This was a challenging case with an unhappy and demanding patient, with high expectations. You may have a patient in your surgery, or in a consultation skills simulated exam, who looks disgruntled when you explain why their request is not appropriate, no matter how hard you try to provide suitable alternative suggestions. If this is the case, question what you may be missing – ICE, impact, experience – and be curious. Verbalise that you have sensed their dissatisfaction, and fully empathise (including repeating the impact of the problem in the context of their life) before you fully explain why you feel their request is inappropriate. Negotiate and take time to educate the patient, which may also demonstrate that you do know what you are talking about! If, at the end of the consultation, the patient remains unhappy, you may still have done everything appropriately. In an exam, it may be that the nub of the case is to see how you manage the challenging consultation. So, don't dwell on it! It is difficult to justify using NHS resources inappropriately simply because a patient has high expectations. E.g. a referral to an endocrinologist for acne without abnormal blood tests.

Some patients have persistent acne lasting up to the age of 30–40 years and sometimes beyond.[1]

Red flags – refer immediately if   Severe psychological distress.

Uncontrolled acne developing scarring.

Nodulo-cystic acne (Rx can be initiated, but refer).

Diagnostic uncertainty.

Refer for oral isotretinoin, if the patient wishes, for moderate/severe or Rx resistant acne or scarring.

On examination   Comedones, papules, pustules and nodules/cysts.

Treatment[1,2]

See reference[2] for an excellent table advising which treatment works best for each grade of acne. E.g. BPO, topical antibiotics, Duac, OCP or oral antibiotics.

PCDS[1] advise:

Topical retinoids should be used for all grades of acne.

Do not combine a topical and oral antibiotic.[1]

Do not use lymecycline alone – combine with BPO or/and a topical retinoid. [1]

Azelaic acid is helpful in darker skin at risk of hyperpigmentation.[1]

Possible regimes

- Azelaic acid 20% – Skinoren.
- Either BPO or Adapalene alone but they work well in combination (Epiduo).
- Topical Retinoid/Antibiotic Combination Treclin (resistance may limit duration of use).[1]
- Epiduo at night + Duac in the morning.
- Lymecycline + Epiduo.
- Combined oral contraceptives containing co-cyprindiol, e.g. Dianette and any of the above.

Avoid pregnancy   With oral tetracyclines, topical retinoids and isotretinoin.

Doctor's Notes

Patient	Francesca Reece	32 years	F
PMH	NVD 1 year ago		
	Migraines		
Medications	No current medications		
Allergies	No information		
Consultations	GP consultation 1 month ago – advised sun protection for melasma.		
Investigations	No investigations		
Household	Oliver Reece	34 years	M
	Jennifer Reece	13 months	F

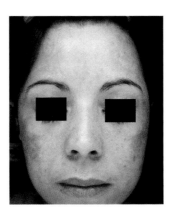

Example Consultation

Open ☐	Tell me about this problem from the beginning. What thoughts have you had about it?
Impact ☐	How has this affected you? Has this changed how you live, your behaviour or mood?
Curious ☐	I see that you saw another GP a month ago. How did that go?
History ☐	Before this, any problems with your skin at all? Have you any other symptoms which cause you trouble? Are you otherwise well? Tell me more about your migraines. Any other medical conditions or skin problems which run in the family? Do you take any medicines? How is Jennifer? Do you have a partner? What does he think? How is your relationship? Have you spoken to anyone else about this? Are you working as well as being a mum?
Risk ☐	Do you spend much time in the sun? Is there stress in your life? How often are you taking ibuprofen for your migraines?
ICE ☐	What do you think has caused this? Is there anything you are worried about? What would be most helpful to you today?
Empathy ☐	This problem is causing you to change your lifestyle and lowering your self-esteem.
Sense ☐	I can see how important this is to you. You look saddened by the change to your skin.
O/E ☐	Thank you for sending a photograph of your face. May I have a close look at this? I can see some pale brown patches on your forehead and cheeks. Everywhere else looks fine.
SummarICE ☐	To summarise, since your pregnancy you feel upset and embarrassed by the uneven pigment on your face. You want to enjoy the outdoors with Jennifer. You feel out of shape, through not running and, therefore your skin is having an impact on your life. You also feel embarrassed and upset that your partner agreed with your comment. You hope a dermatologist can suggest a treatment or a prescription today. Have I got it?
Impression ☐	This is called melasma. Unfortunately, pregnancy can sometimes cause this.
Experience ☐	May I explain about melasma or do you already know about it?
Explanation ☐	Melasma is increased pigment in the skin. The exact cause is unknown but contributing factors are thought to be hormones, stress and sun exposure. There may be a family history. Some perfumed cosmetic products can make it worse.
InCludE ☐	I appreciate you hoped to be seen by a dermatologist; however, I know about treatments for this condition and can recommend something. You were worried this would not go away: hopefully we can improve things but it's important to be realistic. Melasma is difficult to treat and may persist but, gradually, treatments should help to control it. As you are otherwise well, I don't think blood tests will help.
Options ☐	I have some suggestions. Firstly, avoid all things that can make it worse. Ibuprofen can cause a pigment reaction so stop taking this and we could discuss other treatments for migraine on the phone next week? All hormones can make melasma worse. Most of the hormone in the Mirena stays in your womb, but some may be in your bloodstream. You could change to a copper coil which may not make much difference but you could consider the risks and benefits of being hormone free. The copper coil has no hormone but can cause heavier or longer periods and swapping coils is another procedure. Condoms are not as reliable. Could you talk to your partner about this? Finally, wear Factor 50 sun cream 2-hourly throughout the year when outside and use an unperfumed cleanser, moisturiser and make-up.
Recommend ☐	There are lots of creams for melasma. To start with, we could try azelaic acid 15% in the morning and adapalene at night. All creams can cause irritation, so give the skin a break for 1–2 days if this occurs. Perhaps start by using them on alternate days for a week. The risks of creams are that irritation can cause inflammation and make the pigmentation worse. What are your thoughts about this? If this doesn't help, we could try a different combination of creams. These suggestions may start to make a gradual improvement. I do believe this is melasma, but we can do a biopsy to check for other diagnoses if you wish? How do you feel about the suggestions?
Empower ☐	How could you help your fitness? Wear a cap, use sun cream and enjoy running again.
Specifics ☐	Can you please make an appointment to talk to me on the phone next week to discuss your migraines, then for your skin in 3 months? If you are feeling frustrated, see me sooner but, remember, change will take time.
Safety net ☐	If you ever notice any new skin lesions, see a GP straight away.

Dermatology–3

Doctor's notes	Francesca Reece, 32 years. PMH: NVD 1 year ago. Migraines. Medications: none. GP consultation 1 month ago – advised sun protection for melasma.
How to act	Quiet but make it clear that you would be grateful for the doctor's help.
PC	*'My skin around my face still looks brown.'*
History	Since your pregnancy with Jennifer you have had a discoloration around your face. You saw another GP before you moved to the area and felt s/he did not help at all. S/he just suggested sun cream which you used, but this did not help so you now prefer to stay indoors, which is a shame because you would like to spend time outside with Jennifer. You have occasional migraines; you have had a few recently so take ibuprofen several times a week for this, but melasma is your priority today. If the doctor asks questions about your migraine, they are a unilateral headache which takes you to bed, with no raised ICP symptoms. They have been with you since your teenage years and have not changed. You have no features of depression, but the problem does get you down. You have no other symptoms on systemic enquiry. You have no FH of this condition.
Social	You enjoy meeting up with your friends. You work in an office selling online sports equipment and do not smoke or drink alcohol. Your partner once agreed when you said, 'It doesn't look nice, does it?' You know he didn't mean to hurt your feelings but knowing he doesn't like the look of it has made you feel more down. You are already feeling out of shape after the baby and haven't managed to lose much weight. You have a good relationship with your partner who is supportive. He hasn't said anything else that is negative. You have a good group of friends, but it has not happened to them so they don't understand.
	You used to be very active and go running. You don't want to pay for gym membership as you will hardly have the chance to go with the baby and work.
ICE	You are worried this will never go away.
	You don't know what the doctor may be able to do but hope you can see a dermatologist.
	You believe it is your hormones as it started in pregnancy. Do you need a blood test?
	You wonder if going back on the contraceptive pill might help.
	You have the Mirena coil fitted and have had no complications with this.
	If the doctor mentions changing the Mirena, you will consider this.
	You would like, if possible, to be given a prescription to start treatment today.
	Decline a biopsy if offered – you don't like the sound of that.
Examination	Melasma around the forehead and lateral cheeks only.

Dermatology – 3

Learning Points

Ask
Family history (60% report a family history[1]).

Sun exposure.

Contraception.

Impact on life and self-esteem.

Medications can trigger a hyperpigmentation reaction, e.g. NSAID or minocycline.[1]

Blood tests
Thyroid levels if symptomatic.

U&E if suspect Addison's disease.

Advice
Sun protection – hat and factor 50 sun cream, applied 2-hourly – throughout the year.[1]

Avoid perfumed cosmetics, deodorants or soaps.[1]

All hormonal contraceptives can contribute, so discuss the risk/benefit of trying non-hormonal methods.

The response to the advice and treatments can be slow.[1]

Use make-up to disguise and camouflage the pigment.

Pregnancy
Usually melasma will start to fade a few months after pregnancy.[2]

Differential diagnosis
Post-inflammatory pigmentation[1]

Solar lentigines/lentigo[1]

Drug-induced pigmentation[1]

Naevus of Ota and naevus of Hori[1]

Addison's disease

Severity
Melasma Area and Severity Index (MASI).[3]

Refer
For biopsy to confirm the diagnosis if uncertain.

Consider dermatology email advice.

Treatment
'The most successful formulation has been a combination of hydroquinone, tretinoin and moderate potency topical steroid.'[1] This is available in combination as a private prescription called Pigmanorm.

See reference[1] (DermNet NZ) for the full list of treatments.

Risks of treatment
Irritation – see BNF for individual treatment.

Contact dermatitis, further post-inflammatory hyperpigmentation.[1]

Doctor's Notes

Patient	Arthur Miller	12 years	M
PMH	Eczema		
Medications	Eumovate		
	Oilatum		
Allergies	No information		
Consultations	No recent consultations		
Investigations	No investigations		
Household	Anita Miller	45 years	F
	Gary Miller	49 years	M
	Sophie Miller	8 years	F

Open ☐	Thank you for phoning. Arthur, how is your eczema? Mum, what are your thoughts? We can certainly make sure Arthur has a prescription back on repeat.
ICE ☐	I'm just wondering if we can improve things further. What do you think, Arthur? Are you happy with your skin? Why not? What would you like to change? What did you think we may say today? Is there anything else you would like? Mum, what are your thoughts? Is there anything else you thought would be helpful today?
Sense ☐	I can see it is very important that you never run out of creams.
Curious ☐	What do you use for soap, Arthur? And to wash your hair? Is your head itchy?
History ☐	Are you otherwise well? How often do you need to use the Eumovate cream, Arthur? Is that once a day? And in between times how is the skin? Is it completely back to normal? How often do you use the Oilatum? Do you like the Oilatum? Does anyone else in the family have eczema? Are there any other conditions which run in the family? What is the worst your skin has been like? Tell me more about that.
Risk ☐	Do you have any allergies? Pets? Is anything making you unhappy? At school?
Impact ☐	How does your skin impact on your life, Arthur? How about using your medication? How would you feel about using the Oilatum four times a day? What would stop you?
O/E ☐	May I have a look at photographs of your skin now? Please show me wherever it is a problem. Thank you. I can see that there are dry and red flaky patches on the arms and behind the knees. There are no signs of infection. This is mild–moderate eczema.
SummarICE ☐	Arthur, your skin is always itchy but it becomes red every 2 weeks when you need to use the Eumovate, usually twice a day for a couple of days, then it settles down. Mum, we can make sure that you always have cream to use when needed.
Impression ☐	I agree. The eczema is slightly flared up and it is important to make sure it doesn't get worse.
InCludE ☐	It sounds as if the eczema is rarely completely absent and therefore I'd like to help with that, to prevent you needing to use the Eumovate every 2 weeks.
Experience ☐	Arthur, what have you been told about how to use the Oilatum cream? What about the Eumovate? Do you know why we don't suggest using the Eumovate every day?
Explanation ☐	Oilatum is a strong moisturiser. If you use this cream four times a day, it stops the dryness which causes the itching and leads to flare-ups of the eczema. Eumovate is quite a strong steroid cream. The moisturiser won't cause any harm so we can use lots of it, but the steroid creams can cause problems; for example, the skin can get thinner and bruise or it can cause problems inside the body such as weak bones or diabetes. You haven't been using a large amount of steroid, so I am not concerned that you will develop these problems. You are welcome to use the steroid when it flares up, as you have been doing, but I would like to help you to have healthier skin that is less itchy and not so prone to cracks and infection. How does that sound?
Options ☐	I'm wondering what we need to do to help you feel happy with your moisturising creams: change the cream or make it stronger so you need to use it less? Or both? Great – let's do that.
Recommend ☐	Another cream, Doublebase Dayleve, lasts longer. Can we try it every morning?
Empathy ☐	Could you tell your friends about your eczema so they know why you need the cream?
InCludE ☐	Okay, can we be sneaky then and wash out your current shower gel container and fill it with Oilatum? Then your friends won't notice.
Empower ☐	Showering can wash off the morning moisturiser but using Oilatum as a soap will help. Your current shower gel and shampoo strip away all your good work with the moisturiser. There's a better shampoo for eczema – shall we try it? If you can put another layer of moisturiser on after a shower where no one can see, e.g. in the toilet, then do so. Shall I give you a small tube to keep in your bag? If you need the Eumovate, just use this once a day. Mum, what do you think?
Specifics ☐	Shall we speak again in a month and see if that's made a difference? You may find that you no longer need the Eumovate. I will add the creams to your repeat prescriptions. If you also book an appointment for your daughter, we can check how she is getting on.
Safety net ☐	If your skin ever looks red or oozing, see the GP as this may be a sign of infection.

Patient's Story

Doctor's notes Arthur Miller, 12 years. PMH: eczema. Medications: Eumovate and Oilatum.

How to act **Mum** Demanding. Intelligent.

Arthur Articulate.

PC *'We need more steroid cream for Arthur but apparently Arthur needs a medication review.'*

History **Mum** Arthur always responds well to the Eumovate, which he's been using for years. Arthur was born by NVD at term and had no antenatal or postnatal problems. He has had all his immunisations. There is no family history.

Arthur You have no other medical problems. You currently use the Oilatum cream twice a day when the eczema is bad and you don't use it the rest of the time. You have to use the Eumovate every 2 weeks for a couple of days for your arms, wrists and legs. You use it twice a day. In between times it can be itchy, even on the head, but it doesn't always look red. You use Lynx shower gel and Head and Shoulders shampoo. In the past your skin has been cracked and painful and you needed an antibiotic. You have no other medical conditions. You have a younger sister who also has eczema and you have been using her hydrocortisone cream when you ran out of Eumovate.

Social **Arthur** You play sport every day. You are happy at school. You live with your parents and sister. You have no pets.

ICE **Mum** You would like a prescription for the Eumovate to be on repeat so you don't have to keep coming back. You will tell the doctor if there is a problem. You have no concerns.

Arthur Your skin is itchy at times and this bothers you. You don't like using the emollient as it makes you feel sticky. You never take it to school with you and you never apply it after showering after sport. You think your friends would laugh at you putting moisturiser on but it does help. You think the cream works well

Examination Mild–moderate eczema on the arms and behind the knees.

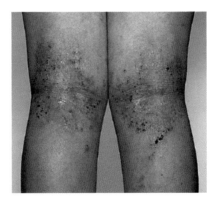

Reproduced from *Common Skin Diseases*, 18th edition (2011), CRC Press. With thanks to the late Ronald Marks and Richard Motley.

Ask	Atopy.
	Family history.
	Impact.
	Compliance and regime with emollients and use of other soaps.
	Stress.
Cause	Genetic and environmental.
	Mutation in the filaggrin gene in atopic eczema causing a defect in the skin barrier layer… 'immunological changes are probably secondary to enhanced antigen penetration through a deficient epidermal barrier. The relevance of this finding is that it reinforces the importance of the regular use of emollients to help manage eczema.'[1]
Flags	Sign of infection.
	Overuse of steroids and underuse of emollients.
	Admit if painful vesicular or ulcerated lesions which may be eczema herpeticum.
Management	Moisturiser '15–20 minutes before applying the topical steroid'.[1]
	Take the time to find out why compliance may be an issue and consider how to adapt the management plan for the individual to increase their emollient use.
	'In both children and adults, it is more effective and safer to "hit hard" using more potent treatments for a few days than it is to use less potent treatments for longer periods of time.'[1]
Other Rx's	Antihistamines for itch.
	Advise emollients as soap substitutes.
	Scalp preparations and shampoos.
	Bandages and dressings.
	Antibiotics – topical or oral.
	Topical immunomodulators – tacrolimus and pimecrolimus.[1]
	Coal tar and ichthammol.
	Salicylic acid.
	Potassium permanganate.

 See the **Link Hub at CompleteMRCGP.co.uk** for helpful links to patient information for eczema
The Primary Care Dermatology Society Website is very helpful. See http://www.pcds.org.uk/clinical-guidance/atopic-eczema for further information.

Doctor's Notes

Patient	Maureen Staples	70 years	F
PMH	Psoriasis		
	Pre-diabetes		
	2 × normal vaginal deliveries		
	Hypertension		
Medications	Dermovate		
	Cetraben		
	Ketoconazole scalp shampoo		
	Amlodipine 5 mg		
Allergies	No information		
Consultations	No recent consultations		
Investigations	18 months ago HbA1c 44 mmol/mol. BP 130/70.		
Household	Brian Staples	72 years	M

Example Consultation

Open ☐ Thank you for coming in to see me. Tell me about you. Tell me about your medical history please. Any problems at all?

Impact ☐ What aspect of the psoriasis troubles you the most? In what way is it a nuisance?

ICE ☐ Is there anything you have been worried about or would like to talk about, as we certainly have time? Is there anything you thought or hoped we may decide today?

History ☐ I'd be interested to know more about your psoriasis from the beginning please. Where is it a problem at present? How bad is it at the moment? And what treatments have you used? How often do you apply the Cetraben? What do you wash with? What shampoo do you use the rest of the time? What do you think about this cream? How often do you apply the Dermovate? Does it make a difference? Every day? How many days within the month would you not apply it? When was the last time you had more than a week's break from it? The scalp shampoo: does this work? How often do you use this? Tell me about a time when your psoriasis was particularly a problem. Do you have any other symptoms elsewhere in the body? Are your eyes and joints okay? How is your general health? Do you have a family history of any medical problems?

Sense ☐ You seem very relaxed about your health. We do like you to see us at least once a year and more often if there are any issues.

Curious ☐ What would you change or try to improve if you could?

O/E ☐ May I have a look at your skin, wherever it is a problem? May I also take your blood pressure. Thank you. May I feel your pulse and listen to your heart? Please step onto the scales, I'd like to check your height and weight.

SummarICE ☐ To summarise, you feel well but the psoriasis has always been a nuisance, rubbing on and damaging clothes and, if you could improve this, it would be helpful. You like the Cetraben which you use twice a day and also in the shower.

Impression ☐ Your psoriasis is moderate in severity. Your high blood pressure is currently under control. I'm wondering how your blood sugars are now and also, because you are a post-menopausal woman, we should have a think about your bones.

Experience ☐ What do you know about psoriasis? Has anyone explained to you the risks of too much steroid cream?

Explanation ☐ Psoriasis is caused by increased cell turnover. The Dermovate is a very strong steroid. You can use this daily for 8 weeks but then you should have a 4-week break as there are risks of too much steroid being absorbed into the body. For example, it can lead to changes in your hormones, a rise in blood pressure, diabetes and thinning of the bones.

Options ☐ I wonder if we can take this opportunity to look at your general health to aim for improvements as well as changing your treatment for psoriasis.

InCludE ☐ I notice that last year's blood test showed that your blood sugar was in the range of pre-diabetes. Was this explained to you? That is correct.

Future ☐ I will also put your numbers into a calculator to determine risk of frail bones so we can discuss this next time. How does this sound?

Empathy ☐ You've lived with a troublesome condition all your life – it must have been wearing.

Recommend ☐ I recommend that you continue the Cetraben at least four times daily and please now stop the steroid cream for at least 4 weeks and use a cream instead, which contains vitamin D, for the next 4 weeks. It is called Dovonex and you put it on twice a day. How do you feel about this? For the scalp I would suggest trying Cocois ointment at night and wash it off in the morning with Capasal shampoo.

Future ☐ If these don't work, we could try coal tar for the body and a steroid mousse for the scalp.

Specifics ☐ It would be helpful if in 1 month you could please arrange a blood test, followed by an appointment with myself at least 2 days later to discuss the results and response to your treatment. I will be telling the nurse what we are testing for: blood cholesterol, kidney function and sugar. If we are not winning, we can ask the dermatologist to see you – you may be suitable for UV treatment. What are your thoughts about this?

Safety net ☐ If ever the skin looks red and is weeping, it may be an infection, so see a doctor.

Doctor's notes	Maureen Staples, 70 years.
	PMH: psoriasis, pre-diabetes, 2 × NVD and hypertension.
	Medications: Dermovate, Cetraben, ketoconazole shampoo and amlodipine.
	Investigations: 18 months ago. HbA1c 44 mmol/mol. BP 130/70.
How to act	Polite and playing down symptoms.
PC	*'I have come for my annual review please.'*
History	You do not like to bother the doctor.
	The pharmacist told you that you are due for your medication review.
	The psoriasis has been present all your life. You do not think about the impact it has on your life as you are used to it. But it does bother you: *'It is a nuisance.'* By this you mean it itches, rubs against clothes and the dry skin ruins your clothes.
	You use the Dermovate most days so you are unsure if it makes a difference. Your last steroid break was 4 months ago. You apply this to your elbows and knees.
	You like the Cetraben and use this in the shower and morning and night.
	Your head irritates you the most. It is itchy. You use the shampoo twice a week and OTC antidandruff shampoo the rest of the week.
	You have taken your blood pressure in the waiting room: it is 120/60.
	No family history.
Social	You have not worked since you were married. Your husband is well.
	You are a proud grandmother of seven grandchildren.
	You enjoy a whisky with your husband every night. You have never smoked.
ICE	Your psoriasis has been with you ever since you can remember. You remember the doctor saying last year that pre-diabetes means nearly diabetes. Since then, you cut out sugar and swim most days. You were very interested in the psoriasis in your 20s and read all about it – but you have forgotten most of it now. You have no concerns. You expect the doctor will just give you the same creams. You are interested in any suggestions the doctor has.
Examination	The psoriasis plaques are moderate in severity. There is psoriasis on the scalp. HS normal. HR 70 bpm regular. BMI 20. BP 120/60.

The 2020 RCGP curriculum reminds us about 'Associated morbidity; physical such as cardiovascular disease and psychological such as depression.'

Ask/triggers	Trauma, infection, pregnancy, sunlight, drugs, stress, alcohol, smoking and HIV.[1]
Associations	Autoimmune conditions.
	Psoriatic arthropathy 'In 30%... early intervention can reduce joint damage.'[1]
	Cardiovascular disease.
	Venous thromboembolism.
	Depression.
Examine	Joints and nails, BP, BMI.
Investigate	CVD: BP, lipids and HbA1c.
NICE suggest	Explain the risks of steroid Rx. Stop steroids when the skin is nearly clear. Prescribe a maximum of 8 weeks of topical potent or very potent steroids, followed by a 4-week break. Encourage emollients. Offer referral with second and third line treatments if required.[2]

For limb/trunk psoriasis:[2]

> 1st – 4 weeks of a potent steroid a.m. and vitamin D/or analogue (e.g. Dovonex) p.m.

> 2nd – Continue the steroid for a maximum of 8 weeks.

> 3rd – Continue vitamin D (or analogue) twice daily until 8–12 weeks.

> 4th – Either a potent corticosteroid BD for 4 weeks or coal tar (e.g. Exorex) BD or combined steroid/vitamin D (Dovobet or Enstilar foam) daily for 4 weeks.

Very potent corticosteroids only if:

> 'In specialist settings under careful supervision when other topical treatment strategies have failed for a maximum period of 4 weeks.'[2]

'Do not use very potent corticosteroids in children and young people.'[2]

Scalp psoriasis

NICE suggests:[2]

- 1st – Commencing with a potent corticosteroid daily for up to 4 weeks.
- 2nd at 4 weeks – Change preparation or add ointments to remove scale. Apply before the steroid.
- 3rd at 8 weeks – Combined calcipotriol + steroid or if mild/don't tolerate, a vitamin D product alone.
- 4th at 16 weeks – A very potent steroid for 2 weeks or coal tar or seek advice.

If mild – an example regime as advised by a dermatologist

Start with	Ointment at night and wash off with a shampoo in the morning.
	Ointment: Sebco™ scalp ointment (coal tar, salicylic acid, sulphur) or Cocois.
	Shampoo: Capasal shampoo (coal tar 1%, coconut oil 1%, salicylic acid 0.5%), T gel or Polytar.
No improvement	Above plus steroid and vitamin D preparation.
	Steroid: betamethasone valerate (Bettamousse) 0.1% (potent).
	Vitamin D: calcipotriol scalp solution.
When improved	Stop the Sebco and continue shampoo and the Bettamousse.
When controlled	Stop the steroid (Bettamousse) and continue antipsoriasis shampoo PRN.

ENT, Speech and Hearing

	Cases in this chapter	Within the RCGP 2020 curriculum: ENT, Speech and Hearing	Learning points in this chapter include:
1	Facial Nerve Palsy	'Cranial nerve disorders such as Bell's palsy'	Causes, natural history and management of facial nerve palsy (Bell's palsy)
2	Acute Otitis Media	'Ear disorders: earache and discharge including otitis externa and media with and without effusion'	Management of otitis media and externa
3	Deafness and Tinnitus	'Hearing problems including deafness such as occupational, presbycusis, otosclerosis, tinnitus and associated speech or language disorders' 'Ensure that a patient's hearing impairment or deafness does not prejudice the information communicated or your attitude as a doctor towards the patient and be able to communicate effectively'	Deafness and tinnitus Weber and Rinne's test
4	Sinusitis	'Sinus problems including acute and chronic infection'	Management of sinusitis
5	BPPV	'Vertigo – including BPPV' 'Dix–Hallpike test to diagnose BPPV' 'The Epley manoeuvre'	Causes and management of BPPV Assessment using Dix–Hallpike test Epley manoeuvre
Extra Notes	ENT 2WW and Emergencies	'Relevant local and national guidelines including fast track referral guidance for suspected cancer' 'Upper respiratory infections including… epiglottitis'	Suspected cancer Referral criteria Unilateral deafness Epiglottitis

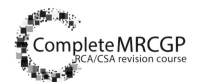

CompleteMRCGP
RCA/CSA revision course

CHAPTER 5 REFERENCES

Facial Nerve Palsy

1. NICE CKS. Bell's palsy. http://cks.nice.org.uk/bells-palsy. May 2019.
2. http://patient.info/health/bells-palsy
3. Margabanthu G., Brooks J., Barron D, Miller P. Facial palsy as a presenting feature of coarctation of aorta. *Interact Cardiovasc Thorac Surg* 2003; 2: 91–3.
4. Peitersen E. The natural history of Bell's palsy. *Am J Otol* 1982; 4: 107–11.

Acute Otitis Media

1. NICE CKS. Otitis media – acute. http://cks.nice.org.uk/otitis-media-acute. Jan 2021.
2. NICE CKS. Analgesia – mild-to-moderate pain. https://cks.nice.org.uk/analgesia-mild-to-moderate-pain#!scenario:5. Aug 2020.
3. https://gpnotebook.com/simplepage.cfm?ID=-1576665032

Useful Resource

Patient information leaflet: https://patient.info/ears-nose-throat-mouth/earache-ear-pain/ear-infection-otitis-media#nav-2

Deafness and Tinnitus

1. NICE Guideline NG98. Hearing loss in adults. https://www.nice.org.uk/guidance/ng98. Jun 2018.
2. NICE CKS. Tinnitus. https://cks.nice.org.uk/tinnitus#!scenario. Mar 2020.

Useful Resource

Patient information leaflet: https://www.tinnitus.org.uk/pages/category/information-leaflets

Sinusitis

1. NICE CKS. Sinusitis. http://cks.nice.org.uk/sinusitis. Mar 2021.

Useful Resource

Patient information leaflet: http://patient.info/health/acute-sinusitis

BPPV

1. NICE CKS. Benign paroxysmal positional vertigo. http://cks.nice.org.uk/benign-paroxysmal-positional-vertigo. Oct 2017.
2. http://patient.info/doctor/vertebrobasilar-occlusion-and-vertebral-artery-syndrome
3. http://www.thebsa.org.uk/wp-content/uploads/2014/04/HM.pdf

Useful Resource

Patient information leaflet: http://patient.info/health/benign-paroxysmal-positional-vertigo-leaflet

ENT 2WW and Emergencies

1. NICE Guideline NG12. Suspected cancer: recognition and referral. Jan 2021.
2. NICE CKS. Hearing loss in adults. https://cks.nice.org.uk/hearing-loss-in-adults#!scenario. Sept 2019.
3. NICE Guidelines. Sore throat – acute. http://cks.nice.org.uk/sore-throat-acute#!diagnosisadditional:6. Jan 2021.

Information taken from NICE guidelines with kind permission. Please note the guidelines change frequently and you should ALWAYS check for the latest updated guidance. Remember that NICE guidance is only applicable to patients in the UK.

ENT, Speech and Hearing

Doctor's Notes

Patient	Mike Williams	55 years	M
PMH	Hypertension		
Medications	Ramipril 5 mg daily		
Allergies	No information		
Consultations	Recent consultation with PN – BP well controlled.		
	Calculated CVD risk 12% – statins discussed but patient declined.		
	Medication reauthorised for 3 months.		
Investigations	3 months ago. Normal U&E. Total cholesterol 6.1 mmol/L, ratio 2.2.		
Household	Barbara Williams	55 years	F

Example Consultation

Open ☐ Mr Williams, it's good to meet you. I'm sorry to see you looking so concerned and with this weakness in your face. Tell me how it started. Have you noticed anything else? How is your health generally?

History ☐ Any earache? Any deafness or dizziness? I notice you have high BP. Can I check if you've been taking your medication? And tell me more about you. Do you have family or friends around you? Tell me about your work.

Sense ☐ I can see how concerned and upset you are and understandably so.

ICE ☐ You are worried this is a stroke. Do you have any other thoughts or worries? Did you have anything in mind you hoped I might be able to do for you today?

Flags ☐ I need to ensure this problem is confined to the nerve in your face. Are your arms and legs feeling and working normally? Any problems with your vision? Are you able to wrinkle your forehead? Any problems with your speech?

Curious ☐ Have you known this happen to anyone else? Were your father's symptoms the same or different?

Impact ☐ I understand you want this to resolve as quickly as possible. How might this problem affect you?

SummarICE ☐ To summarise, you woke up this morning with a lopsided face, blinking is difficult and you have been drooling from your mouth. You are worried it might be a stroke due to your BP and your father's history, but also because you don't take medication for cholesterol. You fear how this looks to others and want to do whatever is required to help you return to work as soon as possible. Have I missed anything out?

O/E ☐ I would like to check your BP, examine the nerves in your face, both ears and your mouth and check for lumps around the ear. Is that okay?

Empathy ☐ I appreciate this is distressing. It's very unpleasant for you to have your face affected like this.

InCludE ☐ I understand why you questioned a stroke, but thankfully it isn't.

Impression ☐ We call this Bell's palsy – it's a temporary weakness of the face nerve.

Experience ☐ Have you heard of Bell's palsy? Do you know anyone who has had it?

Explanation ☐ In Bell's palsy, the facial nerve suddenly stops sending normal electrical impulses to the muscles in the face so they can't work normally. We don't know what causes it, although it may be a virus. Most people make a full recovery over a period of weeks or months and only a few are left with any lasting weakness. If there were 100 people like you, 71 would make a full and complete recovery, 13 would have a little weakness and just 16 would have lasting facial weakness.

Recommend ☐ We know that taking steroid tablets for about 10 days may help this to get better quicker. This is what I would suggest. How do you feel about that? I recommend prednisolone 50 mg daily for 10 days.

Options ☐ You are correct – steroids may increase your BP temporarily. Like any treatment, we need to weigh up the benefits against the risks. Your BP is nicely controlled so I am happy for you to take the steroids. What do you think? We also need to protect your eye as the surface of the eye can become too dry. I'm going to prescribe some lubricants and an eye pad to use at night.

InCludE ☐ Antivirals? A good thought, but unfortunately it's been found that they don't work.

Empower ☐ I'm going to give you a leaflet to read about Bell's palsy.

Future ☐ Come back and see a GP in a week when you have finished the tablets.

Safety net ☐ If you feel you are getting worse, or if the eye becomes sore or if the other side of your face becomes affected, see the GP the same day or ring 111 if it is out of hours. I don't think this will happen, but if your arm, leg or other parts of your body become weak, call 999 straight away.

ENT, Speech and Hearing – 1

Doctor's notes	Mike Williams, 55 years. PMH: hypertension. Medication: ramipril. All well at a routine check with the nurse 3 months ago. Medication renewed. Statins declined.
How to act	Very worried.
PC	*'I woke up this morning and my face is lopsided. Have I had a stroke?'*
History	You realised you are drooling at the mouth and can't move the left side of your face. You have no other neurological symptoms and you feel well in yourself.
	You were diagnosed with hypertension 5 years ago. You mostly (but not always) remember to take ramipril. The nurse discussed statins but you had read they cause leg cramps and didn't think you needed them.
	Family history of stroke – father died of this 2 years ago.
Social	You live with your wife. You have no children. You work at a local stately home, showing visitors around. Money is tight as your wife lost her job. Never smoked. Minimal alcohol.
ICE	You believe you have had a stroke. You have no other thoughts of what may be causing this. You are angry at yourself for declining the statin.
	Before your father died you saw a change in him mentally as well as physically, which was upsetting to see.
	You work with the public and you fear what people may think. Whatever is wrong you want to get back to work soon. You don't think you get sick pay.
	If the doctor mentions this might be 'a virus' you will ask for antiviral drugs to get better as quickly as you can. If the doctor mentions steroids, you would be concerned they would push your BP up.
Examination	CN VII – asymmetry visible. Left side – face drooping and cannot close eye or blink.
	Only if specifically asked, left side of forehead is affected – does not wrinkle when asked to 'screw up face or raise eyebrows'.
	BP 130/70.
	Ears and mouth – NAD.
	No parotid swelling.
Questions	*'Will this get better? Will the other side of my face go the same way?'*

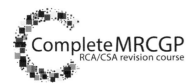

CompleteMRCGP
RCA/CSA revision course

Learning Points

The most common cause of facial weakness. Unilateral, comes on rapidly. Can make the diagnosis on symptoms/signs **if no other medical cause can be found.**[1]

Cause A problem with facial (VII) nerve at the geniculate ganglion. Cause unknown but ?viral ?reactivation (herpes or varicella).

Epidemiology Typical age group: 15–45. Equally common in men and women.[1]

Risk factors Diabetes, hypertension or obesity. Also, if pregnant or immunocompromised. Upper respiratory tract infections.

Symptoms Rapid onset of a unilateral facial weakness with drooling and excessive tears.

Investigations No routine tests needed for new onset Bell's palsy in primary care.[1]

Prognosis Recovery generally starts in 2 weeks, but may take up to 12 months to fully resolve.[2]

Treatment 1. Reassure that the outlook is good. Likely to recover fully within 3–4 months.

2. Corneal protection essential – lubricant drops/ointment at night/eyepatch.

3. Consider prednisolone, if patient presents within 72 hours. Options:

50 mg for 10 days

60 mg for 5 days, then taper down by 10 mg each day for 5 days

4. Antivirals not recommended as no evidence that they make any difference.

Differential diagnosis – rare but serious conditions

Stroke Remember that in an UMN lesion, the forehead is generally spared due to dual innervation.

Cancer Consider tumours of brain, facial nerve, parotid gland, skin tumour, facial nerve, malignant otitis externa.

Cholesteatoma Hearing loss + foul smelling discharge from the ear.[1]

Trauma E.g. after surgery, or fracture of the base of the skull.

Coarctation Raised BP, high level of suspicion in children.

Reports of Bell's palsy + HTN leading to detection of underlying coarctation of aorta.[3]

Lyme disease If a rash or symptoms of Lyme disease has been present.

Referral To neurology or ENT if: any doubt about diagnosis, neurological symptoms getting worse or no improvement within 3 weeks or if suspect serious underlying problem such as parotid tumour or cholesteatoma.[1]

To ophthalmology: if the person has troublesome eye symptoms (for example, pain, itchiness or irritation.[1]

A study of 1011 patients[1,4] 71% complete recovery

84% complete or near complete recovery

16% permanent deficit of facial function

Doctor's Notes

Patient	Sarah Smith	5 years	F
PMH	None		
Medications	No current medications		
Allergies	No information		
Consultations	No recent consultations		
Investigations	No recent investigations		
Household	Darren Smith	34 years	M
	Natasha Smith	33 years	F
	Charlie Smith	9 years	M

Sarah attends the GP with her mum today.

Open ☐	Hello Sarah, hello Mrs Smith. Oh, I'm so sorry to hear you've got earache – that's horrid isn't it? Sarah, tell me how it feels. Mum, can you tell me more about her earache? Anything else that you have noticed?
History ☐	Have you tried any medicine? How is Sarah's health? Any problems at birth? Any concern in the past with hearing or development? Is she fully immunised? Is she allergic to any medicines? Who is at home? What do you both do for a living?
Flags ☐	Is Sarah drinking okay? Any signs that she can't hear so well? Has she had a high temperature? When did this start? Do the fevers go down with pain relief? Is she moving her neck and looking at lights okay? Any concerns with her breathing? Rashes? Good, it sounds like the rest of you is okay, Sarah, but we need to look at your ears!
Risk ☐	Does anyone in the family have any ear problems?
Sense ☐	It's rare that you need to bring Sarah to see us and I sense you must be concerned about her.
ICE ☐	May I ask if you've come across ear infections before? Did anything particularly worry you about Sarah? Did you have anything in mind that I might be able to prescribe or do for Sarah today?
Impact ☐	Has Sarah needed time off school? Has that been difficult for you, for example with your own work?
Curious ☐	You mentioned that you are not keen at all on antibiotics. May I ask why you prefer to avoid them? I'm sorry to hear about Charlie's experience but I can tell you that allergies don't normally run in families.
SummarICE ☐	To summarise so far, Sarah is healthy but has had earache for 5 days. You were hoping to avoid antibiotics due to previous experience. You feel this is likely to be a virus but you would like to check there are no complications developing, like mastoiditis which you have read about. Have I understood correctly?
O/E ☐	I'd like to check Sarah's temperature and pulse, look at the throat and ears, check she has no swellings and listen to her chest. Is that okay with you, Sarah? Would you like to sit on Mum's knee while I have a look?
Empathy ☐	The ear drums are red and look sore. There is pus in the left ear suggesting the eardrum may have popped due to the infection. The mastoid bone is not painful, which is reassuring.
Impression ☐	My impression is that she has a middle ear infection causing a temperature.
Experience ☐	What is your experience of ear infections…or with friends' children?
Explanation ☐	The fact that Sarah has had a cold for 2 weeks and now earache for 5 days with no improvement despite regular pain relief, and the discharge in her ear canal, makes me think it is more likely a bacterial infection.
InCludE ☐	Therefore, although I know you aren't keen on antibiotics, they should help. Thankfully the mastoid bone does not appear affected. What are your thoughts? Grommets may be inserted with repeated ear infections where the fluid build-up may prevent hearing development.
Recommend ☐	Like you, I'm keen to only use antibiotics when they are really needed but I do think that Sarah needs them and this is what I would suggest.
Options ☐	Research suggests that after 4 days of symptoms antibiotics are more likely to be necessary. A fever and pus also suggest it is not clearing. What are your thoughts now? Okay, I will issue amoxicillin.
Empower ☐	Please give this antibiotic three times a day for 5 days. Here is a leaflet on children's ear infections.
Future ☐	I expect her to start getting better in a couple of days. It would be helpful to see her again in about 6 weeks to make sure the eardrum has healed. In the meantime, don't put anything into the left ear and keep it dry.
Safety net ☐	If, however, she gets worse please bring her back.
Specifics ☐	For example, a fever which does not come down with paracetamol/ibuprofen or ongoing symptoms after completion of the antibiotics, a swelling behind the ear, pain moving the neck, breathing problems suggesting a chest infection or hearing problems.

Patient's Story

Acute Otitis Media

Doctor's notes	Sarah Smith, 5 years. Attending with mum, Natasha Smith, aged 33 years.
	PMH: none. Medications: none.
How to act	Caring, articulate, sure of yourself and going to stand your ground.
PC	*'She's had earache for the past 5 days. I just wanted you to check her out, please.'*
History	Sarah can tell you it hurts but then looks to Mum.
	Sarah has had a cold for a couple of weeks and started with bilateral earache about 5 days ago, L>R. You thought this might be something she had caught at school. You have been giving her regular paracetamol and ibuprofen but with no real improvement. You noticed some discharge in her ear canal this morning. She has had a fever since last night but it settled with analgesia.
	There are no lower respiratory symptoms.
	She is a little miserable and off food but drinking and passing urine.
	No symptoms of meningitis.
	She seems able to hear normally but keeps pulling at her ears.
Social	Two-parent family. Dad is an accountant and mum is a part-time teacher. One older child: Charlie, aged 9 years.
ICE	Most ear infections are viral. Antibiotics should be avoided because they interfere with your immune system. Charlie got a rash with amoxicillin and is now 'allergic' to it. It didn't seem to make him any better.
	Sarah has never had antibiotics and you don't intend her to start now.
	Deep down you believe she is fine, you have experience with children, but when it's your own you doubt your judgement and want an opinion. You looked on the internet and started reading about the mastoid bone. You would like reassurance this bone is okay.
	If antibiotics are offered, you will refuse them. *'Are you sure? She's never had antibiotics and I don't want her to have them now.'*
Understanding	You have read that it is much better for children to make their own antibodies to infections.
	You have known some children tell you they have had an operation for grommets.
Ask the doctor	*'When is the grommet operation necessary?'*
Examination	Temperature 38.5°C. HR 100 bpm. Throat red, both ear drums very red, discharge in left ear canal, chest clear.

Learning Points

Managing patients who present with ear infections[1,2]

Advice for everyone with acute otitis media

- Reduced hearing may be present for a few days.
- High temperature is common.
- Symptoms usually last 3 days but can be up to 7 days.
- Use regular paracetamol or ibuprofen – appropriate for age.
- Drink plenty of fluids, eat normally, if you can.
- Decongestants and antihistamines probably don't work.

If unwell:

Think about admission

- Under 3 months of age or 3–6 months of age with a temperature of >39°C – hot and irritable.

Immediate admission

- If very unwell, e.g. severe systemic infection.
- If you suspect complications:
  - Infective – intracranial abscess, meningitis or mastoiditis.
  - Neurological – facial nerve paralysis.
  - Vascular – sinus thrombosis.
- Children <3 months with temperature >38°C.

Antibiotics[1,3]

Note that crying and pain are often a lot less from day 2, regardless of treatment with antibiotics.

Use immediately – very unwell, symptoms of a more serious illness or complication, or high risk of complications.

Consider antibiotics if age <2, symptoms for more than 3 days or otorrhoea but remember possible adverse effects of antibiotics. Options are:

- No antibiotic + advice to seek help if symptoms worsen, not improving in 3 days or becomes very unwell.
- Prescription for antibiotic to get if needed + above advice.
- Immediate antibiotic + above advice.

Antibiotic of choice: 5–7day course of amoxicillin, or erythromycin if allergic to penicillin. Note erythromycin less effective against *H. influenzae*. Can also use azithromycin or clarithromycin – effective against all main bacteria that cause acute otitis media.[1,3]

If symptoms worsen, think about:

- Resistance to antibiotic – has one been used previously?
- Could this be glue ear?
- Are there symptoms or signs that might suggest a more serious diagnosis?

Note there is some evidence that use of antibiotics is linked to reduced middle ear effusions after 3 months.[3]

Follow-up

Routine follow-up is not required.

Learning point – making assumptions about expectations

It is easy to jump to assumptions; for example, that the mum of a hot poorly child is wanting antibiotics but, as in this case, that is not always the situation. Always keep an open mind and check the patient's thoughts, fears and hopes (ICE) so that you are informed rather than surprised and you can tailor your explanation and shared management plan appropriately.

ENT, Speech and Hearing – 2

Doctor's Notes

Patient	Anthony Warren	52 years	M
PMH	Vasectomy 5 years ago		
Medications	None		
Allergies	None		
Consultations	Nil recent		
Investigations	None		
Household	Julie Warren	45 years	F
	Emma Warren	12 years	F
	Daniel Warren	9 years	M

Open ☐	Hello Mr Warren – I'm very sorry to hear that. Please tell me more about your hearing. And tell me what others have noticed – for example your wife and children.
ICE ☐	What has your wife noticed? And what worries you most? Did you have anything in your mind you thought I might be able to do today?
History ☐	A few questions about the deafness. How did this start? When are you most affected? Any situations when it seems particularly bad? Any ringing in the ears? What is it like? When do you notice this?
Flags ☐	Are both ears affected or just one? Any discharge or pain in the ears? Has your nose been blocked? Have you had any nose bleeds? Any episodes of dizziness or loss of balance? Any blurring of vision or weakness or numbness of arms and legs?
Impact ☐	Tell me how this is affecting you – in your job at school and your home life.
Risk ☐	Please tell me about your work over the years. Have you ever worked in a noisy environment? Do you have any hobbies that involve noise? Do you scuba dive? Do you take any medications? Anyone in the family with hearing problems?
Experience ☐	I'm interested to know more about your father.
Empathy ☐	I'm sorry to hear that – he must have felt very isolated.
Curious ☐	What do you know about deafness? Are there any students at school who are deaf?
Sense ☐	I sense you are embarrassed about this as well as frustrated at how it affects you.
O/E ☐	First, I would like to look in both ears with a special torch called an otoscope. Thank you. Both ears look normal, there is no wax and the drums are shiny and healthy. Now I want to do two tests with a tuning fork. I'm going to make the fork ring and then put it on the middle of your forehead. Please tell me whether you hear it louder on the left or on the right, or both the same. Thank you. Now I'm going to ring the fork again and place it on your mastoid bone on each side, here. Please tell me when it stops ringing. I'm then going to put it next to your ear. If you can still hear it, please show me by raising your hand and then tell me when it stops.
SummarICE ☐	To summarise, for several years you have noticed a bit of a problem with your hearing, but others have noticed it more and you feel it's time to get some help.
Impression ☐	I think you have what we call sensorineural hearing loss.
Explanation ☐	This means that the tiny hairs in the ear, or the nerves to the ear are not working well so that the nerve signals that transmit the sound are weaker, causing deafness. The ringing in your ears is called tinnitus and it is very common in sensorineural deafness.
Empathy ☐	It must be very upsetting – your work is affected and you are worried you may go very deaf and become isolated like your father. And children can be so cruel.
Recommend ☐	I recommend that we refer you to get a hearing assessment called an audiogram. The hearing technicians will be able to recommend and prescribe a hearing aid for you.
InCludE ☐	I know this isn't what you hoped for but modern hearing aids are small and discrete. How do you feel about this now? It will take some getting used to but try and persist – it should really help.
Options	For the tinnitus, I would like to give you a PIL from the British Tinnitus Association. There are lots of suggestions to try, such as having a little background noise at night, e.g. the radio at very low volume. I would also like to check your BP, cholesterol and blood sugar – please see the PN for this.
Empower ☐	There are some things you can do to help. Please protect your hearing by always using good ear protection in a noisy environment, for example when playing at concerts.
Future ☐	Please come back to see me after you have been to audiology and we can discuss their findings.
Safety net ☐	If you have a sudden change in hearing or develop severe earache, discharge, nosebleeds, dizziness or any weakness or numbness in your face or limbs, please see a doctor straight away.

Patient's Story

Doctor's notes   Anthony Warren, 52 years. PMH: vasectomy. Medications: none.

How to act   Concerned, embarrassed. If the doctor does not face you and speak clearly, you will struggle to hear what he or she says and will need to ask him or her to repeat themselves.

PC   *'The wife thinks I'm deaf. She's wondering if something can be done.'*

History   For the last few years you have noticed increasing problems with your hearing. At home you have to have the TV louder than everyone else would like. Your wife remarks that you often don't hear her and are always saying 'Pardon?' At school the classroom can be noisy and you don't always hear what the students say. Your daughter Emma recently started at the school and has told you that other students laugh and snigger about your hearing and call you *'Dodo'*, or *'Deaf as a dodo'*. She is embarrassed about this. Your father went very deaf at a relatively young age and you remember how socially isolated he became, almost a recluse and cut off from the family. You also have bilateral tinnitus and notice this especially at night when it's quiet and trying to sleep. In fact, you wondered if it was the neighbour's burglar alarm, but your wife couldn't hear it at all.

Social   History teacher at local comprehensive school. Enjoyable but really tough school with challenging students. You live with your wife and two children. She is a hairdresser. Social drinker, never smoked. Hobbies – play guitar with a local band. Gigs once a fortnight, often noisy.

ICE   Ideas – *'I am going deaf like my father. It must be inherited. There's probably nothing that can be done to help.'*

Concerns – *'How am I going to do my job? I don't really want to wear a hearing aid as I fear the students would tease me about this.'*

Expectations – Possibly a referral to ENT.

Examination findings   Both ears – no wax, canals clear, ear drums normal and shiny. Weber's and Rinne's show sensorineural deafness, bilateral. No neck lumps.

> Weber's – the tuning fork is heard equally loudly in both ears.
>
> Rinne's – can hear the tuning fork after it is removed from the mastoid, but only for a few seconds. L=R.

Learning Points

Deafness

Red flags	Unilateral.
	Sudden onset.
	Fluctuating hearing levels.
	Persistent tinnitus, especially if pulsatile or causing distress.
Immediate referral	NICE advise if:
	• Sudden onset (3 days or less) severe sensorineural deafness. May be viral but oral steroids may be needed.
	• Hearing loss with facial droop – urgent admission ENT, or stroke pathway if stroke suspected.
	• Immunocompromised + deafness + otalgia + discharge with no response to 72 hours of treatment.
2WW referral	Unilateral progressive deafness especially with vertigo and/or tinnitus.
	Nasal obstruction and epistaxis with persistent unexplained hearing loss may mean post-nasal space tumour.
	Adults of Chinese or Southeast Asian heritage with hearing loss and middle ear effusion not associated with infection.
Adults with dementia, learning disability, cognitive impairment	Consider audiology referral for assessment then every 2 years for hearing test.
Examination	Ear drums and canals, palpate neck for lumps. Use Weber's/Rinne's to differentiate sensorineural form conductive hearing loss.
Sensorineural hearing loss	Caused by damage to acoustic nerve, the cochlea or the hair cells.
	Risk factors – age, noise exposure, atherosclerosis, smoking.
Conductive hearing loss	Caused by ear wax, perforated ear drum, problems with ossicles.
Weber's	Unilateral conductive loss – sound is louder in affected ear.
	Unilateral sensorineural hearing loss – sound louder in non-affected ear.
	Heard equally in both – normal hearing or hearing loss is bilateral.
Rinne's	Air conduction better than bone conduction (AC > BC) – normal hearing or sensorineural deafness.
	BC > AC – conductive deafness.
Treatment	Encourage early use of hearing aid. May need persistence.

Tinnitus

Urgent referral	Unilateral; pulsatile; associated with unilateral hearing loss; associated with persistent otalgia.
Treatment	Reassure, treat cause if possible, check medications and review, discuss sound therapy, refer for counselling or CBT.

Doctor's Notes

Patient	Jennifer Richards	39 years	F
PMH	Two normal vaginal deliveries		
	Upper respiratory tract infection		
Allergies	No known drug allergies		
Medications	Rigevidon		
Consultations	Routine pill check with practice nurse 2 months ago – all well		
Investigations	BP 2 months ago 102/60		
Household	Alan Richards	30 years	M
	Louis Richards	10 years	M
	Amy Richards	8 years	F

Open ☐	Hello Mrs Richards. Oh, I am sorry to hear that. Please tell me more about how your sinusitis started this time and what symptoms you are getting.
History ☐	Tell me about the nasal discharge. Clear? Green? Any headaches – whereabouts? Has this happened before? Please tell me about any medical problems in the past. Have you tried any medication for this?
Flags ☐	Does the light bother you? On a scale of 1–10, how bad are the headaches? Do you feel ill? Any double vision? Have you had a fever?
Sense ☐	You sound quite tense and upset at the moment. Tell me what's going on in your life as well as the sinus pain?
Impact ☐	How is the sinusitis affecting you at home and work?
Curious ☐	Tell me about school and the pressures at work. What do you teach? How long for? Are you busy at home too? Do you have support there?
ICE ☐	You mentioned you had sinusitis before and it didn't get better with a normal antibiotic and you were prescribed a powerful one. Tell me – what worries you about the sinusitis? As well as antibiotics, was there anything else you were hoping I could do to help?
SummarICE ☐	To summarise so far, you had a cold for about a week and now facial pain and discharge for 3 days which is not getting better with paracetamol. There's pressure in your face and pressure in your life too as Ofsted are coming in 3 days and it's important to be at your best and do well.
O/E ☐	Do you have a thermometer? Could you check your temperature for me? Could you press over your forehead and cheeks and either side of your nose? Any soreness? Could you bend forward and see if this makes the pain worse?
Empathy ☐	Feeling lousy with facial pain and headaches must be pretty miserable, especially with the stress of an imminent Ofsted visit.
Impression ☐	From what you've told me, I think you are absolutely right – you have sinusitis.
Explanation ☐	To be honest, it's far more likely to be viral than bacterial and there is no evidence that antibiotics make any difference for people like you who are normally fit and well.
InCludE ☐	I suspect that last time you got better despite the antibiotics rather than because of them. Let's talk about how we can have you feeling better as soon as possible.
Options ☐	I will talk you through some self-help measures. I don't want to prescribe antibiotics because all the evidence suggests that they will make no difference and they may give you diarrhoea and contribute to drug resistance.
Empower ☐	I will text you a link to a PIL that describes things you can do that will make a difference.
Recommend ☐	My recommendation is regular fluids and pain relief, warm facial compresses, salt solution for your nose, and a decongestant spray. Breathing in steam probably doesn't help. You may wish to try nasal douching. People either love it because it flushes out the sinus passages or hate it because squirting salty water into your nose isn't pleasant.
Future ☐	This should get fully better within 2–3 weeks and, with the treatment, you should start to feel better soon.
Specifics ☐	If you are not fully better in 2–3 weeks or if you get bad headaches, a temperature or feel really ill, book an appointment to see me straight away.
Safety net ☐	If this happens out of hours, phone 111.

Doctor's notes	Jennifer Richards, 39 years. Two pregnancies and URTI in past. On combined pill for contraception (Rigevidon).
How to act	Anxious, demanding.
PC	*'I won't keep you long, Doctor. It's my sinusitis again – I just need antibiotics.'*
History	Sore throat and runny nose for a week, self-medicated with paracetamol. Last 3 days, increasing nasal discharge (sometimes clear, sometimes green) and facial pain. Some headaches: frontal, worse when you bend your head forwards. You've had headaches for a few weeks anyway and think it is work stress.
	Paracetamol has been useless.
Social	Married with two children. English teacher at local secondary school. Ofsted inspection in 3 days' time – school was 'failing' last time, pressure to do better this time, otherwise the school might close and you could lose your job.
	You rarely drink alcohol and do not smoke.
ICE	You know that doctors are reluctant to prescribe antibiotics but you don't ask for them often and this time you really need them as you believe they will make you better quicker. Last time you had amoxicillin and it didn't do anything and you had to come back for stronger ones (cefalexin) which made the sinusitis better after a week.
Ask the doctor	If refused antibiotics: *'What can I do? I need to be on top of this in 3 days when the inspectors come.'*
	If given antibiotics: *'What do I need to do about contraception? Will they interfere with my pill?'*
	If offered amoxicillin: *'It does not work and I need cefalexin.'*
Examination	Temperature 37.2°C. Tender in forehead and cheeks, worse when you bend forward.

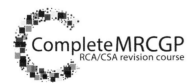

CompleteMRCGP
RCA/CSA revision course

ENT, Speech and Hearing – 4

Acute sinusitis[1]

'Acute sinusitis usually follows a common cold, and is defined as an increase in symptoms after 5 days, or persistence of symptoms beyond 10 days, but less than 12 weeks.'[1]

Usual management[1]

Paracetamol and/or ibuprofen (relieve symptoms by reducing pain and temperature).

Consider irrigating nose with saline solution.

Some may wish to try intranasal decongestant, e.g. spray (OTC) – but no evidence to support use. Oral decongestant not recommended.

No proven benefit[1]

Steam inhalation, antihistamines, mucolytics, warm face packs.

Antibiotics

Not needed if symptoms for <10 days unless patient is systemically very unwell, has symptoms and signs of a more serious illness or condition, or is at high risk of complications.

May consider if symptoms >10 days, but remember adverse effects of antibiotics and that antibiotics makes little difference to how long symptoms last.

Adults: phenoxymethylpenicillin 500 mg QDS for 5 days, or co-amoxiclav 500/125 TDS for 5 days or doxycycline or clarithromycin if allergic to penicillin.

Children and young people <18 – choice of antibiotic as above in age-appropriate dose but doxycycline contraindicated in <12 years.

Nasal corticosteroids (see NICE guidance for further details)

After 10 days of symptoms, consider prescribing high-dose nasal corticosteroid for 14 days, e.g. mometasone 20 mg BD (off label use) in adults and children >12 years.

Rare but important complications needing admission[1]

Severe systemic infection.

Orbital involvement (double vision, oculomotor nerve paralysis, eyeball displaced, new ↓visual acuity).

Intracranial involvement with symptoms/signs of meningitis, frontal bone swelling, severe fontal headache or focal neurological signs.

Chronic sinusitis[1]

Consider if nasal blockage/discharge with facial pain/headache and/or loss of smell for >12 weeks.

Associated with atopy, asthma, immunosuppression.

Manage with above measures but also consider 3 months of intranasal corticosteroids.

Consider referral to ENT if:

- 3 months' trial of intranasal corticosteroids + above measures are ineffective.
- Unilateral symptoms.
- Nasal polyps especially in children.
- Recurrent episodes of otitis media + pneumonia in children.
- Unusual opportunistic symptoms.
- Symptoms interfering with quality of life.
- Allergic or immunological risk factors that need investigation.

ENT, Speech and Hearing – 4

Doctor's Notes

Patient	Freda White	60 years	F
PMH	Type 2 diabetes		
Medications	Metformin, gliclazide		
Allergies	No known allergies		
Consultations	Diabetes check 1 month ago – all well		
Investigations	1 month ago HbA1c 54 mmol/mol. Lipid profile normal.		
	U&E normal		
	BP 130/70		
	No microalbuminuria		
Household	Raymond White	70 years	M

Open ☐	I'm sorry to hear about that. Please tell me more about the dizziness from the beginning. Tell me how and when this started.
ICE ☐	What thoughts have you had about this? Did you worry it may be from the cruise? Did anything make you worry that there might be something significant going on?
History ☐	By dizzy do you mean lightheaded or is the room spinning? Do you still have symptoms now? How long did it last? Have you noticed any triggers? Have you had this before? Apart from the diabetes, do you have any other significant medical problems?
Sense ☐	I sense you are very concerned about this and perhaps, particularly, about whether there is something seriously wrong with you.
Impact ☐	Tell me about work. What do you do? Do you need to drive to get to work? How has the dizziness been affecting things that you normally do at home?
Empathy ☐	It must be very unpleasant feeling dizzy and sick so much. I understand your fears about what this could be and the consequences that not working would bring for your family. No wonder your husband is concerned.
Curious ☐	I'm wondering why you think it may be a tumour; have you read something online?
Flags ☐	Have you had any headaches? Have you vomited? Any deafness or ear problems? Any other symptoms in the chest like pain or palpitations? Any symptoms of the arms or legs not feeling or working normally? Any ringing in your ears? Does your coordination seem normal?
Risk ☐	How is your diabetes? Blood sugars at home? Has the dizziness made you fall?
SummarICE ☐	To summarise, for the last few weeks you have had episodes of the room spinning lasting a minute or so, worse in bed and in the mornings. You have felt sick but not been sick. You wondered if it might be a hangover from the cruise or even a brain tumour.
Impression ☐	I think your dizziness is coming from the inner ear where there is fluid which tells your brain which way up you are. Sometimes crystals form in the fluid which then causes confusing messages to be sent to the brain. The conflicting messages from your ears and eyes causes dizziness, particularly when you change position. We call this benign paroxysmal positional vertigo. Benign means it's nothing serious, paroxysmal means it comes and goes, positional means when you move your head and vertigo means spinning dizziness. We call it BPPV for short.
Experience ☐	Have you known anyone with vertigo or dizziness when they move their head?
Explanation ☐	I know that your symptoms are distressing but I don't think it's anything serious and it will get better whatever we do. Most people get better within a few weeks.
Options ☐	So we could do nothing, and this will most likely settle on its own, or we could try to get rid of the crystals by performing a series of neck movements. This can make you feel better very quickly. At least two-thirds of people get better with this treatment. There are some medications which can help with the dizziness, such as cinnarizine, which we could use short term?
Empower ☐	I will text you an information leaflet to read about the problem and the treatment, which is called the Epley manoeuvre. We can do this at the surgery. Let me know and I'll book you in. Think it over and perhaps talk to your husband. Until then, take care in the mornings and get up slowly. Be careful on stairs. You can drive once you feel safe and the dizziness stops.
Safety net ☐	I would expect the dizziness to start improving – longer intervals between episodes and the dizziness becoming less severe – but, if for any reason you start to feel worse or something new happens, please see the doctor.

Doctor's notes	Freda White, 60 years. PMH: type 2 diabetes. Diabetes check 1 month ago, all well. Medications: metformin, gliclazide. HbA1c 54 mmol/mol. Lipid profile normal. U&E normal. BP 130/70. No microalbuminuria.
How to act	Concerned.
PC	*'I woke up feeling dreadfully dizzy and sick this morning. It isn't the first time.'*
History	For the last few weeks you have had frequent episodes of suddenly feeling dizzy. If asked more about the dizziness – the room is spinning. The episodes last less than a minute each but are unpredictable. However, you have noticed that it comes on when you roll over in bed. Your house has stairs and you nearly fell down them this morning as you were going down to make a cup of tea. It seems to be worse in the morning. You have never had serious problems with your neck. You have always been well.
	You have no cardiac or neurological symptoms. You have not vomited. You have no ear symptoms including pain or discharge.
Social	Cleaner at the local primary school. Husband older and retired factory worker. No alcohol and never smoked.
ICE	You are worried this is a brain tumour. One of the children at school had one and died recently and this was very sad for everyone. You think she had dizziness too.
	Could it also be to do with getting seasick on a recent cruise (your first, to celebrate 40 years of marriage)? Your husband is very worried about you. You want to know what this is and how to make it better. You are not sure you can work like this and you rely on your wage to supplement his pension.
Ask the doctor	*'Is it a brain tumour?'*
	'Will it get better?'
Examination	Dix–Hallpike test positive with nystagmus on turning head in each direction. No cerebellar signs. BP 128/66 sitting and 130/70 standing.

Learning Points BPPV

Benign paroxysmal positional vertigo (BPPV) is a common cause of recurrent dizziness.[1]

Who? Middle-aged (usually >50 years) and older people. Women:men = 2:1.

Symptoms Severe dizziness and nausea when head in certain positions (e.g. lying on one side, or face up in bed). Can feel off balance for several hours after the dizziness has gone.

Cause Otolith particles fall into semicircular canals (especially posterior canal – 85%) and cause fluid in inner ear to move.

Precipitating factors Spontaneous; ear surgery; head injury; bedrest; post-viral.

Children – migraine.

Diagnosis Confirm symptoms of dizziness that are related to the position of the head. Note that attacks last 20–30 seconds but get better if the head is kept still.

Differential Ménière's disease, anxiety, postural hypotension, viral labyrinthitis, vestibular neuritis, acoustic neuroma, chronic otitis media, MS, CVA, vertebrobasilar occlusion (patient.co.uk has a useful description for the doctor[2]), brain or nasopharyngeal tumours.

Examine Tailor the examination to the symptoms. Consider: BP, ears, Dix–Hallpike manoeuvre, cerebellar signs + full neurological assessment to rule out differentials.

Treatment May resolve with no treatment. Epley manoeuvre, Brandt–Daroff exercises.

Contraindications for Dix–Hallpike manoeuvre, Epley manoeuvre and Brandt–Daroff exercises

Absolute 'Fractured odontoid peg, recent cervical spine fracture, atlanto-axial subluxation, cervical disc prolapse, vertebro-basilar insufficiency that is known and verified, recent neck trauma that restricts torsional movement.'[3]

Relative 'Carotid sinus syncope (consider if history of drop attacks or blackouts), severe back pain, recent stroke, cardiac bypass within the last 3 months, severe neck pain, rheumatoid arthritis affecting the neck, recent neck surgery, cervical myelopathy, severe back pain, severe orthopnoea may restrict duration of test.'[3]

Additional learning point

How much can you do in 10–12 minutes? Taking a history from a patient, using the Dix–Hallpike test as a diagnostic tool and then treating the patient using an Epley manoeuvre is not realistic in a normal 10–12-minute consultation. Use the opportunity to give the patient a leaflet to read about your proposed treatment and book them in for a separate appointment for treatment sometime soon.

ENT, Speech and Hearing – 5

2WW referral criteria for suspected ENT, oral and facial cancer

Suspected cancer pathway

Laryngeal[1] Age >45 with persistent unexplained hoarseness or unexplained neck lump.

Oral[1] Unexplained ulcer in the oral cavity lasting more than 3 weeks or persistent or unexplained lump in neck.

Thyroid[1] Unexplained thyroid lump.

Consider urgent referral (for an appointment within 2 weeks) to a dentist for assessment of possible oral cancer if persistent red or red and white patch in the mouth or a red or red and white patch in the oral cavity consistent with erythroplakia or erythroleukoplakia. If assessed by the dentist as having any of these, the dentist should refer via suspected cancer pathway (2WW).

Emergency ENT problems

Unilateral deafness[2] Sudden onset (over 3 days or less) of unilateral deafness that has occurred within the last 30 days and cannot be explained by external or middle ear causes, may have treatable causes, including autoimmune disease, chronic infection, vestibular schwannoma and stroke. Early intervention may significantly improve symptoms.

EMERGENCY: refer within 12 hours as possibility hearing may be restored.

Epiglottitis[3] Now more common in adults than children. DO NOT examine the throat – send to hospital 999. Risk of complete airway obstruction.

Adults	Severe sore throat with painful swallowing. Predictors of airway obstruction are sitting upright, stridor and breathlessness.
Children	Tentative, careful breathing (normal respiratory rate).
	Tachycardia.
	Cry and voice muffled – reluctance to talk.
	May have inspiratory stridor and hoarseness.
	Drooling.

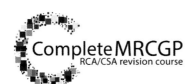

CHAPTER 6 OVERVIEW

Eyes and Vision

	Cases in this chapter	Within the RCGP 2020 curriculum: Eyes and Vision	Learning points in this chapter include:
1	Blepharitis	'Eyelid problems such as blepharitis' 'Conjunctivitis including infectious causes (bacterial, viral, parasitic, chlamydial and allergic causes)'	Management of blepharitis
2	Squint	'Squint – childhood and acquired due to nerve palsy, amblyopia, blepharospasm'	Causes and management of squint
3	Acute Glaucoma	'Glaucoma – acute, closed angle and chronic open angle'	Presentation and management of acute angle closure glaucoma
4	AMD and Cataract	'Recognise how sight loss can interfere with mobility and lead to social isolation and difficulty in communication (such as use of telephones or computers) as well as the impact of poor eye health on loss of confidence, mental health, activities of daily living, independent living and ability to work'	Presentation and management of AMD and cataract
5	Retinal Detachment	'Retinal problems including detachment'	Presentation and management of retinal detachment
Extra Notes	The Red Eye	'Red eye – differential diagnoses and appropriate management including timescale and urgency'	Differential diagnosis of the red eye

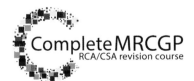

CompleteMRCGP
RCA/CSA revision course

CHAPTER 6 REFERENCES

Blepharitis

1. NICE CKS. Blepharitis. http://cks.nice.org.uk/blepharitis. Apr 2019.
2. http://patient.info/doctor/blepharitis-pro. Dec 2014.
3. Patient information leaflet: https://www.moorfields.nhs.uk/condition/blepharitis-0

Squint

1. http://patient.info/doctor/strabismus-squint. Jun 2015.
2. http://patient.info/doctor/amblyopia-pro. Jun 2015.
3. http://www.nhs.uk/conditions/Squint/Pages/Introduction2.aspx – includes a video of an ophthalmologist describing squint and its treatment for patients/carers.
4. https://www.moorfields.nhs.uk/sites/default/files/Atropine%20treatment%20for%20Amblyopia.pdf

Acute Glaucoma

1. NICE CKS. Glaucoma. http://cks.nice.org.uk/glaucoma. Nov 2020.

Useful Resources

Patient information leaflet: http://patient.info/health/acute-angle-closure-glaucoma. Jul 2018.
Patient information leaflet: http://patient.info/health/glaucoma-chronic-open-angle. Jul 2018.

AMD and Cataract

1. NICE CKS. Cataracts. http://cks.nice.org.uk/cataracts. Mar 2020.
2. NICE CKS. AMD. https://cks.nice.org.uk/macular-degeneration-age-related. Oct 2020.
3. http://patient.info/doctor/age-related-macular-degeneration-pro. May 2021.
4. DVLA. https://www.gov.uk/driving-eyesight-rules. Contains public sector information licenced under the Open Government License v3.0.

Useful Resources

Patient information leaflet: https://nei.nih.gov/health/maculardegen/armd_facts (available in auditory form and large text).
Patient information leaflet: http://www.rnib.org.uk/eye-health-eye-conditions-z-eye-conditions/cataracts

Retinal Detachment

1. NICE CKS. Retinal detachment. http://cks.nice.org.uk/retinal-detachment. Aug 2019.

Useful Resources

Patient information leaflet: http://patient.info/health/retinal-detachment-leaflet. May 2021.
Patient information leaflet:http://www.rnib.org.uk/eye-health-eye-conditions-z-eye-conditions/retinal-detachment.
Patient information leaflet: http://www.moorfields.nhs.uk/condition/retinal-detachment.

Information taken from NICE guidelines with kind permission. Please note the guidelines change frequently and you should ALWAYS check for the latest updated guidance. Remember that NICE guidance is only applicable to patients in the UK.

Eyes and Vision

Doctor's Notes

Patient	Alison Hughes	50 years	F
PMH	NVD aged 31 and 33 years		
Medications	No current medications		
Allergies	No information		
Consultations	No recent consultations		
Investigations	No recent investigations		
Household	John Hughes	52 years	M
	Sally Hughes	19 years	F
	Louise Hughes	17 years	F

Open ☐   I'm very sorry to hear that. Please tell me more about your eyes; how did this start and how long have you had problems?

History ☐   Are your eyes sticky all day or just in the mornings? Do you wake up and find that they are closed shut? Any problems focusing? Have you tried anything so far? Do you wear contact lenses? What sort of lenses are they? Tell me about work. What do you do and where do you work – is it an air-conditioned environment?

Curious ☐   I can see you aren't wearing your contact lenses today; tell me, why that is? (F2F)

Flags ☐   Are both eyes equally affected? How is your eyesight? Any changes recently? Have you seen your optician for a sight check? Are your eyes sensitive to light?

Risk ☐   Does anyone in the family have eye problems? Any skin problems such as dry, red or flaky skin on your face?

Impact ☐   Tell me how this is affecting you each day so I can fully understand your situation.

Sense ☐   I sense that this is embarrassing, working in the fashion industry where appearances matter.

ICE ☐   You wondered if this was conjunctivitis. Did you have any other concerns? Or worries about your eyesight? You wondered if I could give you antibiotics; was there anything else you thought might help?

SummarICE ☐   To summarise, for a few weeks you have had recurrent stickiness and discharge from both eyes. You've had to leave your lenses out. Your sight is fine. You tried antibiotics but they did not work. This is important to you, and for you at work. It is uncomfortable and unpleasant to wake up with sticky eyes but, in addition, working in the fashion industry means you need to look your best and resolve this as soon as possible. You would prefer to wear contact lenses if possible.

O/E ☐   Thank you for sending the photo. I can see the edges of your eyelids are red and flaky, but the white of your eye looks normal.

Empathy ☐   It must be embarrassing and difficult having sticky eyes that you have to clean at work.

Impression ☐   My impression is that you have an inflammation of the eyelid margin, which we call blepharitis. The eyes are fine and, in particular, the white part of your eye is not inflamed or infected.

InCludE ☐   I don't think this is conjunctivitis. Also, conjunctivitis would probably have got better with antibiotic ointment and, as your symptoms haven't, I don't think more antibiotics would help.

Experience ☐   Have you heard of blepharitis or known anyone who has had this?

Explanation ☐   Blepharitis is common and can be managed at home by careful cleaning of the eyelids. You will need to use warm compresses and buy some baby shampoo to use every day. Try to avoid eye make-up, if possible. If you must, please use water-soluble products that you can easily remove. I'm sorry, but you should probably leave your contact lenses out for the moment. Thankfully, this condition does not put your eyesight at risk.

Options ☐   I would like to send you a leaflet about blepharitis which gives you advice on how to clean the eyes. Could I text you the link? I recommend arranging an appointment with your optician to check for dry eyes and for their professional advice about your contact lenses.

Empower ☐   It can be persistent so you will need to continue for a number of weeks or even longer. How do you feel about what I've suggested? Do you have any questions?

Safety net ☐   Please come back in 2–3 weeks if this is not working. If you have any new eye symptoms or are concerned, please come back at any time, or see your optician/contact lens practitioner.

Patient's Story

Doctor's notes   Alison Hughes, 50 years. PMH: NVD aged 31 and 33 years. Medications: none.

How to act   Worried but expecting to be cured with some drops or ointment.

PC   *'I keep getting conjunctivitis. My eyelids are stuck together every morning. Do I need antibiotics?'*

History   For the last few weeks you have woken up on most days with sticky eyes. You are usually a contact lens wearer but have left them out. This has not helped. You went to the chemist and got ointment (antibiotics) but this did not make much difference. Comments have been made at work both about you wearing glasses and also about the appearance of your eyes.

Social   You live with your husband and work as a PA to a fashion editor of a newspaper where it is important to look good at work. It is an air-conditioned office.

ICE   You believe this is conjunctivitis (your children have had this) and understand it is an infection. Worried about the appearance of your eyes, you need and expect the doctor to give some stronger antibiotics to sort this out quickly. You are slightly worried about your eyesight long term.

You have not come across blepharitis.

Keen to continue to wear contact lenses, you respond negatively if the doctor suggests leaving them out long term and react with incredulity if doctor suggests baby shampoo.

Examination or photo sent   Wearing glasses. Eyelid margins are red and crusty. No redness of conjunctiva.

Questions   *'Will this get better? How quickly will this happen?'*

'Could it affect my sight?'

'Do I have to stop wearing contact lenses?'

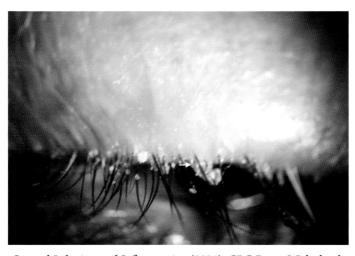

Reproduced from *Corneal Infection and Inflammation* (2021), CRC Press. With thanks to Rashmi Singh, Ritika Mukhija, Alisha Kishore, Noopur Gupta and M Vanathi.

Learning Points

Common eye problem in general practice.

Age	Typically >40 years, but can be younger.
Symptoms	Eyelids stuck together in the morning. Eyelashes sticky, greasy or crusty. Gritty sensation in eyes. Eyelids feel sore. Unable to tolerate contact lenses. Light sensitivity.
Differential diagnosis	Other infections, e.g. conjunctivitis, impetigo or cellulitis. Skin problems such as dermatitis or psoriasis. Rarely – tumours such as actinic keratosis, BCC or SCC.
Two types	Anterior blepharitis = the base of eyelashes affected.
	Posterior blepharitis = Meibomian glands affected.
	…but it can be difficult to distinguish between the two types.[1]
Aetiology	*Staphylococcus*. Can be associated with seborrhoeic dermatitis or rosacea. May be linked to demodex (microscopic mites) – possibly causing sensitivity or irritation to eyelids.[2]
Management	Chronic condition, so management rather than cure.

1. Warm compresses to the eyes for 5–10 minutes.
2. Massage the eyelids with a cotton wool bud to loosen oils and crusts.
3. Clean the edge of the eyelids with warm water and a little baby shampoo (1:10 dilution). Diluted sodium bicarbonate solution is not recommended because it is more likely to cause irritation.

Recommend the above steps twice daily at first, then once daily as it improves.

If the above steps do not work, topical antibiotic ointment or cream for 6 weeks can be prescribed.

1st line – chloramphenicol. 2nd line – fusidic acid. 3rd line – oral tetracycline or doxycycline for 6–12 weeks.[2] There is no clear evidence for steroid drops.

If linked with seborrhoeic dermatitis or dandruff, an antidandruff shampoo for hair and eyebrows may be needed. If linked with dry eyes, lubricant drops or artificial tears may be required.

Advise avoiding contact lenses during acute episodes.

Blepharitis and conjunctivitis are two of the most common eye conditions in primary care. Be sure that you can distinguish between the two and that you can explain about treatment options.

Always ask about contact lens wear as those who do are more prone to get Gram-negative infections. Do not assume that the patient in front of you always wears glasses!

Remember that a 'minor' problem is not necessarily trivial to the patient.

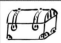 See the **Link Hub at CompleteMRCGP.co.uk** for useful links to **Moorfield's Eye Hospital PILs**[3]

Doctor's Notes

Patient	Amena Khalil	4 years	F
PMH	No information		
Medications	No current medications		
Allergies	No information		
Consultations	No recent consultations		
Investigations	No recent investigations		
Household	Lilia Khalil	28 years	F
	Ahmed Khalil	29 years	M

Open ☐	How can I help?
History ☐	Oh I see. I'm very sorry to hear that. Please tell me more about her eyes. For example, how did you first notice this?
Flags ☐	Has this stayed much the same or has it got worse? Does she seem to see okay? Can she run around without tripping and falling? Can she look at books with you?
ICE ☐	Do you know anything about eye problems like this? Is there anything you've been worried might be wrong or that you hoped we might be able to do to help?
Risk ☐	Has anyone in the family had eye problems? Did Amena injure her eye as a baby?
Sense ☐	I sense you are worried about how she looks, about her eyesight and about whether not being able to get her to a doctor has made things worse.
Impact ☐	Tell me what's been happening in your life recently.
Curious ☐	I see you've only recently registered with us. How are you getting on in the UK?
SummarICE ☐	So, to recap, Amena was fine at birth but, quite soon after she had an illness with a temperature, you noticed that her eyes were not straight and this has continued, not getting any better. You are worried about her vision and whether this can be corrected.
Empathy ☐	You must have been through such a lot in the last few months; I can't imagine how difficult it must have been for you.
O/E ☐	Thank you for sending the photo. I can see what you mean as Amena's right eye is turned in.
Impression ☐	Mrs Khalil, looking at the photo I suspect Amena has a convergent squint.
Experience ☐	Can I check that you understand this word 'squint'? Have you heard about this before? Squints are very common, about 1 in 20 children have a squint and the good news is that we should be able to help. Convergent means pointing inwards.
Options ☐	I would like to see Amena in the surgery to fully examine her eyes, to check the back of her eyes, her light reflexes and how her eyes move. If this confirms a squint, it would be helpful get her eyes tested by our eye specialist team at the hospital. They may suggest that she needs to wear glasses or might suggest she wear a patch on one eye to make the weak one stronger. This may well be all she needs but it is possible she might need a small operation in the future to straighten the eyes.
InCLudE ☐	Mrs Khalil, this is not your fault. There's nothing you've done wrong or neglected to do, it's just bad luck. You haven't left it too late for us to help Amena.
Empower ☐	We can sort this out for you and there will be nothing to pay; treatment in the UK is free of charge. You can best help Amena by taking her to her appointments and following the treatment plan, for example by making sure she wears her glasses and uses an eye patch if that's what is recommended for her.
Future ☐	Can I make an appointment for you to see me tomorrow? Then we can decide about the eye referral. Remember that NHS treatment is all free; there will be nothing to pay. I would also like to offer the support of a Health Visitor. Every child in the UK has a Health Visitor from birth until they attend school to support the mum and child. Often, they weigh the child and answer any questions or concerns you may have. May I ask Julie, our Health Visitor, to make contact with you? Is there anything else you need? There is also a local organisation called Asylum Welcome, which you may be interested in. There are also Children's Centres where you can meet other mums with small children. I'll give you contact details for all of these tomorrow.
Safety net ☐	If for any reason you are unable to make her appointment, please let us know. If her eyes change, or her sight seems to get worse, please contact a doctor or an optician. Opticians are available locally, usually at the shopping centres and are also free for children – there is nothing to pay to have your child seen and tested.

Patient's Story

Doctor's notes	Amena Khalil, 4 years. New patient. PMH: none. Medications: none.
How to act	[Mum] Worried, ground down, sad.
PC	*'Her eyes are crossed, Doctor; she cannot look straight. Can anything be done?'*
History	Amena is your first child. Quite soon after her birth, your village was overrun by terrorists. You stayed in increasingly bad conditions for some months and then fled with just a few possessions and eventually went to a refugee camp, where you have been for 2 years. There was no medical help. You were one of the first families to be evacuated to the UK. You are very grateful to be safe but conscious of all the family you have lost and left behind in Syria: your parents, brothers, sisters, nephews and nieces. You have a university degree and speak good English.
Social	You, your husband and daughter Amena (the patient) are Syrian refugees. You are staying in temporary housing. A helper there suggested booking a GP appointment.
ICE	Amena appeared normal at birth but developed 'crossed eyes' a few months after birth, after a febrile illness. You knew there was a problem but could not afford medical help and then there were no doctors in the refugee camp. You fear that not being able to feed her properly may have made it worse, especially a lack of vitamins. You are worried you have left it too late – that she will look like this forever and may not see straight. A friend said that, at 4, Amena may be too old to have surgery and may not be able to see properly. You have little money and are unsure whether you will have to pay.
Ask the doctor	*'Can anything be done?'*
	'Is it my fault?'
	'Can she see out of that eye?'
	'Will an operation put things right?'
	'Will I need to pay?'
Examination	PERLA. Convergent squint or see photograph: right eye turned in.

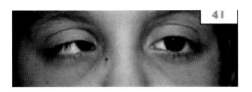

Reproduced from *Pediatric Clinical Ophthalmology* (2012), CRC Press. With thanks to Scott E. Olitsky and Leonard B. Nelson.

Learning Points

Terminology   Strabismus – any misalignment of the eyes. AKA 'squint'.[1]

Amblyopia – decrease in vision caused by an abnormality of vision during eye development (i.e. first 2–3 years of life). Common causes are strabismus, congenital cataract and refractive error. AKA 'lazy eye'.[2]

Incidence[3]   Squint (strabismus) is common – incidence about 1:20.

Who to refer[3]   It is 'normal' for eyes not to move together for a few weeks after birth but, if persisting longer than the age of 3 months, this needs a referral to a paediatric orthoptist.

Cause[3]   Squint can appear from birth or may be acquired later.

There can be a genetic link.

Sometimes appears after febrile illness; however, would have happened anyway.

Complications[3]   Often associated with refraction problems such as long or short sight.

Convergent squint is linked with long sight.

Treatment objectives[3]

1. Good sight in both eyes.

2. Both eyes working together (3D, stereoscopic vision).

3. Both eyes appear 'straight'.

Children often need glasses, then 'patching' of the good eye to make the weaker one stronger. If non-compliant, can use atropine drops to blur vision in the 'good' eye.[4]

Surgery is often needed to straighten the eyes. One or more muscles are tightened or detached/reattached.

This is generally very successful day-case surgery and recovery is quick. The eye can feel itchy or sore for a few days afterwards. Treatment is best started as early as possible and, beyond age 6–7 years, it is difficult to achieve optimal results. 3D vision is essential for some occupations such as a fire fighter or airline pilot.

Social prescribing

Social prescribing recognises the positive impact that voluntary services can have on a patient or their family.

For example, a patient suffering with depression who is under housing, financial and emotional stress may benefit more from community advice and support than a doctor's pill. Social prescribing is a service becoming increasingly available in GP practices and the GP often refers to a Social Prescribing Coordinator employed by the practice and commissioned by the PCN. The idea behind this is to recognise the social and psychological needs of the patient and direct patients to available community services with the aim of increasing quality of life. Local services may include: Citizen's Advice, Age UK, MIND, Asylum Services, Children's Centres, Women's Centres and hundreds/thousands more. A GP should be aware of the services available locally (community orientation).

The patient in this case is an asylum seeker who is not well versed in the structure and processes of the NHS. It is worth spelling out what may appear obvious to you but not to the patient – for example, that NHS treatment is free. If the patient is worrying about cost, this may inhibit him or her from attending the specialist appointment.

Doctor's Notes

Name	Abida Khan	70 years	F
PMH	No information		
Medications	No information		
Consultations	Routine elderly person review with nurse – BP 140/90.		
	Recent consultation with viral URTI – advised to get OTC preparations from the chemist.		
Investigations	None		
Household	Rashid Khan	72 years	M

Example Consultation

Open ☐ — Hello Mrs Khan. I'm very sorry to hear that. Please tell me more about your eye and the sickness.

History ☐ — Have you had this before? How is your vision just now? Are there haloes around lights? Have you been sick or just felt queasy?

ICE ☐ — What thoughts have you had about this? Any other worries? Did you have anything in your mind you thought I might be able to do today?

Impact ☐ — Tell me a bit about yourself. How has this affected you today, up until coming to see me?

Flags ☐ — Has anyone in the family had eye problems?

Risk ☐ — Are you long-sighted or short-sighted? Have you taken any medication at all lately? Do you ever wear contact lenses? Do you have a history of any bowel or joint problems?

Sense ☐ — You mentioned your father's blindness. Are you worried that might happen to you?

Curious ☐ — You thought you needed antibiotics for your recent cold. Were you annoyed that they weren't prescribed?

SummarICE ☐. — You went out to the cinema last night and eye symptoms that you've had to a lesser extent for months came on really severely. You fear you have an infection which may harm your eyesight and are worried you might go blind like your father.

O/E ☐ — I want to have a good look at both eyes. I need to feel the eyes with your lids closed, shine a light in both eyes to check the pupils, test how well you can focus with a chart and look at the back of the eye. This will mean I need to come quite close to you, is that okay?

Empathy ☐ — I can understand how worried you are, particularly with your father going blind.

InCludE ☐ — You wondered if this was an infection, but I don't think it is.

Impression ☐ — My impression is that there may be a build-up of fluid pressure in the eye, which we call glaucoma.

Experience ☐ — Have you heard of glaucoma or know anyone who has it?

Explanation ☐ — In glaucoma, the eye fluid can't circulate as it should and pressure tends to build up, giving you pain and sickness. Left untreated it can be very serious. It's not an infection but it is possible that the decongestant tablets may have contributed to bringing this on. Being long-sighted and from SE Asia are also risk factors. Being in the near darkness of the cinema may have been the final trigger.

Options ☐ — It is really important that we get you to the hospital to be seen by a specialist eye doctor as soon as possible. I will phone the emergency eye clinic now to arrange this. Have you got someone who can drive you to the hospital? Whilst you are waiting, you may be more comfortable lying flat on your back on my couch, face up with no pillow. Would you like some painkillers and something to take away the sickly feeling?

Empower ☐ — I am going to print off a PIL about glaucoma so that you understand what has happened and what to expect.

Future ☐ — I think the doctors at the hospital will give you some eye drops and medicines to reduce the pressure in your eye so that you are more comfortable. It is likely that they will suggest a small operation on your eye with a laser to make a wider passage for the fluids in your eye to move around.

Safety net ☐ — If for any reason you are not seen at the hospital, please let me know and I will sort this out. Please call or see me next week to tell me what is happening.

Eyes and Vision – 3

Doctor's notes	Abida Khan, 70 years. PMH: routine elderly person review with PN 4 weeks ago – BP 140/90. Recent GP consultation: viral URTI. Advised OTC preparations. Medications: none.
How to act	Very worried. In discomfort. Annoyed (you think you should have had antibiotics recently and that you are ill now because you weren't prescribed them).
PC	*'I was watching the new James Bond film at the cinema last night when I started to feel sick and my left eye became sore. It's no better today.'*
History	You were out at the cinema last night with family for a birthday celebration when you noticed your left eye starting to ache. You were all right when you set out from home but your sight became blurred and there were haloes around the street lights when you went home. You have had a few similar but very mild episodes, but they passed quickly. Things are no better today – you feel sickly and unwell. You have recently had a cold that was troublesome. You came to the doctor for antibiotics but were told you did not need them and that you should go to the chemist. This annoyed you because you are entitled to free prescriptions. Nevertheless, you went to the supermarket and bought some decongestant tablets (Sudafed Blocked Nose).
	You have always been long-sighted and wear glasses. You remember that your father had very poor eyesight in later life (although you are not sure why) and he was blind for the last few years. He lived with you and you had to look after him with this disability.
	You have no fever or symptoms of a lung infection. Your cold is better but you feel sick and disorientated.
Social	Housewife, married to an accountant. Lives with husband. Grown-up children. Never smoked and no alcohol.
ICE	What is happening? Why do I feel so ill? Has the cold affected my eye – an infection perhaps? Will I go blind like my father?
Ask the doctor	*'What is happening?'*
	'Have I got an eye infection because you wouldn't prescribe antibiotics?'
	'Am I going blind like my father?'
Examination	Right eye normal. Left eye – pupil does not react to light. VA 6/9 right eye, 6/60 left eye. Left eye red.

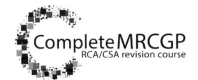

Eyes and Vision – 3

In presentations of acutely red and painful eye, suspect acute angle closure glaucoma, particularly if risk factors present:

- Female, older, long-sighted and Asian heritage or Black ethnicity. (Other risk factors are DM, myopia, steroid use, including inhaled and topical, if high dose.)
- History of similar problems – headache, blurred vision, nausea, eye pain, haloes around lights.
- Recent use of antimuscarinic (e.g. amitriptyline) or adrenergic (e.g. phenylephrine).

Symptoms   Headache, nausea and vomiting, blurred vision and haloes.

Signs   Eyeball feels hard to the touch. Pupil fixed and semi-dilated.

Reduced VA. Optic disc abnormal – engorged vessels (difficult for non-specialist to detect).

Management[1]

Medical emergency. Refer immediately to ophthalmologist for admission. If this is not immediately possible:

- First aid – lie patient flat (no pillows) face up – may reduce pressure.
- Give pain relief and antisickness drug.
- If available – pilocarpine 1 drop 2% in blue eyes and 1 drop 4% in brown eyes (evidence based).
- Acetazolamide 500 mg orally if no contraindication.

Secondary care management[1] – topical and IV drugs to reduce pressure then usually laser surgery to iris. Initial treatment is usually iridotomy – to make a hole in the iris to let aqueous humour flow through. Other options are:

- Iridoplasty – helps the iris to shrink from the trabecular network.
- Peripheral iridectomy – to remove small section of the iris.
- Cataract removal – if appropriate and indicated.
- Ongoing use of eye drops to reduce the pressure.

The unaffected eye is treated too as it is also at risk – generally laser iridotomy.

Always ask about OTC medications and do not assume that they are benign products with few relevant side effects. The product bought by this patient contained phenylephrine which may well have contributed to the sudden onset of acute glaucoma.

Doctor's Notes

Name	Fred Scott	81 years	M
PMH	Hypertension		
Medications	Atenolol 100 mg daily		
Consultations	BP check with nurse 2 months ago – all well		
Investigations	U&E, cholesterol normal 2 months ago		
Household	Daisy Scott	84 years	F

Example Consultation

Open ☐ Hello Mr Scott – thank you – let me just have a moment to read the note. Did the optician explain to you their concern?

History ☐ Okay, now was this a routine check or had you noticed any problems with your sight? Tell me what problems you had noticed, for example with reading or distance vision.

Risk ☐ Are you driving? How about at night? Have you had any near misses?

Flags ☐ Can I check if you smoke? Do you eat a good diet? Fruit and veg?

Sense ☐ I sense that you have had some concerns yourself about your sight and whether it's safe to drive, even before you saw the optician.

Impact ☐ Tell me about your home situation. How far are you from the shops? Does anyone else drive? Any family nearby? Can you use internet grocery shopping?

Curious ☐ You mentioned your father went blind; can you tell me about that?

ICE ☐ What thoughts have you had since you saw the optician? Tell me what worries you about your sight or not driving. Was there anything you were hoping I might suggest?

SummarICE ☐ After the near miss you were worried about your sight and your optician has confirmed your worst fears and told you not to drive, which is a real blow.

Empathy ☐ It must have been a shock for you being told that you had some problems. The car is a lifeline for you and being told not to drive is worrying.

Impression ☐ The optician says you have two problems: one is that you are developing cataracts and the other is age-related macular degeneration or AMD.

Experience ☐ I know your father had eye problems; have you heard about cataracts or AMD?

Explanation ☐ Cataracts are a cloudiness of the eye lens so the light can't pass through it so well. The other problem means that the most sensitive and the important area of the back of the eye is becoming worn and less sensitive, so your sight will not be as sharp as it used to be.

InCludE ☐ You mentioned vitamins. Eating a balanced diet is important but there is some evidence that supplements with vitamin C and antioxidants can slow AMD.

Options ☐ Controlling your BP well may also help and we should recheck that in a couple of weeks. It's good that you don't smoke. Surgery will cure the cataracts and I can refer you for this, if you like. There is no need to wait until the cataracts are worse. It will not help the AMD but your sight could be reassessed after the operation and it might mean you can drive for a while longer. Your vision may deteriorate with time but this can be quite a steady change.

Empower ☐ How do you feel about this? Would you like me to refer you? Would you like me to send you a PIL about AMD? I will print it off in large print so it is easier to read. If your children can help you with the internet, you can also listen to the leaflet being read out loud.

Future ☐ May I book you in for a BP check in 2 weeks? We can do some blood tests to make sure everything else is okay, e.g. your blood sugar. You shouldn't drive for now – your insurance would not cover you if you had an accident. Could one of your children help with shopping for now? Could they shop on the internet for you and get groceries delivered to your home?

Safety net ☐ If your sight deteriorates further whilst waiting for the appointment, please call.

Patient's Story

Doctor's notes	Fred Scott, 81 years. PMH: hypertension. Medication: atenolol.
How to act	Polite, concerned about your eyesight.
PC	*'I went to the optician this morning and she wrote a note for you – I handed it in this morning.'*
History	You went for an eye check today and the optician told you that you are developing cataracts and AMD. She said your sight was borderline for being able to drive and suggested you stop. She told you to see your GP to discuss this. You had noticed that your sight seemed a bit worse than usual and troublesome 'haloes' around street lights had already made you give up night-time driving. You had a near miss last week when you did not see a car and pulled out of a junction. You have had to stop buying a newspaper as you cannot read the print anymore.
Social	You are a retired teacher and live with your wife who is also retired. You live quite a way from the shops and rely on being able to drive to do the shopping and get out and about. The car is your 'lifeline'. Your wife has never driven; you have always been the family 'chauffeur'. There are no family members close by. Your father went blind in later life, when he was about 83. You remember how he struggled and became virtually housebound before he fell over at home, fractured his hip and died shortly afterwards. You have never smoked and eat a balanced diet. You are a basic computer user, not internet literate.
ICE	You are now very worried about your sight.
Understanding	You have never heard of AMD and will react badly to the use of this acronym that means nothing to you (unless described). You saw your father lose his independence once he started to lose his sight and are worried you are going the same way. You are sure you are still safe to drive to the shops – it's not far and you know the way.
Ask the doctor	*'What is AMD? Is it okay to drive short distances?'*
	'Am I going blind?'
	'Will an operation help?'
	'Why can't I have an operation now?'
Optician's note	*'… I have advised him to see you for referral to an ophthalmologist for treatment of his AMD and cataracts. His sight is below the legal level for driving.'*

Cataract[1]

Epidemiology	Mainly >60. Men and women equal risk.
Aetiology	Changes in proteins that make up lens.
Symptoms	Cloudiness. Especially night vision with haloes around lights.
Risk factors	FH, diabetes, eye surgery or injury, uveitis, prolonged or high-dose steroids. Other risk factors: smoking, alcohol, poor diet, sunlight, myotonic dystrophy, neurofibromatosis type 2, atopic dermatitis (independent of possible risk factor from use of topical corticosteroids).
Treatment	Surgery. No need to wait 'until cataract is ripe' anymore. Usually LA, go home same day. Lens removed and replaced with plastic one. May still need glasses for near vision. Clarity and colour vision should be improved.
Consider	How the cataract affects vision and quality of life, what surgery involves including risks and benefits, whether the patient wants surgery, if they can co-operate with eye examinations, surgery and post-operative care.

Age-related macular degeneration (AMD)[2]

Epidemiology	Women > men. More common in people of Caucasian ethnicity.
Symptoms	Affects central but not peripheral vision. Reading, facial recognition more difficult. Size or colour of objects may appear different with each eye.
Risk factors	FH, age (>50), smoking, alcohol, poor diet, sunlight, long-sightedness, hypertension, history of CVD, lack of exercise.
Referral	Urgently to be seen in 1 week, especially if rapid onset of symptoms. Advise patient that if there is a delay >1 week or symptoms deteriorate whilst waiting for appointment, they should attend Eye casualty.
Dry AMD	Most common type, macula cells become damaged by build-up of drusen deposits. Visual loss gradual, over many years.
	Treatment: diet rich in vitamins A, C, E may help. Consider antioxidants (AREDS2 combination).* Stop smoking, modify CV risk factors.
Wet AMD	10% people with dry AMD may develop wet AMD.[3]
	Abnormal blood vessels develop beneath the macula and damage the cells.
	Much more serious than dry AMD – vision can deteriorate in days.
	Treatment: injections of antivascular endothelial growth factor. Laser treatment largely superseded but may be suitable for some.

Also consider – referral to low vision services, group-based rehabilitation programme, eccentric vision training, support with depression and psychological problems.

*AREDS2 = vitamin C 500 mg, vitamin E 400 IU, lutein 10 mg, zeaxanthin 2 mg, zinc 25 mg, and copper (cupric oxide 2 mg).

DVLA driving requirements

No need to tell DVLA if only affects one eye, providing still meet visual standards for driving. Must tell DVLA if both eyes affected.[4]

Visual standards:[4]

- Vision at least 6/12 using both eyes.
- Adequate field vision.
- Read number plate from 20 m.

When a patient has sight problems, think about how you can give them accessible patient information, e.g. auditory leaflet or print off in large type. Remember that older people may be highly internet literate or may have a basic level of skills – don't make assumptions, check it out.

Eyes and Vision – 4

Doctor's Notes

Name	Eric Johnson	61 years	M
PMH	Type 2 diabetes diagnosed 10 years ago		
Medications	Metformin 500 mg TDS		
	Gliclazide 160 mg daily		
	Blood glucose testing strips		
Consultations	Annual diabetes review with practice nurse 1 month ago		
Investigations	HbA1c 59 mmol/mol. BP 150/80 (recheck booked). Foot check normal. Diabetic eye check at hospital – mild retinopathy.		
Household	Kathleen Johnson	61 years	F

Open ☐	Hello Mr Johnson. I'm very sorry to hear that. Please can you tell me more about the blurred vision, starting from when you first noticed it?
History ☐	Does the vision fluctuate or is it just as bad all the time? Any pain in the eyeball? Any redness? Any other eye symptoms? Has it affected your driving? Tell me about your work.
Flags ☐	Any floaters? Anything that appears to be like a curtain coming across your vision? Any flashes?
ICE ☐	What thoughts have you had about this? What concerns you most? Tell me, did you have any thoughts yourself about how I might be able to help you best today?
Risk ☐	You wear glasses – are you short-sighted or long-sighted? Do you ever wear contact lenses? Did you have any eye problems when you were a baby? Has anyone in the family had anything similar? Have you been hit in the eye recently?
Sense ☐	I sense this is very worrying for you and understandably so.
Impact ☐	Your sight is really important and you need to be able to drive safely to do your job. With diabetes, you need to be able to see well to check your blood sugars so that you can monitor your control. Diabetes, as you know, can affect eyesight so it is especially important to get your blood sugars under control.
Curious ☐	You mentioned being stressed; please tell me a bit about that. What is stressing you?
SummarICE ☐	To summarise, for the last couple of weeks the sight in your right eye has got worse – it is now blurred and you had a near miss in your car. You have had some understandable stress at work and I hear that it feels very important to fly to the USA next week.
Empathy ☐	It's very scary noticing that your vision is blurred for no apparent reason.
Impression ☐	I don't think it's likely this is caused by your diabetes but the squash ball may possibly have had a role. Being very short-sighted is another risk factor.
InCludE ☐	As this is only affecting one eye and not the other, I don't think it's likely to be caused by diabetes.
Explanation ☐	I think it is very likely that the membrane at the back of the eye, which we call the retina, has come unstuck and this is why you have had these symptoms. Another possibility is bleeding into the jelly part of your eye – this can also cause floaters.
Experience ☐	This is called a detached retina; is this something you have heard of before?
Options ☐	I'd like to thoroughly examine your eyes by checking your sight using a chart, checking your fields of vision and looking at the back of the eye. Would you be able to come down to the surgery this morning for an examination? It's likely that after examining you I will recommend we get you assessed by an expert as soon as possible because this condition can get worse if left untreated. I would ring and speak to the on-call doctor for eye problems at the local hospital. I would expect them to examine you and they may want to treat you today either with laser treatment or by putting a gas or oil bubble into the eye to help hold the retina back in place.
Future ☐	I'm sorry but I think it is unlikely that you will be able to fly to the USA next week as this could prevent healing of the retinal problem and could be very risky for your eyesight. You must not drive while your vision is a concern. Who can drive you to the surgery? Good.
Specifics ☐	Important, although less urgent than your eye problem, is that your diabetes control is not optimal and your HbA1c level at 59 is higher than it should be. Let's also make an appointment with the diabetes nurse to help get that sorted out.
Safety net ☐	If for any reason you aren't able to get to the surgery today, please phone me at the surgery to let me know so that I can see if I can sort out an alternative.

Doctor's notes	Eric Johnson, 61 years. PMH: type 2 diabetes.
	Medications: Metformin, gliclazide, blood glucose testing strips.
How to act	Very concerned.
PC	*'My vision's gone blurred in my right eye.'*
History	You are a 61-year-old businessman with diabetes that you struggle to manage well. Over the last couple of weeks, you have noticed a slight reduction in VA in your right eye. You put this down to stress at work (financial viability of your company – selling tractors) or the diabetes being not well controlled, but last week you realised you couldn't see a car that was on your right-hand side when driving and had a near miss. This was very scary. You have also noticed a few flashes and floaters in your right eye over the last couple of weeks. You have always been short-sighted and wear quite thick lenses and contact lenses for sport. You try to keep fit by playing squash and were hit in the eye by a ball a few weeks ago. The eye was a bit sore for a few hours but then okay. You did not seek help at the time because you were busy and it is always hard to get an appointment at the doctors.
Social	Married, with grown-up children. Businessman, working long hours. Important business meeting in the USA next week – crucial you get to this as there is potential for a big order that could make or break the company.
ICE	You are unsure what is causing it but wonder if it was the eye injury with the ball. You suspect your diabetes may be another possibility. You think the doctor will tell you off about your diabetes or tell you not to get so stressed (and this would annoy you). You are worried that either your vision is deteriorating or the doctor will say you can't fly.
Ask the doctor	*'Am I going blind?'*
	'Is it the diabetes?'
'	*Was it the squash ball injury?'*
	'If treated today, can I go to the USA next week?'
Examination	VA left eye – 6/9, right eye – 6/60. Reduced visual field – lateral vision right eye.
	Fundoscopy – difficult and retina not seen clearly.

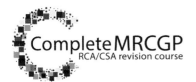
CompleteMRCGP
RCA/CSA revision course

Learning Points

Epidemiology	1 to 1.5/10,000 people per year.
	(One or two new cases per year in a medium-sized practice of 10,000 patients.)
	Risk increases with increasing age: lifetime risk = 3% at 85 years.
	Average age of occurrence = 60 years.
	Male = female.
Risk factors	Short-sightedness, FH, eye trauma, previous cataract surgery, diabetes (proliferative retinopathy), inflammatory eye problems, e.g. uveitis, scleritis, malignancy (secondary deposit or ocular melanoma primary), congenital eye disease (glaucoma, prematurity, cataract).
Symptoms	New onset of floaters (lines, haze, dots).
	New onset flashes of light.
	Sudden onset loss of vision – starts at edge of vision and progresses to centre. Often described as a 'curtain'.
	Reduced visual acuity – blurred vision.
	Contralateral eye affected in 10%.
Examination	Visual acuity – may be reduced to 'counting fingers'.
Management	Of new onset floaters/flashing lights:

1. Urgent (same-day ophthalmology) – if 'curtain', visual field loss, blurred vision, abnormal fundoscopy.

2. Less urgent (slit lamp within 24 hours) – if no reduction in VA, no field loss, fundoscopy normal.

Either case: PIL produced by RCO and RNIB – 'understanding retinal detachment'.

Hospital treatment

There are various ways of closing the hole and holding the retina against the eye wall. Surgeons often use a gas or oil bubble, then laser or cryotherapy to 'stick' it in place. The patient has to lie in a particular 'posture' to get the bubble in the right place. No air travel is permitted if gas has been used as the gas could expand and cause glaucoma and/or blindness.

When a patient has a chronic illness as well as the acute presentation (diabetes in this case), think about how the new problem will impact on their ability to manage their chronic illness. In this case, problems with sight could make it difficult to use and read a blood sugar monitor, with implications for diabetic control, ultimately risking further sight damage.

Extra Notes

The primary care dilemma is to be able to confidently differentiate mild benign conditions (e.g. conjunctivitis) from those that need urgent referral.

What to ask	When did it start?
	How did it start – quickly or gradually?
	What eye symptoms (blurred vision, pain, photophobia, discharge)?
	One eye or both eyes?
	Contact lens wearer?
	Any general symptoms (headache, nausea, fever, rash)?
	Possible injury, foreign body or trauma?
PMH – eyes	Has it happened before?
	Any eye operations? Any conditions associated with eye conditions, e.g. IBD, inflammatory arthritis.
Impact	Work? Driving? Reading?
Examination	VA, pupils, fundoscopy.

	Age	Pain	Symptoms	Signs	Urgent referral
Conjunctivitis (Most are viral. Antibiotics do not significantly shorten bacterial conjunctivitis)	Any	No	Itchy, gritty, discharge	Redness, watering Sticky discharge. VA normal	No, but refer if not settling/responding over 7–10 days or if suspect herpes. Swab for chlamydia in neonates
Subconjunctival haemorrhage	Older people	No	May start after coughing. Sometimes the eye aches	Deep redness Usually unilateral VA normal	No, but refer if >1 week, check BP
Episcleritis	Any	No	Mild discomfort	Defined wedge of redness VA normal	No, but refer if >1 week
Trauma/FB	Any	Yes	Pain. Usually unilateral	Depends on trauma	Depends – immediate if penetration Slit lamp needed
Acute glaucoma	Older, usually >50	Yes	Pain, haloes around lights, blurred vision, feels sick, ill, headache	Severe redness, ↓VA, pupil fixed, semi-dilated	Yes – immediate
Acute anterior uveitis	Usually 20–50 years	Yes	Blurred vision, headache, light sensitive	Severe redness, ↓VA	Yes – urgent same day
Corneal ulcer (ulcerative keratosis)	Any	Yes	Photophobia, watering, blurred vision	Stains with fluorescein	Yes – urgent same day
Scleritis	>50	Yes	'Boring' eye pain + photophobia and ↓VA. Usually systemic disease, e.g. gout, herpes zoster, connective tissue disorder	Depends. Anterior = deep injection. Posterior = minimal signs	Yes – 24–48 hours
Endophthalmitis (inflammation of ocular cavities)	Any	Yes	Red eye, ↓VA, recent surgery, IVDU, trauma, immunocompromised	Hypopyon in anterior chamber, eyelid oedema	Yes – immediate. Rare condition but significant++

Table adapted from http://patient.info/doctor/red-eye

Eyes and Vision

CHAPTER 7 OVERVIEW

Gastroenterology

	Cases in this chapter	Within the RCGP 2020 curriculum: Gastroenterology	Learning points in this chapter include:
1	Abdominal Pain	'Abdominal pain including differential diagnoses' 'Acute abdominal conditions: ...cholecystitis'	Differential diagnosis of abdominal pain
2	Dyspepsia	'Common and important conditions: dyspepsia, GORD'	NICE Guideline CG184. Gastro-oesophageal reflux disease and dyspepsia in adults: investigation and management. October 2019 Gallbladder polyp
3	Irritable Bowel Syndrome	'Irritable bowel disease [is a] common condition affecting a significant proportion of the population' 'Functional disorders: irritable bowel syndrome' 'Stool tests including faecal calprotectin'	NICE guideline CG61. Irritable bowel syndrome in adults: diagnosis and management. April 2017 Faecal calprotectin
4	Change in Bowel Habit	'Gastrointestinal malignancies including... colorectal'	Colorectal cancer red flags NICE Guideline NG12. Suspected cancer: recognition and referral. January 2021
5	Inflammatory Bowel Disease	'Inflammatory bowel disease such as Crohn's disease, ulcerative colitis'	Assessing severity Drug monitoring
Extra Notes	Management of Abnormal LFTs		Fatty liver

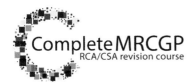

CompleteMRCGP
RCA/CSA revision course

CHAPTER 7 REFERENCES

Abdominal Pain

1. http://patient.info/doctor/acute-abdomen. Aug 2019.

Dyspepsia

1. NICE Guideline NG12. Suspected cancer: recognition and referral. Jan 2021.
2. NICE Guideline CG184. Gastro-oesophageal reflux disease and dyspepsia in adults: investigation and management. Oct 2019.
3. NICE CKS. Dyspepsia – unidentified cause: Proton pump inhibitors (PPIs). https://cks.nice.org.uk/topics/dyspepsia-unidentified-cause/prescribing-information/proton-pump-inhibitors-ppis/. Oct 2018.
4. NHS West Midlands. West Midlands Cancer Alliance Hepatobiliary Gallbladder Polyps Management Guidelines. Apr 2020.

Irritable Bowel Syndrome

1. NICE Guideline CG61. Irritable bowel syndrome in adults: diagnosis and management. Apr 2017.
2. Spiller R., Aziz Q, Creed F. et al. Guidelines on the irritable bowel syndrome: mechanisms and practical management. *Gut* 2007; 56: 1770–98.
3. NICE Diagnostics Guidance DG11. Faecal calprotectin diagnostic tests for inflammatory diseases of the bowel. Oct 2013.
4. Van Rheenen P.F., Van de Vijver E., Fidler V. Faecal calprotectin for screening of patients with suspected inflammatory bowel disease: diagnostic meta-analysis. *BMJ* 2010; 341: c3369.

Change in Bowel Habit/Colorectal Cancer

1. NICE Guideline NG12. Suspected cancer: recognition and referral. Jan 2021

Inflammatory Bowel Disease

1. Ford A., Moayyedi P., Hanauer S.B. Ulcerative colitis. *BMJ* 2013; 346: f432.
2. NICE Guideline NG130. Ulcerative colitis: management. May 2019.
3. Truelove S.C., Witts L. Cortisone in ulcerative colitis: final report on a therapeutic trial. *BMJ* 1955; 2: 1041–8.
4. NICE Guideline NG129. Crohn's disease: management. May 2019.

Management of Abnormal LFTs

1. Collier J., Bassendine M. How to respond to abnormal liver function tests. *Clin Med (Lond)* 2002; 2: 406–9.

Information taken from NICE guidelines with kind permission. Please note the guidelines change frequently and you should ALWAYS check for the latest updated guidance. Remember that NICE guidance is only applicable to patients in the UK.

Doctor's Notes

Patient	Rosie Carpenter 40 years F
PMH	Irritable bowel syndrome
Medications	Desogestrel
Allergies	No information
Consultations	1 month ago renewal of repeat contraception. No problems.
Investigations	BP 116/62
	BMI 31
Household	No household members registered

Sense ☐ I can hear you are in a lot of pain. We do not have morphine at the surgery but as soon as we get to the bottom of what is causing your pain we will arrange urgent treatment.

Open ☐ Can you describe the pain? Please take me through your symptoms from when you first noticed something wasn't right. Anything else that you have noticed?

Flags ☐ Have you had a high temperature? Have you vomited? Did you see any blood or black when you vomited? Any problems passing urine? What are your stools like? Have you noticed any blood or black colour in your stools? Have you been able to keep fluids down?

Risk ☐ Any history of tummy ulcers or gallstones? Have you noticed any symptoms of acid going up the gullet or pain after meals in the past months? When was your last period? Is there any chance you could be pregnant? Do you have a thermometer? Could you check your temperature for me and count your pulse for 1 minute? 38.4 and 114 – thank you. Both of those are higher than normal.

History ☐ What medical problems have you had in the past? Do you take any medicines? Alcohol? Ibuprofen?

ICE ☐ Have you had thoughts about what could be causing this? What are you most worried it could be? Apart from morphine, is there anything else you thought I may suggest?

Curious ☐ Has a doctor given you morphine in the past?

SummarICE ☐ So, for 24 hours you have had a pain which is severe. You have noticed stomach pains following eating. You vomited once and have had a fever. You fear this could be similar to the problem your father had when he died of a bleed in the stomach. I am sorry to hear that. Thankfully, I do not believe the same is happening to you.

O/E ☐ I'd like to ask you to come to the surgery now so that I can examine you, recheck your temperature, breathing and heart rate, blood pressure in both arms and feel your stomach, as well as listen to your chest and heart if I may. Although all sounds normal with urination and periods, I would also request you provide a urine sample so we can exclude a urine infection and pregnancy.

Impression ☐ From what I've heard so far, I believe you may have a gallbladder infection. The other possibility is a tummy ulcer but, due to the location of your pain and your fever, I believe a gallbladder infection is more likely.

InCludE ☐ I don't think this is a rupture of your stomach or a blood vessel like your father because you have seen no blood and you do not drink alcohol which is likely to have led to his bleed. What are your thoughts?

Experience ☐ Do you know anything about gallstones?

Explanation ☐ The gallbladder releases a liquid – I always compare it to Fairy Liquid – to help sort out the fat in our food. This liquid can turn into stones called gallstones which can then lead to a blockage. This blockage may cause intermittent pain, like the pain you have been experiencing after food. I think the pain you have been getting over the past few months is gallstones. The blockage from gallstones can also result in an infection.

Empathy ☐ It is extremely painful and makes you feel terribly unwell.

Recommend ☐ If I'm right, and this will be clearer when I've examined you, we need to get you to hospital and I would contact the Surgical Admission team. My other thoughts are that there is the possibility of an infection elsewhere, for example the pancreas, but I think a gallbladder infection is more likely. What's going through your mind?

Future ☐ At the hospital, I expect they will give you painkillers and antibiotics and fluids so that you will soon start to feel better. They will also do blood tests and possibly an ultrasound scan to confirm the diagnosis. Thankfully, most cases of gallbladder infection get better quickly with this treatment but, if the diagnosis is confirmed, and once you are more comfortable, the doctors may talk to you about having your gallbladder removed at some point in the future.

Specifics ☐ Can your husband drive you here straight away? Please don't eat or drink anything until I have seen you.

Safety net ☐ There is always the possibility you may become more unwell en route. If this happens your husband would have to stop the car and call 999.

Patient's Story

Doctor's notes	Rosie Carpenter, 40 years. PMH: irritable bowel syndrome and BMI 31.
	Medication: Desogestrel.
	POP checked 1/12 ago and no problems.
How to act	Keep putting pressure on the doctor. He/she needs to do something!
PC	*'What's going on? I've never been in this much pain. I need morphine.'*
History	The pain started yesterday and has gradually been getting worse. 10/10 severity.
	It is in your upper stomach and radiating to the back and feels sharp.
	It is worse after eating. You have had a fever.
	You have no reflux symptoms and your bowels are normal.
	You have been sick with the pain earlier this morning. You feel nauseous and unwell.
	You have been getting pain in the upper abdomen over the past few months whenever you eat. You have not lost weight and have seen no melaena. You have no dysphagia.
	You have no cardiac or respiratory symptoms.
	You have no urinary symptoms. LMP was normal 2 weeks ago.
	You have never had morphine but the paracetamol and ibuprofen you have taken have not helped.
Social	You don't drink alcohol as your dad was an alcoholic. You don't smoke.
	You work in publishing. You are married and live with your husband. You take no drugs.
ICE	You fear this is an ulcer and that the ulcer may burst which you presume is what happened to your father when he died of a stomach haemorrhage. You expect the doctor to give you pain relief straight away and you want reassurance.
Examination	Abdomen tender RUQ, Murphy's positive, normal bowel sounds. No abdominal masses or organomegaly or ascites.
	HR 114 bpm regular. Temperature 38.4 °C. BP 138/84 in both arms. RR 18. HS normal and chest clear.
	Your husband is at home with you and can drive you to the surgery.

Gastroenterology – 1

Differential diagnosis of abdominal pain[1]

Acute pancreatitis	Tender, distention, fever and tachycardic. Causes include gallstones, alcohol and raised cholesterol.
Peptic ulcer	Reflux symptoms (belching, heartburn, nausea) ± melaena.
Acute cholangitis	Charcot's triad (presents in <1/3) = fever, jaundice, RUQ pain (usually mild).
	Usually in older adults, e.g. secondary to a cancer obstructing the bile duct.
Cholecystitis	Murphy's sign (RUQ pain) or mass + fever or raised CRP/WCC ± vomiting, radiation to back, distention. Usually from gallstones.
	RFs = raised BMI/women/diabetes. Can be more severe in men.
Acute biliary colic	RUQ pain (with radiation to scapula) secondary to gallstones.
	Local tenderness but no fever.
Mesenteric ischaemia	Possible vascular history. Sudden onset. Systemically unwell.
	May appear SOB or vomit.
Appendicitis	Initial generalised pain before localising to RLQ + peritonitic.
Bowel obstruction	Vomiting + constipation + distended + not passing flatus. Peritonitic if perforated.
Renal colic	Severe loin to groin pain ± haematuria (macroscopic or microscopic).
Pyelonephritis	Urinary symptoms + loin pain + febrile + positive dipstick ± rigors.
Ectopic pregnancy	Lower abdominal pain (may radiate to shoulder) + β-hCG positive ± systemically unwell.
Ovarian cyst torsion	Severe pain radiating to iliac fossa or flank usually with nausea and vomiting.
Ovarian cyst rupture	May be peritonitic or haemodynamically unstable.
PID	Adnexal tenderness or cervical excitation + negative β-hCG ± history of STI. May be systemically unwell.
AAA rupture	Pain (abdominal or back) + haemodynamically unstable.
MI	Crushing central chest pain may radiate to arm or jaw (may present as abdominal pain) with SOB, nausea or vomiting and sweating. May be haemodynamically unstable.

Advice

β-hCG in any female (of reproductive age) despite recent LMP or contraception.

If for good reason (e.g. not had sexual intercourse for a year), history is 'taken in good faith'.

Most of the differential diagnoses listed require admission. Biliary colic and renal colic management will depend on the severity of the pain and your local access to scans. If there is no haematemesis/melaena and the patient is well, suspected peptic ulcer disease can be referred routinely (if not meeting 2WW guidelines) for endoscopy via local protocols.

Pyelonephritis can be treated in the community if the patient is afebrile and doesn't have significant pain, but be aware of pyelonephritis complicating renal colic – this is a urological emergency! PID may be managed in the community if the patient is systemically well. If the patient is managed at home, provide careful safety netting advice and consider admission if there is no improvement in 48 hours.

This case is assessing your ability to manage a patient's demands and make a thorough assessment. It would be reasonable, in a face-to-face consultation and if you felt the patient was very unwell, to check their observations first, explaining that you will return to ask them questions about the problem once you are happy they are not in immediate danger.

Even if you are unsure of the cause, a febrile, tachycardic patient with abdominal pain warrants urgent further investigation.

Due to the regulation of controlled drugs, it is unusual for practices to keep morphine. If being pressured, as the patient is focused on morphine, address this then take the full history.

Doctor's Notes

Patient	Daniel Hernandez 38 years M
PMH	None
Medications	No current medications
Allergies	No information
Consultations	New patient check last week with HCA.
	Smoker 15/day. Alcohol 25 units/week. BP 124/75. BMI 32.
	Mentioned abdominal pain, advised to see GP.
Investigations	No investigations
Household	No household members registered

Example Consultation

Open ☐ Can you tell me more about this pain? When did you first notice it? Is there a pattern?

History ☐ What brings it on? Does anything make it worse? Or better? Where do you feel the pain? Does it go anywhere else? How have your bowels and waterworks been? Tell me a little about yourself; where do you work? Who's at home? A food magazine – do you eat a healthy diet, would you say? Have you noticed any particular meals which make the pain worse? Have you noticed a cough at night or first thing in the morning?

Risk ☐ Do you smoke? How much alcohol do you drink? Is there a family history of stomach problems? Have you been taking any painkillers, for example ibuprofen, for anything?

Flags ☐ Have you lost weight? Vomited blood? Passed black stools? Does it cause any other symptoms like nausea, sweating or breathlessness? Have you had any difficulty swallowing?

ICE ☐ You've had this pain a while now; have you had any thoughts what it could be? What worries have crossed your mind? Was there anything specific you were expecting me to do today?

Sense ☐ I sense you are anxious about what happened to your mum.

Curious ☐ Please share your mum's experience. Are you worried?

Impact ☐ How has this pain affected you? Has it stopped you doing anything?

SummarICE ☐ So, you have been getting pain in your lower chest and upper tummy for 2 months, worse at night and after large meals or alcohol. You thought it could be gallstones as your mum had this problem. You are worried about needing an operation or blood tests.

Impression ☐ From listening to your symptoms It sounds to me as if you might well have acid reflux rather than gallstones. Thankfully there are no worrying symptoms. But to be sure about this I would like you to come to the surgery this morning so I can examine you: I'd like to feel your tummy to check for any tenderness, in particular the upper part of your tummy and around your gallbladder area. If I am right, there might be a little tenderness in the upper tummy but none around the gallbladder. I would also check your heart rate. I expect this to be normal but if it was raised it would make me think again. I can see your blood pressure and BMI have been checked last week. Would that all be okay? Is 11 a.m. today convenient? Great – I'll see you then.

InCludE ☐ I know you were concerned about needing blood tests or an operation but this is unlikely.

Experience ☐ Have you heard of reflux? Do you know anything about it?

Explanation ☐ Reflux is when stomach acid comes out of the stomach and into the food pipe. This causes pain as the acid irritates the food pipe. It can go up to your throat and cause soreness there too.

Empathy ☐ Reflux is common but can be uncomfortable. I hear it has affected your enjoyment of food.

Recommend ☐ Thinking ahead – if we confirm the diagnosis of acid reflux, thankfully it is treatable. A tablet called omeprazole, which you take every morning for a month, reduces the build-up of stomach acid. Most people don't have any side effects. Rarely it can cause a nasty diarrhoea and if taken long term it can affect vitamin B12 levels and bone strength, but used in the short term and from time to time it works really well. How do you feel about trying omeprazole?

Future ☐ In most cases, symptoms will settle but, if not, there are other tests we can do. For example, some people have a bacterial bug in their stomach which can cause reflux. If your pain is still there after the treatment, I would like to test for this with a stool or breath test.

Empower ☐ Diet and lifestyle can cause acid reflux so changing this can both treat and prevent it. Let's consider what triggers the stomach acid. Avoiding large meals at the end of the day, reducing alcohol and caffeine, avoiding spicy food, raising the head of your bed and losing a bit of weight can all help. What are your thoughts? I recommend stopping smoking altogether. Would you like to see our nurse for support and help with this?

Specifics ☐ Okay I'll see you at 11 a.m. Just to let you know that it may take 3–4 weeks of treatment before the pain fully resolves. If it hasn't fully gone by this time, I'd recommend you book another telephone call with me. If it returns in future, please let me know.

Safety net ☐ If at any point in the future your symptoms change or are any worse, for example you start vomiting, the pain worsens or you pass blood or black stool, see a doctor straight away.

Doctor's notes	Daniel Hernandez, 38 years. PMH: new patient. BP 124/75. Smoker 15/day. Alcohol 25 units/week. BMI 32. New patient HCA consultation last week. Mentioned abdominal pains, advised to see GP. No investigations. No household members registered.
How to act	Relaxed but anxious if tests are mentioned.
PC	*'Doctor, I have a pain in the stomach.'*
History	For the last 2 months you have been getting stomach pains intermittently.
	The pain can be sharp or burning and is located in your upper abdomen/lower chest.
	The pain starts in the lower chest but radiates up, sometimes to your throat.
	You feel you have been belching more too with some nausea.
	The pain is worse at night after a large meal. It tends to be worse at the weekends when you have been out with your friends.
	You have not been sick, you have normal bowel motions and no black stools. You have not lost any weight, although you have been trying to.
	You have tried Gaviscon which did help a bit. You have since been trying to avoid foods you would normally enjoy. You have taken no other medicines.
Social	You came to the UK from Spain 20 years ago to study at university.
	You got a good job as a graduate journalist so decided to stay. You write for a food magazine and enjoy going out for meals.
	You will often have a few glasses of wine with your meals. When you saw the nurse she told you that you were drinking too much, so you have tried to cut down.
	You do smoke but know you should stop! You're thinking about trying an e-cigarette.
	You live alone but have some good friends and colleagues with whom you socialise.
ICE	You are worried about gallstones. Your mother had an operation to remove her gallbladder and you remember her getting abdominal pains when eating. She still lives in Spain so you haven't had chance to ask her more about her symptoms.
	You have a needle phobia so worry you may need blood tests or surgery.
	You expect the doctor to examine you and possibly order blood tests.
Examination	Abdomen soft and non-tender. Observations normal.

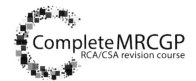

The decision about how to manage these conditions is based upon the presence or absence of 'red flag' symptoms and whether the patient has had an endoscopy before.

NICE criteria for 2WW referral for urgent direct access gastrointestinal endoscopy[1]

Either – dysphagia.

Or – age ≥55 years with weight loss AND one of: upper abdominal pain or reflux or dyspepsia.

NICE criteria for non-urgent direct access upper gastrointestinal endoscopy[1]

Either – haematemesis (if, however, it is an acute presentation or the patient is haemodynamically unstable, then admit to hospital).

Or – age ≥55 years with either:

- Treatment-resistant dyspepsia.
- Upper abdominal pain + low haemoglobin.
- Raised platelet count + one of nausea or vomiting or weight loss or reflux or dyspepsia or upper abdominal pain.
- Nausea or vomiting + one of weight loss or reflux or dyspepsia or upper abdominal pain.

If no red flags are present

Has the patient had upper GI endoscopy before?

YES – be pragmatic – if the endoscopy was recent or the symptoms have not changed since the endoscopy you may decide to follow conservative Rx as indicated on the endoscopy.

NO – termed 'uninvestigated dyspepsia' give a trial of treatment.

Dyspepsia treatment[2]	1st PPI for 4–8 weeks.
	2nd H2 receptor antagonist (H2RA) therapy.
Lifestyle factors	Always remember to modify lifestyle factors: caffeine, alcohol, spices.
Check drug history	E.g. NSAID, SSRI, bisphosphonates, calcium antagonists, nitrates, corticosteroids.
***Helicobacter pylori* testing**	NICE advise test if status unknown or uncertain.[2]
	If dyspepsia is likely to be secondary to a reversible lifestyle factor – consider avoidance of the precipitant and a treatment trial first.
	Either a carbon-13 urea breath test, a stool antigen test or validated laboratory serology testing.[2]
	If retesting, only use the breath test.[2]
Return of symptoms	Consider a low-dose maintenance dose as required.[2]
	However, continue to review PPIs. Long-term risks include bone fracture, vitamin B12 deficiency or *Clostridium difficile*.[3]
	Remember PPIs must be stopped 2 weeks before *H. pylori* testing and endoscopy.[2]
Differential diagnosis	Biliary, pancreatic and cardiac disease.
Gallbladder polyp[4]	Refer for cholecystectomy if >1 cm or <1 cm and symptomatic or gallstones present or polyp increasing in size at surveillance follow-up or in any patient with PSC.
Surveillance	If polyp 6–9 mm – repeat USS in 6 months. If ≤5 mm repeat USS in 12 months. See algorithm in reference 4.

Doctor's Notes

Patient	Rebecca Short	23 years	F
PMH	Anxiety		
Medications	Sertraline 50 mg OD		
Allergies	No information		
Consultations	No recent consultations		
Investigations	No investigations		
Household	No household members registered		

Example Consultation   Irritable Bowel Syndrome

Open ☐ Can you tell me about your symptoms from the beginning? Can you describe your bowels? Do you have any pain? Where do you feel the pain?

History ☐ Does anything make it better? Does anything make it worse? Do any particular foods make the symptoms worse? Do you feel bloated? Is that persistent or intermittent? Do you have any other symptoms such as vomiting? Tell me more about yourself.

Risk ☐ Do you have a family history of bowel problems? Any bowel or ovarian cancer in the family? Do you smoke? Do you drink alcohol? Any foreign travel? Do any foods make it worse?

Flags ☐ Have you lost any weight? Have you passed any blood? Have you passed any black stools? Do you need to open your bowels at night? Have you had any incontinence of stools? That must have been upsetting; tell me more about what happened.

ICE ☐ Have you had any thoughts about what is causing them? Is there anything that has been troubling you? Were you hoping I would do anything specific today?

Sense ☐ I sense that you have been feeling stressed recently. Is there anything which is causing you stress? How is life at home? How is life at work?

Curious ☐ You mentioned your mother told you to come. Did she have any particular worries?

Impact ☐ How have these symptoms affected you at home and at work?

SummarICE ☐ So, you have been having a mixture of loose and hard stools and you get abdominal cramps which improve when you open your bowels. The symptoms tend to be worse when you are most anxious. You haven't lost weight, passed blood or black stools. You are worried that you may have Crohn's as your cousin has it, and you are concerned you may need time off work.

Impression ☐ It sounds to me more likely that you have irritable bowel syndrome rather than Crohn's disease.

O/E ☐ To confirm this, though, I would like to see you at the surgery to feel your tummy, later this morning if that's convenient? I would ask you to lie on the couch so I can feel for any tenderness in your tummy, check your pulse and temperature, then measure your BP and weight. If I am right about IBS, I would expect to find that your pulse and BP are normal and that there is little if any tenderness in your tummy. This would help confirm what I am thinking.

Experience ☐ Have you heard of irritable bowel? Do you know anyone with it?

Explanation ☐ Irritable bowel syndrome is a condition in which the bowel becomes oversensitive and can cause pain, wind, diarrhoea or constipation, and often a mixture of all of these.

Empathy ☐ It is harmless but can be uncomfortable, embarrassing and a real nuisance.

Recommend ☐ Thinking ahead, I would recommend that it would be sensible to do some tests to rule out any other causes of your symptoms. We can check blood tests for coeliac disease (wheat allergy), thyroid, kidney and liver abnormalities and inflammatory markers to help rule out conditions like Crohn's disease. How does that sound?

Empower ☐ If these tests are all normal, we can be fairly confident that you have IBS. There are several treatment options including medication and a special diet. Let me tell you about these so you can have a think about what you might like to try first. The diet is related to avoiding the foods which are high in FODMAPs, which are a type of carbohydrate poorly absorbed by the intestines. FODMAPs can make you feel full of gas. I will print off a list of all the foods to avoid. The medication is called mebeverine. You take it three times a day, about 20 minutes before meals. It helps to relax the muscles in the gut so that you don't get painful cramps. You can buy it from the pharmacy or I can prescribe it for you. Most people have no side effects, but a few people may get an itchy rash that is a nuisance, but usually settles with antihistamines.

Future ☐ May I see you at 11.30 a.m.? We can check you over, feel your tummy, and take the blood tests. We could talk again on the phone soon, go through the results and perhaps discuss your anxiety further? When I see you today I'll give you information on a helpful therapy called CBT.

Specifics ☐ I've booked your appointment for today but please can you book a follow-up telephone call with me in a week – whenever is convenient for you.

Safety net ☐ In the future, if the symptoms get worse, you pass blood or black stools, or you have any concerns please call the surgery. If you ever have severe stomach pain, see a doctor straight away, phoning 111 if it is out of hours.

Gastroenterology – 3

Patient's Story

Irritable Bowel Syndrome

Doctor's notes	Rebecca Short, 23 years. PMH: anxiety. Medication: sertraline.
How to act	Anxious.
PC	*'I have been having a lot of diarrhoea recently, Doctor.'*
History	You have been having intermittent loose stools for around 9 months. You get cramping abdominal pain which is relieved by opening your bowels and an intermittent feeling of bloating. You sometimes pass mucus. At other times you feel that you get bunged up. You have not lost any weight; you have not passed any blood. No vomiting. No black stools. The symptoms do seem to be worse when you are stressed or worried. At times you have had to rush to the toilet at work which has caused you to get in trouble for leaving your phone.
	No foreign travel. No pattern with foods.
	You have not needed to open your bowels in the night.
	You are ashamed to say that once you were caught short and had some faecal incontinence.
	Only disclose this if the doctor asks.
Social	You work in telephone sales. You have been put under a lot of pressure recently by your manager. You have targets to meet all the time and this has been difficult. If you don't meet your targets you get paid less and sometimes struggle to pay your rent. You have had some time off recently with anxiety but went back to work when your job was threatened. You don't get sick pay. The sertraline does seem to help. You live with your boyfriend. Your parents are local. Your mum encouraged you to 'get checked out' as your cousin has Crohn's disease.
	Non-smoker.
	Social drinker.
ICE	You are worried that you may have Crohn's disease too. You worry you will need to take time off work, which may lead to you being sacked.
Examination	Abdomen soft, generalised mild tenderness. BMI 21. HR 88 bpm. BP 110/70. Temperature 36.8 °C.

Diagnosis (symptoms must be present for at least 6 months)[1]

'Abdominal pain or discomfort, that is either relieved by defaecation or associated with altered bowel frequency or stool form.'[1] In addition, two of the four following symptoms:

Altered stool passage (straining, urgency, incomplete evacuation).

Abdominal bloating, distension, tension or hardness.

Passage of mucus.

Symptoms made worse by eating.

Extra features which make IBS more likely:[1,2] 'Lethargy, nausea, backache and bladder symptoms.'[1]

Red flags

- Any signs or symptoms in line with the NICE guidance on recognition and referral for suspected cancer. For example: change in bowel habit, rectal or abdominal mass, unintentional or unexplained weight loss, or PR bleeding.
- Fever.[2]
- Diarrhoea waking the patient from sleep.[2]
- Inflammatory markers for inflammatory bowel disease.[1]

Refer to NICE guidance Suspected cancer: recognition and referral. Jan 2021.

Social history

Travel, mood, stress, diet and alcohol.

Investigations to rule out other causes

FBC (suspicious if raised platelet count or anaemia), ESR and CRP (IBD), coeliac screen.

NICE state NO need to do: USS, sigmoidoscopy, colonoscopy, barium enema, TSH, faecal ova/parasites, FOB, hydrogen breath tests for people who meet the IBS diagnostic criteria.[1]

Faecal calprotectin

When to test?	After ruling out red flags, to differentiate between IBS and IBD, if specialist assessment is being considered.[3]
What is it?	A protein secreted from inflammatory cells in the gut.[4]

Differential diagnosis of IBS where the main symptom is diarrhoea (IBS-D)

'Microscopic colitis, coeliac disease, giardiasis, lactose malabsorption, tropical sprue, small bowel bacterial overgrowth, bile salt malabsorption, colon cancer.'[2]

Management[1]

General lifestyle, physical activity, diet and symptom-targeted medication.

Dietary changes	Regular meals, restricting caffeine, fizzy drinks and alcohol, avoid insoluble fibre and artificial sweeteners, a trial of probiotics for 4 weeks.
Low FODMAP diet	But only if advised by health professional with dietary expertise.
Pain	Trial of antispasmodics (e.g. mebeverine, hyoscine).
Bowels	Laxatives but avoid lactulose. Loperamide for diarrhoea.
Others	Relaxation/activity. Low-dose TCA, SSRIs, linaclotide (constipated patients) – See NICE summary Irritable bowel syndrome with constipation in adults: linaclotide. Apr 2013.

Classification[2]

IBS-D (diarrhoea predominant)	IBS-C (constipation predominant)
IBS-M (mixed)	Alternators (switch subtype over time)

Doctor's Notes

Patient	Emmanuel Adebayo 71 years M
PMH	Osteoarthritis of right knee
	Hypertension
	GORD
Medications	Co-codamol 30/500 PRN
	Amlodipine 10 mg OD
	Ramipril 5 mg OD
	Lansoprazole 15 mg OD
Allergies	No information
Consultations	No recent consultations
Investigations	No investigations
Household	No household members registered

Open ☐	Please take me back to the start and talk me through what you noticed and when. Anything else? How do you feel in yourself?
Flags ☐	Have you lost weight? Passed any blood? Any fevers?
History ☐	Are your bowels currently either hard or watery? Have you had any other symptoms. Or pain? Where do you feel the pain? How long does it last? Does anything make it worse? Or better? Have you felt sick? Have you actually vomited? Have you had trouble with your bowels in the past? As we've not met before, could I just clarify your past health problems and which medications you take? Does anyone live with you at home? I'm sorry to hear that. Do you have any other family or friends around you?
Risk ☐	Do you have a family history of bowel problems? Do you smoke? Or drink? Have you travelled abroad recently? Have you taken any antibiotics?
ICE ☐	Have you had any thoughts about what could be causing these symptoms? Have you been worrying about anything in particular? You've mentioned that you would like some laxatives; was there anything else that you were hoping for today?
Impact ☐	What is it like living with this problem?
SummarICE ☐	So, you have had erratic bowel movements for 8 weeks and with some blood and lost a little weight. You thought you may have constipation and piles and would like some laxatives.
O/E ☐	May I see you today at 11:30 a.m. to examine you? I would check your weight and then ask you to undress behind a curtain and then lie on the couch. It would be really helpful if I could feel and listen to your tummy and also examine inside your bottom. This would involve putting one finger into your bottom to feel for any lumps or bumps and to check for blood. I would ask one of our nurses to chaperone.
Impression ☐	Although constipation and piles may explain some of your symptoms, with weight loss and blood in the stool it is important we find out what is causing this. There may be something more serious going on. I think it's really important that we consider all causes from inflammation to bowel cancer. (Pause). What is going through your mind? I'm sorry to steer you down the road of investigations and worry but I will support you through this.
Sense ☐	I sense the possibility of cancer has come as a shock to you. How do you feel about this examination?
InCludE ☐	It is of course possible the codeine has made you constipated with intermittent overflow where only loose motions can get around the hard stools. Bleeding can occur when you are constipated. Another possibility is diverticular disease – which is not a cancer. Diverticulae are little pouches in the bowel which can become infected.
Explanation ☐	However, neither of these possibilities explains the weight loss. Would you like me to discuss the next steps that we should take to rule out a condition like bowel cancer? We refer patients to the hospital urgently so they can be seen within 2 weeks. The hospital doctor will talk to you, examine you and offer you a test where a thin flexible tube with a light is passed through the back passage to look for any abnormal areas of bowel.
Empathy ☐	This must be worrying after your wife's experience. What is going through your mind?
Recommend ☐	My recommendation would be that I see you this morning and then, based on what you've told me, refer you to see the hospital specialists urgently. I would also like to do a blood test today to check your blood count, and kidney and liver function, which will help us and the specialist at the hospital.
Future ☐	After this morning's appointment you will be seen by the specialist within 2 weeks. Your bowel motions are formed and normal consistency today but if they become watery, we may need a stool sample to check for infection. I'll give you a pot in case this happens. Also, lansoprazole can sometimes affect the bowels – could you manage without it?
Safety net ☐	Should you feel unwell before you are seen at the hospital, develop severe tummy pain, vomit or pass a lot of blood, please let a doctor know straght away and if the surgery is closed this means calling 111.
Specifics ☐	Could you please ask reception for an appointment with me in 2–3 weeks after your appointment with the hospital so that we can discuss what has happened and what is planned?

Gastroenterology – 4

Doctor's notes	Emmanuel Adebayo, 71 years. PMH: OA, HTN, GORD. Medications: co-codamol 30/500, amlodipine 10 mg OD, ramipril 5 mg OD, lansoprazole 15 mg OD.
How to act	Relaxed.
PC	*'Good morning Doctor. I was wondering if you could prescribe me some laxatives?'*
History	You have been taking co-codamol on and off for a few years for knee pain; recently your bowels have been playing up. For the last 8 weeks or so you have noticed your bowels have been erratic. Some days you have been rushing to the toilet with diarrhoea and other days you have had sluggish bowels. You have been getting abdominal pain on the left side too. You have read the drug leaflet with co-codamol and wonder if you could be constipated. You have lost your appetite and your trousers have become looser. You aren't sure how much weight you have lost. A couple of times you have noticed a bit of dark blood mixed into your stools but wondered whether this was just due to piles, which you had a long time ago. You feel generally okay, slightly lacking in energy. You have had no fevers. The bowel motion this morning was formed.
Social	You originally moved to the UK from Nigeria in the 1970s. You were an engineer and looking for better job prospects. You are retired now and live alone as your wife passed away 3 years ago from breast cancer. You have some good neighbours who take you shopping because you struggle to get about with the knee pain. You have a son who works in London so you don't get to see him much. You don't smoke, but do drink a couple of whisky and waters in the evening. You don't know of any family history of health problems.
ICE	You don't have any particular concerns, but you would like your symptoms sorted out. The pain is sometimes bad and opening your bowels at night is a nuisance. If the doctor mentions bowel cancer, seem surprised. This wasn't what you were expecting but, if the doctor offers urgent referral, then accept this.
Examination	Normal abdominal and rectal examination. BMI 24.

Refer via 2WW colorectal cancer pathway[1]

- Aged ≥40 years with unexplained weight loss and abdominal pain.
- Aged ≥50 years with unexplained rectal bleeding.
- Aged ≥60 years with either: iron-deficiency anaemia or a change in bowel habit.
- Tests show occult blood in their faeces.

Consider cancer pathway referral

- Rectal or abdominal mass.
- Anal mass or ulceration.
- <50 years and rectal bleeding with any of the following unexplained symptoms or findings:
  - Abdominal pain
  - A change in bowel habit
  - Weight loss
  - Iron-deficiency anaemia

Offer FIT to people who have unexplained symptoms but who do not meet the criteria for a suspected cancer referral, specifically without rectal bleeding and:

≥50 with unexplained: abdominal pain or weight loss

Or

<60 with changes in bowel habit OR iron-deficiency anaemia

Or

≥60 and have anaemia even in the absence of iron deficiency.

This case challenges you to discuss a cancer pathway referral sensitively with a patient who was not expecting a potentially serious diagnosis. It also checks your ability to look for serious pathology even if the presenting complaint seems minor or the patient minimises their symptoms. By taking a thorough symptom history and checking for risk factors and red flags you should be able to spot these cases. Use pauses and give the patient opportunities to ask questions before continuing, to ensure you are going at the right pace for that patient. Many clinicians use the word 'camera' when describing an endoscope. Be clear this is a thin tube with a light.

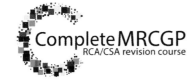

Doctor's Notes

Patient	Anthony Carlisle	26 years	M
PMH	Ulcerative colitis		
Medications	Mesalazine SR 500 mg capsules – 2 g OD		
Allergies	No information		
Consultations	No recent consultations		
Investigations	No investigations in the past year		
Household	No household members registered		

Letter from Gastroenterology Consultant 6 months ago:

RE: Anthony Carlisle
1 Woodland Avenue, Warwickshire
NHS No: 1234567890

Diagnosis: ulcerative colitis (in remission). Diagnosed 3 years ago.

I have reviewed Mr Carlisle in clinic today. I was pleased to find that his ulcerative colitis is well controlled on a maintenance dose of Pentasa. He has suffered very little abdominal pain and diarrhoea and has not had PR bleeding for several months. His weight is stable and he has had no systemic complications. Blood tests done before clinic were satisfactory. His full blood count and inflammatory markers were both normal. I have arranged to see him again in 12 months but would be happy to see him sooner should he run into difficulty.

Yours sincerely,

Dr S. Patel

Example Consultation   Inflammatory Bowel Disease

Open ☐   Could you tell me more about your symptoms? How do you feel in yourself?

History ☐   Have you had any other symptoms such as vomiting? Are you managing to eat and drink? How well controlled is your UC do you think? Have you had many flares in the past? What usually works? Have you needed hospital admission in the past? Have you had any change in your vision? Any joint pains? Have you noticed any rashes?

Flags ☐   How often are you opening your bowels? Is there any blood in your stools? Do you think that you have had a fever? Are you able to check your temperature now for me with a thermometer? 38 degrees – thank you. And could you count your pulse for 1 minute? 110 – again, thank you. Both of those are higher than normal.

Risk ☐   Have you been taking your medication regularly? Has anyone else had similar symptoms? Do you think you could have got food poisoning or a bug from anywhere? Any recent travel abroad?

ICE ☐   You feel that you have a flare of UC and wish to have a prescription for mesalazine; was there anything else you have been wondering about? Is there anything in particular that has been worrying you?

Sense ☐   I sense that you are very keen to get treatment from the surgery; are you concerned that you may need to go to hospital?

SummarICE ☐   So, you have been feeling unwell for 3 days and have bloody diarrhoea. You have been opening your bowels around seven times a day. You are known to have ulcerative colitis and, in the past, enemas have helped settle your symptoms. You need to get better quickly as you have a wedding to go to at the weekend but you don't want to go to hospital as you are looking after the family dog whilst your parents are away.

Impression ☐   I agree with you that this is probably a flare of UC. However, due to the number of times you are opening your bowels, the presence of blood in your stools and your high temperature and raised pulse rate, I feel it would be better if you are checked out in hospital. What do you think?

Explanation ☐   There is a scoring system which helps us decide how severe a flare of colitis is. Your symptoms and examination indicate that this is a severe attack of colitis. Severe colitis usually needs intravenous treatment which can only be done in hospital. You may need antibiotics and fluids as well as medication to settle down the colitis.

Empathy ☐   It must be frustrating and worrying to become ill when you have exciting plans and a dog to care for, but it's likely that the fastest way to get you better is to go into hospital and follow the specialist's recommendations.

Recommend ☐   I would advise going into hospital. You could become seriously ill without the right treatment.

Options ☐   Could you ask a neighbour, friend or your girlfriend to look after your dog?

Specifics ☐   I will phone the on-call medical team to arrange admission and give you a letter to take with you. Do you have someone who could drive you?

Future ☐   After you have been discharged from the hospital, please arrange a call with the GP if we need to change your prescriptions or if you have any further problems.

Safety net ☐   If you become more poorly on the way to hospital, stop and phone an ambulance.

Doctor's notes	Anthony Carlisle, 26 years. PMH: ulcerative colitis. Medication: mesalazine SR 2 g daily.
	Letter from consultant – all well 6 months ago.
How to act	In discomfort, impatient for a script.
PC	*'Doctor, I'm having a flare-up of my ulcerative colitis. Please can I have some more mesalazine enemas?'*
History	Three days ago you started with some left-sided abdominal pain and your stools became looser. Yesterday you opened your bowels seven times and passed bloody diarrhoea. You are feeling unwell this morning and have already opened your bowels three times. When you have had minor flares in the past, you have responded well to topical treatment (mesalazine liquid enemas). You have not been eating well recently and have forgotten a couple of tablets since your mum has been away and not checking up on you. You have not been admitted to hospital since the UC was first diagnosed.
Social	You live with your parents as you are saving up for a deposit to buy a house with your girlfriend.
	Your parents are away on holiday at present; you are looking after the family dog.
	You work in a restaurant as a barman. You have had to phone in sick for the last couple of days. You are supposed to be attending a family wedding at the weekend so are really keen to get some treatment so you can go.
ICE	You are concerned that you will miss the wedding; you have been looking forward to going for months. You want the doctor to give you a prescription. You are not keen on the idea of going to hospital. You are supposed to be looking after the family dog. If the doctor is helpful, interested and explains their concern to you, accept admission.
Examination	Abdomen very tender on the left side, no peritonism. HR 110 bpm. BP 126/74. Temperature 38.0 °C. RR 16. Sats 99%.

Learning Points

Ulcerative colitis[1,2]

Inflammation/ulceration starts in the rectum and extends proximally to different degrees in different patients.

Incidence	Two peaks of incidence – 15–25 years and 55–65 years.
Common symptoms	Rectal bleeding or bloody diarrhoea, abdominal pain, frequency, urgency and tenesmus.
Associated conditions	Primary sclerosing cholangitis, autoimmune liver disease, seronegative arthritis, ankylosing spondylitis, sacroiliitis, scleritis, episcleritis and anterior uveitis, erythema nodosum and pyoderma gangrenosum.
Investigations	FBC, U&E, LFT, ESR, CRP, stool culture, faecal calprotectin.
	Referral for imaging/endoscopy and biopsy.

The severity of UC in adults

Feature	Mild–Moderate	Severe
Bowel movements/day	<6	≥6 +feature of systemic upset
Blood in stool	Small amount or intermittent	Yes
Pyrexia	No	Yes
HR >90 bpm	No	Yes
Anaemia	No	Yes
ESR (mm/hour)	≤30	>30
Abdominal tenderness	No	Yes

The table is adapted from Truelove and Witts' Severity Index.[3]

Crohn's disease[4]

Can affect any part of the GI tract from the mouth to the rectum, most commonly the ileum.

Incidence	Two peaks of incidence: 16–30 years and 60–80 years.
Presenting symptoms	Diarrhoea, blood or mucus in stools, weight loss, lethargy, abdominal pain.

Managing IBD – specialist led

For both UC and Crohn's, most management decisions will be made in secondary care. However, see the link below.

Monitoring and shared care protocols

The drugs most frequently used require monitoring. Be aware that shared care protocols for these may exist in your area. We suggest medication review dates should not be reset for more than 3–6 months and, when you are issuing medications, recent blood test results should be checked.

 See the **Link Hub at CompleteMRCGP.co.uk** for a useful link to:
Monitoring guidance for immunomodulators
The management of UC according to the severity of the acute illness (a useful article which includes a helpful algorithm)

Extra Notes

The diseases in the table below will require referral to the liver team.

Disease	Suspect when
Alcoholic liver disease	AST > ALT, macrocytosis, low platelets, raised GGT
Chronic hepatitis B/C	Risk factors: IVDU, blood transfusion, tattoos/piercings especially abroad, unsafe sexual practices or paying for sex. HBsAg positive or HCV antibody positive. Then check HBeAg/eAb, HBV DNA, HCV RNA
Haemochromatosis	Raised ferritin and transferrin saturation Low TIBC
Wilson's disease	Neurological signs (e.g. tremor, involuntary movements) Kayser–Fleischer rings caused by raised copper Low ceruloplasmin
Autoimmune hepatitis	Anti-smooth muscle antibodies and anti-nuclear antibodies are present. Anaemia. Raised: bilirubin, IgG, ESR, ALT and AST and prothrombin time Associated with other autoimmune conditions
Primary sclerosing cholangitis	Raised ALP, AST and bilirubin Associated with IBD
Primary biliary cirrhosis	Consider if high ALP, raised IgM and anti-mitochondrial antibodies AST/ALT may rise in the later stages

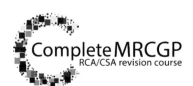
Complete MRCGP
RCA/CSA revision course

CHAPTER 8 OVERVIEW

Genomic Medicine

	Cases in this chapter	Within the RCGP 2020 curriculum: Genomic Medicine	Learning points in this chapter include:
1	Down Syndrome	'Emotional, psychological and social impact of a genetic diagnosis on a patient and his/her family' 'Antenatal and newborn screening programmes (e.g. Down syndrome...)'	Notes on Down syndrome The patient breaks bad news
2	Cystic Fibrosis	'Take and consider family histories in order to identify families with, or at risk of, genetic conditions' 'Principles of assessing genetic risk, including principles of risk estimates for family members of patients with single gene disorders'	Learning points for CF
3	Familial Adenomatous Polyposis	'Systems to follow up patients who have, or are at risk from, a genetic condition and have chosen to undergo regular surveillance (e.g. endoscopy for colon cancer)' 'Manage the day-to-day care of patients with genetic conditions, even if the patient is under specialist care'	Learning points – FAP
4	Breast Cancer	'Identify patients and families who would benefit from being referred to appropriate specialist services' 'Eligibility and referral pathways for genetic and genomic testing' 'Spectrum of risk-reducing measures, from lifestyle modification to target treatments for certain conditions, e.g. mastectomy and/or oophorectomy for *BRCA1/2* mutation carriers'	Notes on the genetics referral criteria for breast cancer
5	HOCM	'Assessing genetic risk' 'Difficulties in determining the exact genomic cause of a condition' 'Emotional, psychological and social impact of a genetic diagnosis on a patient and his/her family'	Notes on HOCM
Extra Notes	How to explain common genetic conditions to patients		Autosomal-dominant and autosomal-recessive, X-linked and chromosomal conditions that are listed in the new curriculum with two to three sentence explanations for patients

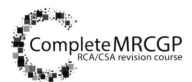

Complete MRCGP
RCA/CSA revision course

CHAPTER 8 REFERENCES

Down Syndrome

1. http://patient.info/health/downs-syndrome-leaflet. Oct 2016.
2. http://www.nhs.uk/Conditions/pregnancy-and-baby/pages/screening-amniocentesis-downs-syndrome.aspx
3. https://www.downs-syndrome.org.uk/about-downs-syndrome/pregnancy-and-baby/screening-diagnosis-and-support/

Cystic Fibrosis

1. https://patient.info/doctor/cystic-fibrosis-pro. Jul 2020.
2. NICE Guideline NG78. Cystic fibrosis: diagnosis and management. https://www.nice.org.uk/guidance/ng78. Oct 2017.

Familial Adenomatous Polyposis

1. https://www.macmillan.org.uk/cancer-information-and-support/worried-about-cancer/causes-and-risk-factors/familial-adenomatous-polyposis-fap

Useful Resource

Patient information leaflet: https://www.ouh.nhs.uk/patient-guide/leaflets/files/10057Pfap.pdf Useful explanation in straightforward language for children who may be affected.

Breast Cancer

1. NICE Guideline CG164. Familial breast cancer: classification, care and managing breast cancer and related risks in people with a family history of breast cancer. https://www.nice.org.uk/guidance/cg164. Nov 2019.
2. https://patient.info/doctor/familial-breast-cancer. Jul 2016.
3. NICE CKS. Breast cancer – managing FH. https://cks.nice.org.uk/topics/breast-cancer-managing-fh/management/. Dec 2018.

Useful Resource

https://www.cancer.org/cancer/breast-cancer/risk-and-prevention/breast-cancer-risk-factors-you-cannot-change.html

HOCM

1. https://patient.info/doctor/hypertrophic-cardiomyopathy-pro. Jan 2021.

Information taken from NICE guidelines with kind permission. Please note the guidelines change frequently and you should ALWAYS check for the latest updated guidance. Remember that NICE guidance is only applicable to patients in the UK.

Doctor's Notes

Patient	Heather Mumford	33 years	F
PMH	NVD aged 33 years		
Medications	No current medications		
Allergies	No information		
Consultations	No recent consultations		
Investigations	No recent investigations		
Household	David Mumford	35 years	M
	Emma Mumford	2 weeks	F

Example Consultation

Open ☐   I'm so sorry to hear that. How is Emma doing? And you? What have the hospital doctors said? How do you feel about this diagnosis? Were you given any warning?

Empathy ☐   It is a huge worry when a new baby needs an operation.

ICE ☐   When you booked the phone call, was there anything else you were hoping we would discuss? I'll take note of everything you wish to talk about then we'll go through it. What other questions do you have? What else has been going through your mind? What worries you most? Anything else you're wondering?

History ☐   I haven't met you before and it's the first time we've spoken. Please tell me more about you. Where is Emma now? Have you always been well? And during the pregnancy? Who are you close to? Do you feel you are receiving much support? What do you do for a living?

Empathy ☐   It must be upsetting when others are not getting in touch.

Impact ☐   Has this news changed you or your relationship? How is your bond with Emma?

Sense ☐   I'm hearing from you that you have unanswered questions and lots on your mind.

Impression ☐   Have you had a talk with a doctor about what this means? Shall we do that today?

Curious ☐   What do mean when you say you feel guilty?

SummarICE ☐   To summarise, you have bonded very well with Emma. Your immediate family are supportive. Your main concern is Emma's health and you are especially worried about the heart operation and any other medical problems Emma may develop. You feel guilty for thinking about the impact on your own life. You have questioned how independent Emma will be and whether she has the potential to live a long life. You would like to discuss how this has happened and whether it is likely to happen in a future pregnancy. Have I got it? Is there anything else you were hoping for today?

Empathy ☐   It is natural to hope that you will have a healthy baby. If there are any problems, it is normal to consider how this will impact on your own life.

Experience ☐   What is your understanding of Down syndrome?

Explanation ☐   At conception, genetic instructions are passed from parent to child within genes and chromosomes. To help understand the difference, if you imagine an instruction manual, all the words in a book are the genes. The genes are grouped into chapters, chromosomes. In Down syndrome, an extra chromosome is made during the transfer of genetic instructions, so you have not necessarily passed down a faulty gene. There is about a '10 times increased risk'[1] of having a baby with Down syndrome in another pregnancy. However, overall, your risk may still be small. There is a new test which is more accurate for Down syndrome which you may think about at the time.

Future ☐   What do you know about an AVSD? It means there is a hole in the muscle in the heart. Therefore, blood with and without oxygen is mixed up. Emma may also have other medical problems such as altered vision and hearing. There is an increased risk of problems later in life like diabetes.

InCLudE ☐   There may be tough times ahead and Emma may have more challenges than most. However, Emma may live happily until a fine old age and she has a loving family on her side. Regarding Emma's future independence, the range of learning difficulties is very variable, but we hope Emma will find her own path. Often personalities are naturally very warm, cheerful and gentle, and so Emma may soon win the hearts of everyone she meets.

Specifics ☐   Shall we catch up again after you have had a chance to talk to your husband and absorb what we have talked about? Is there anything else you would like to talk about next time? Please phone reception to book an appointment with me, a day or two after you have seen the consultant. I look forward to meeting Emma. She'll be a delight I'm sure.

Patient's Story

Doctor's notes	Heather Mumford, 33 years. PMH: NVD 2 weeks ago. Medication: none.
How to act	Anxious. Upset.
PC	*'Doctor, Emma was born with Down syndrome.'*
History	You had a normal delivery 2 weeks ago following a normal pregnancy.
	Emma is doing okay and she is breastfeeding nicely.
	After testing during pregnancy, you were told your risk of a baby with Down syndrome was low.
	You and your husband, David, are currently at home with Emma. He is looking after her in a different room.
	Both you and David have quickly become very fond of Emma.
	You have always been well. You take no medicines.
Social	You are an actuary. Your husband is a 35-year-old lawyer.
	You have never smoked or taken drugs. You used to drink occasionally.
	You have a strong relationship. You have a couple of close friends who have been very supportive but most others have not been in touch and you have only received a couple of baby cards. Your parents died when you were a child but David's parents are supportive.
ICE	You are trying to read about Down syndrome but caring for Emma takes up your time. You are aware that in Down syndrome there are additional genes and another chromosome, although you are a little confused between genes and chromosomes.
	You are mainly concerned about Emma's future health.
	You've been told she has a heart condition called an AVSD and you have an appointment with a cardiologist next week to discuss an operation. You can't bear this thought.
	You stay awake wondering if Emma will have a normal life.
	If the doctor explores your thoughts, you confide in the doctor that you feel guilty when you think about what this means for you and David. By this you mean that you always presumed you would have successful and independent children and you took for granted that you would have a normal family life.
	You fear that only you and David will ever love Emma.
	You are hoping today that the doctor can explain what Down syndrome is, why this has happened and what this means for Emma and your family.
Questions	Have you or your husband passed down a faulty gene?
	Would a second child also have Down syndrome?
	Will Emma die young? What else is Emma at risk of?
	Can the doctor explain the AVSD again?

Genomic Medicine – 1

Learning Points

Down Syndrome

Genetics	Trisomy 21 (in most cases).
Risk	Of having a baby with Down syndrome

Aged 20 years = 1/1500. Aged 30 years = 1/800. Aged 40 years = 1/100[1]

Screening for Down syndrome

Stage 1

Combined test At 11–14 weeks' gestation.	Nuchal translucency (fluid collection measurement at the neck) + hormonal levels + mother's age. This screens for Down syndrome, Edwards' syndrome and Patau's syndrome.[2]
Quadruple test	Around 14–20 weeks' gestation – only screens for Down not for Edwards' or Patau's syndromes. Only done if nuchal translucency not possible.[2]

If more information needed, can do NIPT (to detect Down syndrome, Edwards' syndrome, Patau's syndrome and Turner's syndrome). NIPT analyses the cell-free DNA in the mother's blood[3] rather than hormone levels.

Advertised as >98% sensitivity.

It is also therefore a screening test and women should be counselled regarding the benefits and limitations.

Stage 2

If high-risk result, i.e. if initial tests estimate a risk of >1/150, diagnostic testing will be offered.[2]

Chorionic villous sampling	Around 11–14 weeks' gestation.[2]
Amniocentesis	Around 15 weeks' gestation.[2]

Other Learning Points

The start of a new relationship

What was achieved within this consultation was predominantly support at a time of need, providing a confidante to share thoughts and fears. Normalising the mother's emotions was important to offer relief from feelings of guilt. This consultation provided an introduction to a connection and relationship with the GP which is likely to be ongoing as Emma grows.

The patient breaks bad news

A patient may walk through the door and they break their bad news, without a warning shot and often the discharge letter hasn't reached you. Have a think about what you may say when you are taken aback. Some things will be upsetting or may even trigger emotions or feelings from your own experiences. Show your interest and concern; however, be careful how you react and avoid judgement. Be guided by the patient.

Making connections

In this case there is a clear resonance between the mum's experience of her own parents dying when she was a child, and her fears about what will happen to Emma when she and her husband die. The skilled clinician notices these connections but chooses wisely and carefully about when (or indeed if) to share them with the patient. Today's consultation would have been too soon.

Doctor's Notes

Patient   Olivia Wales   29 years   F

PMH   No information

Medications No current medications

Allergies   No information

Consultations No recent consultations

Investigations No recent investigations

Household   No household members registered

Example Consultation

Open ☐ Tell me about your niece's experience? How is your niece? Apart from genetic testing, what other thoughts have gone through your mind?

Impact ☐ How has your niece's diagnosis impacted on your family? And you, how has it impacted on you?

Sense ☐ I can hear this is very important to you.

ICE ☐ What do you fear the most? Do you have any other questions? You were hoping we could arrange a genetic test for yourself – is that correct? Is there anything else that is important to you? What would it mean to you if you did have a gene that put you at increased risk of having a child with cystic fibrosis – how would this impact on your life?

History ☐ You have always been well, is that correct? Do you take any medicines? Do you work?

Curious ☐ Does your husband think you should have the test? Are you close to your sister? What does she think you should do?

SummarICE ☐ To summarise what you have said so far, your sister's daughter, Grace, has had multiple chest infections and requires medication to help maintain her nutrition. You have watched the amount of stress your sister has had to go through and this has made you question whether you would like children. You are upset by the arguments you have had with your husband. You feel the test may help you to make the choice whether to have a child.

Empathy ☐ It sounds as if you have watched your sister through many sad and difficult times when Grace has been admitted to hospital. That must be hard.

Experience ☐ What is your understanding of cystic fibrosis? What do you know about what causes cystic fibrosis?

Explanation ☐ In cystic fibrosis there is a build-up of mucus in the chest and difficulty absorbing all the nutrients from the diet because an organ next to the stomach, called the pancreas, is not producing the chemicals needed to break food down so it can be absorbed. Unfortunately, it can also cause fertility problems in later life.

Risk ☐ When a child is conceived, information from both parents is passed to the child. This information is coded in genes, one from each parent. Both parents need to pass on a faulty gene for a child to have cystic fibrosis. Everyone has a 1 in 25 chance of carrying the gene for cystic fibrosis. Your sister must have inherited one faulty gene from your parents, which she unfortunately passed on. You may or may not have a faulty gene. If we take the worst-case scenario and assume that you did inherit the faulty gene too, your chance of passing on the faulty gene would be 1 in 2. However, your child would also need to inherit a faulty gene from your husband, who has the background risk of 1 in 25 and then a 1 in 2 chance of passing it on. So, based on this, your risk would be 1 in 100 of having a child with cystic fibrosis.

InCLudE ☐ We don't know that you have inherited the faulty gene; if either you or your husband doesn't have a faulty gene, there is almost no risk of having a child with cystic fibrosis.

Options ☐ How would you feel about speaking to a counsellor about this?

Specifics ☐ I can write to the genetics team and explain what impact this has had and we can be guided by them. If you don't hear from them in the next 6 weeks, please let me know. They may offer a consultation for you to discuss what options are available. Relationship counselling is another option if you think this may be helpful.

Future ☐ If you decide to start trying for a family, do phone again and we can discuss this in more detail.

Patient's Story

Cystic Fibrosis

Doctor's notes	Olivia Wales, 29 years. PMH: nil. Medication: none.
How to act	Polite and quiet.
PC	*'My husband and I would like to start a family but my niece has cystic fibrosis. I'm wondering if there are any special tests we could have?'*
History	You are well, take no medicines and have been happily married for 2 years. Your sister gave birth to Grace 10 years ago and soon afterwards they were told that she has cystic fibrosis. Your sister decided not to have another child. There have been no other members of the family with this condition. This includes your sister's husband's family. Your sister's spirit seems to have gone over the years. The more Grace attends hospital the more sadness your sister has to go through. You believe the stress of the situation led to the breakdown of your sister's marriage. You worry that your sister will be alone if Grace dies.
Social	You are a teacher. You drink no alcohol and have never smoked.
ICE	You have seen your niece have lots of chest physiotherapy and she has had multiple lung infections requiring hospital admissions. She has to take medicines to help absorb her food.
	A charity is taking her to Disney World. You are aware that Grace may not live long.
	What is your risk of having a baby with cystic fibrosis?
	Is there a test you can have done to make sure you don't have the faulty gene?
	You don't know if you want a child if there is a high risk of bringing a child into the world who has to go through Grace's experience. Your husband is desperate for children. He does not want you to have genetic testing. He believes your chances are low and you should just start trying. This has led to arguments within your relationship. You were very excited when Grace was first born but now, watching your sister's life, you don't think you ever want children. You have not told your husband this.
	It was your sister's idea to have the genetic test.

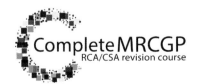

CompleteMRCGP
RCA/CSA revision course

Genomic Medicine – 2

CF is the most common inherited disease in people of White ethnicity, caused by mutations in the CF transmembrane conductance regulator (*CFTR*) gene, on chromosome 7. This affects sodium transport across the cell membrane and antibacterial defences.[1]

Risk factors	Positive FH is the only risk factor.
Carrier frequency	1:25
Systems affected	Respiratory and digestive – pancreatic insufficiency and biliary disease.
Presentation	Usually recurrent LRTI with chronic sputum production. Digestive presentations less common as only 5% pancreatic function necessary for normal digestive function.

Diagnosis[2]

Positive test result in people with no symptoms (e.g. infants screened with blood spot immunoreactive trypsin test) followed by sweat and gene tests for confirmation.

Clinical manifestations, supported by sweat or gene test results for confirmation.

Clinical manifestations alone, in the rare case of people with symptoms who have normal sweat or gene test results.

See NICE guidelines for a full list of who to assess for CF but includes the following:[1]

- FH
- Meconium ileus
- Symptoms and signs that suggest distal intestinal obstruction
- Faltering growth in infants and young children
- Recurrent and chronic pulmonary disease
- Acute or chronic pancreatitis
- Malabsorption.

Management

Patients with CF will be managed in a specialist centre by MDTs but may require GP and/or specialist psychological support particularly at difficult times such as:[1]

- Implications for school and education
- Transition to adult care
- Career planning
- Foreign travel
- Contraception and pregnancy
- Becoming parents
- Organ transplantation
- End of life.

GPs can also help as follows:[1]

- Prescribe cystic fibrosis medicines:
  - In batches of at least 1 month at a time for routine medicines.
  - For longer periods if advised by the specialist team.
  - Following guidance on arrangements for prescriptions of unlicensed medicines.
- Providing routine annual immunisation, including any alterations for people with CF.
- Flu vaccinations for family members and carers.
- Managing health problems unrelated to cystic fibrosis.
- Providing FIT notes as appropriate.
- End-of-life care, working in partnership with cystic fibrosis homecare teams.
- Caring for the person's family members or carers.

Doctor's Notes

Patient	Shane Dickens	23 years	M
PMH	Hay fever		
	Hand injury aged 11 years		
Medications	No current medications		
Allergies	No allergies		
Consultations	No recent consultations		
Investigations	No recent investigations		
Household	No household members registered		

Example Consultation Familial Adenomatous Polyposis

Open ☐	Tell me more about what's led to this. I'm sorry to hear that. How is Darren now?
Impact ☐	How has this affected you? What have you been thinking?
ICE ☐	You mentioned you can't stop thinking about this. What thoughts do you have? What do you think about when you think of Darren?
Sense ☐	I can hear this has come as a shock and you are very worried.
Flags ☐	To help answer your questions I'd like to know more about you, please. Have you had any symptoms – such as changes in the bowel, weight loss or bleeding?
History ☐	Have you had any medical problems? Do you take any medicines? How much alcohol do you drink? Do you smoke or take drugs?
Risk ☐	I would like to explore your family history. Do you have any other brothers or sisters? Do you and Darren share a mum or a dad? Is your mum well? On your mum's side are there any medical conditions? Is your dad well? I'm sorry to hear that. Do you know if he suffered with the same condition? How about your dad's family? Do you know if Darren's mother or family have had bowel problems or young deaths in the family?
Sense ☐	You sound sad. Is there anything else that keeps coming to mind? What do you fear most? Anything else? What did you think I may say today?
Empathy ☐	It must be really hard being such a distance away from your brother at this time.
Curious ☐	You mentioned your mum is worried. What have you talked about? And Darren?
SummarICE ☐	To summarise, Darren has been diagnosed with familial adenomatous polyposis. The news from the surgeon is not clear. You are struggling and feel sad that you have not always been close. Your mum has questioned whether your father and grandmother had the same condition. You would like to discuss this further. You have not had any symptoms and thought I may arrange a telescope test today.
Experience ☐	What do you know about familial adenomatous polyposis?
Impression ☐	Familial means it can run in families, adenomatous relates to the tissue in the gut and polyposis means little lumps, that can turn cancerous, forming from this tissue. This condition can occur randomly with no other family members affected, but usually parents and grandparents have this condition. Let's call it FAP.
Explanation ☐	We call the information which is passed from parent to child 'genes'. There are genes for every part of us. Genes come in pairs. We get one from our father and one from our mother. Which gene is stronger determines what we are like; for example, eye colour. Each parent also has two genes – from their mother and father. If one of their genes is faulty, there is therefore a 1 in 2 chance they have passed a faulty gene on to you. Anyone with this faulty gene will be affected by it. It is possible that your father and his mother had the problem as they both died young. But we don't know. This could have come from Darren's mum's side. If your father did have the gene for FAP, you have a 50% chance of having it. This is a serious condition and the only way to prevent death is to remove the bowel.
InCLudE ☐	It is difficult for me to comment on your brother's chances without having his information with me. If you have the test and it is negative, your risk of bowel cancer is the same as the risk for anyone in the population. You mentioned arranging a telescope test but at this stage we could refer you to the genetics team.
Options ☐	They may discuss having a genetic test. If we find you have the FAP gene, an operation will be stressful and challenging but potentially life saving.
Future ☐	Do you know when you will return? I can arrange the referral today. When you return let's discuss how you are coping. In the meantime, look after your health by avoiding cigarettes and cannabis.
Empower ☐	Or do you wish to have time to think and talk again when you return?
Safety net ☐	If you ever see bleeding from the back passage, do not panic as most of the time this is harmless. However, always see a doctor to check it out.

Genomic Medicine – 3

Patient's Story

Familial Adenomatous Polyposis

Doctor's notes	Shane Dickens, 23 years. PMH: hay fever and hand injury. Medications: nil.
How to act	Concerned. Distracted in thought at times.
PC	*'My brother said I need a colonoscopy for familial adenomatous polyposis.'*
History	Darren is your half-brother, you share the same father. He lives in Australia.
	He has now told you that he had been bleeding from his bottom and thought this was due to haemorrhoids. He kept using haemorrhoid cream but it only got worse when he was opening his bowels and he started to lose weight.
	The doctor sent him for a colonoscopy and it has returned as cancer. Because he was young they did genetic tests and he has the gene for FAP.
	You are healthy. You have had no symptoms. You do not take medicines.
	Your bowels are normal. You have had no bleeding. Your weight is stable.
	You have no other siblings. Darren's mother's side of the family are well.
	Your mother and father were never married, and they separated two years after having you.
	Maternal side: Your mother, maternal grandparents and aunts are well.
	Paternal side: Your father drank a lot of alcohol and committed suicide when he was 39.
	You do not know his medical history.
	You never knew your father's mother. She died young. Your paternal grandfather has dementia. Your father had two sisters who are well. Their children are well.
Social	You have been travelling and finding work as you go in bars or in sports hire shops.
	Last year you completed a Geography degree.
	You have cut your travels short and you flew home once you were given this news.
	You plan to fly out next week to see your brother. You don't know when you will be back so you prefer not to arrange any hospital appointment at present.
	You are not in a relationship. You smoke cigarettes and smoke occasional cannabis.
	You drink alcohol socially but usually no more than 2 pints a night on average.
ICE	You have been reading about FAP and have some questions.
	You understand that you may need your bowel cut out like your brother.
	You are uncertain about Darren's prognosis as you were told 'the surgeons are not sure that they have got it all'.
	1. You are confused by this and keep wondering if this means Darren will die.
	2. *'Mum is worried it'll affect me too.'* She has been reading about the condition and is wondering whether your grandmother and father had the same problem. You want to know if this is likely to be the case. It may explain his suicide.
	3. You feel anxious and are not sleeping well. You have started smoking more cannabis. If the doctor is interested to know what has been on your mind, say, *'I can't stop thinking about Darren'*. If the doctor explores further, say, *'He's such a good guy'* and sound sad and distracted in thought. If the doctor picks up on your cue you can say that you mean you have never been good at communicating with your brother and feel guilty that you did not reciprocate his interest in your life. You think about him often, but he does not know this. You expect the doctor will refer you for a telescope test into the bowel.

Genomic Medicine – 3

Learning Points

What is it?[1]

Rare familial condition that causes many hundreds of polyps to grown in large intestine.

Usually starts in teenage years.

Untreated, at least one polyp likely to become cancerous by age 40.

Other parts of body can be affected:

- Eye – congenital hypertrophic retinal pigment epithelium (CHRPE) – harmless black dots on retina.
- Bones – osteomas (harmless).
- Skin – sebaceous cysts.
- Stomach and duodenum – polyps that may become cancerous.
- Connective tissue – desmoid tumour.
- Other parts of the body – cancer.

Cause[1] Mutation in adenomatous polyposis coli *(APC)* gene. 1:4 people are the first in their family to have the gene mutation. Any children will have a 1:2 chance of inheriting it (autosomal dominant).

Diagnosis[1] Gene testing if first-degree relative has it. From age 12.

Screening[1] Regular colonoscopies from age 12. Gastroscopy from age 25.

Treatment[1] Usually offered aged 16–25. Colectomy or proctocolectomy with stoma.

Genetics Refer for testing of the *APC* (adenomatous polyposis coli) gene, although some may be sporadic.

Symptoms Asymptomatic, rectal bleeding or a change in bowels.

Complications Obstruction, colorectal cancer or other tumours, e.g. thyroid, carcinoid, bone.

Monitoring FBC, CEA, TFT, LFT, FOB, X-rays, advise dental monitoring and colonoscopy.

Also – HNPCC (hereditary non-polyposis colon cancer)

Associations Other cancers, e.g. ovary, prostate and stomach.

Screening Colonoscopy, endoscopy, cystoscopy and pelvic screening.

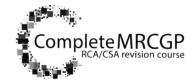

CompleteMRCGP
RCA/CSA revision course

Doctor's Notes

Patient	Nicola Bennett	42 years	F
PMH	Three normal vaginal deliveries when aged 24, 26 and 30 years.		
	Focal migraine 18 years.		
Medications	No current medications		
Allergies	No information		
Consultations	No recent consultations		
Investigations	No recent investigations		
Household	Duncan Bennett	46 years	M
	Arthur Bennett	18 years	M
	Benjamin Bennett	16 years	M
	Elizabeth Bennett	12 years	F

Example Consultation

Open ☐ What has led to this decision? Tell me more about your mother's experience?

Curious ☐ When you say you have built yourself up to this…in what way?

Impact ☐ How has all of this impacted on your life? And on life day to day?

ICE ☐ What goes through your mind? Anything else? Or anything that you particularly fear? What do your family think? How might a positive test for yourself affect your children?

Sense ☐ This has obviously played a large part in your life. It has taken courage to talk to me.

Risk ☐ Has a member of the family already had a worrying gene identified? How old was your mother when she was diagnosed? I'm going to ask about factors which can affect your risk. I see you have had three children, the first when you were 24. Did you breastfeed? What contraception have you used? Did you smoke? Do you drink alcohol? That's all good news. Can you answer these questions about your mother? Do you have Jewish ancestors? Any other cancers in the family?

Flags ☐ How often do you check your breasts? Have you noticed a lump or skin changes?

History ☐ Tell me about your medical history. You mentioned not being able to concentrate…tell me more. Do you work? Is anyone else at home? How is your relationship?

O/E ☐ Would you like me to examine your breasts? We could book an appointment for this today?

SummarICE ☐ To summarise, you would like the genetic test after watching your mother go through breast cancer because you want to protect yourself and your children. Your sleep and concentration is affected. You have thought through potential scenarios and decided you would have a mastectomy. You hope, however, we can reassure you and therefore your children, but you are concerned about how a positive test may impact on them. Have I understood?

Empathy ☐ This is important to you. You've had first-hand experience of the impact of cancer.

Impression ☐ There have been studies looking into when we should do genetic testing. If your mother was over the age of 40 years, with no other cancers in the family, this is reassuring and genetic screening is not recommended. You have also decreased your risk of breast cancer by having three children quite young, all breastfed and you used progesterone-only contraception. Your mother's hormone pattern was quite different and, combined with smoking, she was at increased risk.

Experience ☐ What are your thoughts about what I have just said?

Explanation ☐ You are correct we can never be certain of anyone's genes. We try to use the knowledge we have to base our recommendations on. Positive tests may impact on the mental wellbeing of families. It can be a very difficult decision.

Options ☐ I'd like to help you reach a decision you are comfortable with. May I suggest that we meet again? If you still feel strongly, I can write to the genetics team.

Future ☐ I will email you a link to the public information NICE guidance leaflet which explains further what I have said today.

InCLudE ☐ I recognise that this has had a huge impact on you and made you consider many significant options for your future, including a mastectomy and not having children, so I will contact the genetics team to discuss your personal situation with them. We can then discuss what they suggest. How does this sound?

Empower ☐ Whatever we decide, you will have lots on your mind. I am worried about how this is affecting you day to day. Have you had ideas on how we may be able to help with that? What about CBT? This is a therapy that helps you to work through how to manage powerful thoughts to avoid them impacting on your sleep, mood or concentration. I would recommend this. Have a think about it.

Specifics ☐ We recommend that every woman checks her breasts regularly and I will also send a link for the breast awareness leaflet for you now. Let's talk again in a month – we can book an appointment now. When would suit you?

Safety net ☐ If you feel a lump or you have concerns or questions, don't hesitate to book a face-to-face appointment straight away.

Patient's Story

Doctor's notes   Nicola Bennett, 42 years. PMH: three normal vaginal deliveries aged 24, 26 and 30 years. Focal migraine 18 years. Medication: none.

How to act   Determined and anxious.

PC   *'Doctor, I would like to be referred for the genetic test for breast cancer please.'*

History   You have always feared having breast cancer and it has taken a lot of courage to contact the GP today. *'I've been building myself up to this.'* By this you mean you have had sleepless nights with a lack of concentration at work; however, this has not yet impacted on your ability to work effectively.

Your mother was diagnosed with breast cancer aged 45 years.

You are now aware that you are approaching this age.

Years ago, you decided that you would not worry about this until your 40s.

This has recently been concerning you to the extent that you have played through in your mind all the possibilities which may occur.

Your mother had a mastectomy, chemotherapy and radiotherapy. She remained on tamoxifen but died 10 years later. The cancer had returned and had spread to her bones.

There are no other cancers in the family. Your mother smoked and she only had you aged 37 years. She never breastfed.

Apart from three healthy children who were each breastfed for 1 year, and migraines in your teenage years, you have been healthy. You have used the copper coil as contraception since the birth of your third child. You used progesterone-only contraception prior to this. You started your periods when you were 14 years old.

You are breast aware and check them every day in the shower.

Social   You are a private physiotherapist. You are happily married and your eldest son is about to go to university. You were at university when your mother was diagnosed for the second time and remember feeling so far away at the time. The risk is beginning to feel real. You drink alcohol rarely and have never smoked.

ICE   You expect a referral to a geneticist. You have considered in detail how you may react if the test is positive. You would want a mastectomy. You hope you will be able to cope better with bad news having gone through the possibilities in your mind. You fear how breast cancer may impact on your children. You don't want them to have to go through what you did, watching your mother. You are hoping it will be negative so you can reassure your daughter. You will feel guilty if the test is positive and your daughter will have to go through this. You have been worrying that either your children or your husband are getting fed up with you mentioning it. If the doctor declines a referral, say:

'How can you say I am not at risk? I have the right to be referred.'

If the doctor declines, ask about a private referral. You have not read about the testing in detail, but you read about Angelina Jolie choosing a mastectomy.

If the doctor explores the extent of how this has impacted on your wellbeing and demonstrates an appreciation of this, you acknowledge and respect any advice. If the doctor provides an NHS referral, you are very happy.

Examination   You decline an examination.

Learning Points

Risk factors
Lifestyle: alcohol and smoking. Overweight after the menopause.

Family history: Jewish ancestors and see below.

Hormonal: early menarche.

Nulliparous or late pregnancies.

OCP or HRT.

Limited/no breastfeeding.

Breast screening
Age extension plan = 47–73 years.

Current first invite is before 53 years. Then every 3 years.

Genetics: 'A person who inherits a fault in a *BRCA1*, *BRCA2* or *TP53* gene is at high risk of developing breast cancer…Having a faulty gene is a risk factor but does not automatically mean that you will develop breast cancer…All women who have a faulty *BRCA1*, *BRCA2* or *TP53* gene are at high risk…Women with a high risk have a 30% or greater chance of developing breast cancer in their lifetime.'[1,2]

Referral criteria for specialist assessment, familial breast cancer. NICE[1]

People with a family history of breast cancer but no personal history of breast cancer should be referred from primary care to secondary care according to the following criteria:

Type of cancer in relative	Relatives affected	Age of relatives at diagnosis
Female breast cancer	1 first-degree relative	<40
	2 first-degree relatives	Any age
	1 first-degree and 1 second-degree relative	Any age
	3 first-degree relatives	Any age
Male breast cancer	1 first-degree relative	Any age
Bilateral breast cancer	1 first-degree relative	First primary diagnosed <50
Breast and ovarian cancer	1 first-degree or second-degree relative diagnosed with breast cancer **AND** 1 first-degree or second-degree relative diagnosed with ovarian cancer **ONE SHOULD BE FIRST DEGREE**	Any age

'Advice should be sought from the designated secondary care contact if any of the following are present in the family history in addition to breast cancers in relatives not fulfilling the above criteria: bilateral breast cancer, male breast cancer, ovarian cancer, Jewish ancestry, sarcoma in a relative younger than age 45 years, glioma or childhood adrenal cortical carcinomas, complicated patterns of multiple cancers at a young age, paternal history of breast cancer (two or more relatives on the father's side of the family) (2018).'[3]

Doctor's Notes

Patient	Jason Wright	38 years	M
PMH	No medical history		
Medications	No current medication		
Allergies	No allergies		
Consultations	No recent consultations		
Investigations	No recent investigations		
Household	No household members registered		

Example Consultation

Open ☐	I'm interested to know what has led to this decision.
Empathy ☐	I am so sorry. I understand why you feel the need to be investigated yourself.
Impact ☐	Since your brother's death how has this affected you? Do you feel different? Tell me about other members of the family? How are they doing?
History ☐	Have you noticed any (other) symptoms? And you have no medical problems? Tell me about you…do you work? Do you live with anyone?
Curious ☐	Can you confide in anyone else about how you have been feeling?
Flags ☐	Any pain or palpitations? And during exercise? Any fainting/collapsing episodes?
Risk ☐	Has any other member of the family died suddenly or had a heart condition?
Sense ☐	I feel this is now always on your mind.
ICE ☐	Have you any other fears that have been in your thoughts? You mentioned a referral to a cardiologist. Is there anything else you were hoping I would arrange today?
SummarICE ☐	To clarify what we've discussed so far, you fear you have inherited the same condition as your brother; you have been told this was cardiomyopathy. Since the diagnosis, you have noticed breathlessness at times and you feel you have changed; you have started distracting yourself with work but stopped doing sport. You fear most having to tell your family you have the same condition and feel we need to check your general health and send you to see a cardiologist. Have I understood you correctly?
O/E ☐	Would you be able to come to the surgery so that I could examine your heart, take your blood pressure and feel your pulse? This would help me determine if you might have HOCM because often a murmur is present.
Impression ☐	Whether or not the examination shows a murmur, we should investigate further.
InCludE ☐	From what you have told me so far, however, I don't think that your heart has caused your symptoms. It is very common that when we are very worried about something, we breathe differently and the fingers tingle. This is normal and doesn't mean there is anything wrong with you.
Experience ☐	What is your understanding of your brother's condition?
Explanation ☐	HOCM is a condition that may not give symptoms but can cause SOB, collapses, chest pain or palpitations. The heart muscle is thickened but the vessels are not affected. We don't know what causes it. There is often a family link. In some cases, there is a 50% chance of inheriting the condition. Sudden death is rare but is believed to happen due to abnormal electrical activity causing the heartbeat rhythm to change.
Specifics ☐	I will write today to the cardiology team. I imagine they will first perform a jelly scan of the heart, but I don't think you will hear from them this week. Therefore, we can do an ECG, which is a heart tracing, today. Would that be okay? I will ask the nurse to fit you in this morning and I can also see you to examine your heart, blood pressure and pulse.
Empower ☐	I hope you will soon feel reassured to return to your normal activity.
Future ☐	We can look at the ECG result together. I also wonder if bereavement counselling may help?
Safety net ☐	If ever you experience palpitations, pain or symptoms during exercise, let a doctor know.

Patient's Story

Doctor's notes	Jason Wright, 38 years. PMH: nil. Medications: nil
How to act	Concerned and anxious.
PC	*'I would like a referral to a cardiologist.'*
History	Your brother, Will, died a month ago when he was playing football.

He played at a semi-professional level and collapsed during the match and died at the scene. Lots of people were watching; it was very distressing. The post-mortem diagnosed hypertrophic obstructive cardiomyopathy. You have been advised to 'get checked out'. You are also aware that this has happened to other footballers from news reports.

Since then, you have found that you are breathless.

Your fingers tingle, usually in the evenings or in the car.

You have no medical history. No other family history. No medicines.

You are sad about your brother's death but have no symptoms of depression.

You don't feel that you need any help with your grief.

Social	You are single.

You have a busy work and social lifestyle. Never smoked. Alcohol 20 units/week.

You have returned to work as a barman and you are very busy.

You have no symptoms at work.

You have been taking more on at work as a way of getting on with things.

You have stopped playing football in fear the same will happen to you.

ICE	You were told that Will's heart got bigger.

You then believe the vessel must have burst.

You believe your heart is getting bigger.

You fear having to tell your family you have the same condition.

You just want to see a cardiologist this week before it's too late.

You would like your cholesterol and blood pressure checked also.

Examination	Heart sounds normal. HR 70 bpm regular. BP 120/60.

Learning Points

Cause	Unknown.
Genetics	Usually autosomal-dominant genetic condition with variable penetrance and expressivity.
Physiology	Hypertrophy of the undilated left ventricle with diastolic impairment.
Symptoms	If present (often asymptomatic): angina, dyspnoea, palpitations and syncope.
Examination	Raised JVP, murmur, AF.
Investigations	ECG, CXR, Echo and 24-hour tape.
Management	Control symptoms: heart failure, angina and arrhythmias.
	Consider myectomy and septal ablation.
	Consider an implanted defibrillator to prevent sudden death.
Complications	May cause heart failure, AF, stroke or sudden death (usually from arrhythmia).

There are several aspects to this case. First, dealing with the patient's appropriate concern that he may have HOCM. There is a medical need to assess and refer him for investigation but also to reassure him if he shows no features of the illness at present. If time permits, there may be an opportunity to discuss the genetics of HOCM (autosomal-dominant inheritance) should the patient wish to know. A patient in a simulated surgery-based exam may directly ask you about this, so be prepared to explain patterns of inheritance in layperson's language or with use of diagrams. The patient's false belief that a vessel in his brother's heart had burst should also be sensitively addressed. Lastly, it is very important to acknowledge the devastating loss of his brother and offer support/bereavement counselling should he require it.

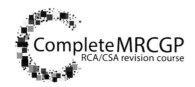

Genomic Medicine – 5

Extra Notes

The new curriculum lists the following genetic conditions. We suggest you should be able to explain each condition in 1–2 sentences as well as being able to explain the probability of each condition being passed on to children.

Autosomal-dominant disorders

Familial adenomatous polyposis

Explanation for patients	*'Familial means it can run in families, adenoma is the tissue in the large bowel and polyps are lumps in the bowel which can turn cancerous.'*
Genetics	Refer for testing of the *APC* (adenomatous polyposis coli) gene, although some may be sporadic.
Symptoms	Asymptomatic, rectal bleeding or a change in bowels.
Complications	Obstruction, colorectal cancer or other tumours, e.g. thyroid, carcinoid, bone.
Monitoring	FBC, CEA, TFT, LFT, FOB, X-rays, advise dental monitoring and colonoscopy.

Polycystic kidney

Explanation for patients	*'Poly means many, cysts are fluid-filled sacs and kidneys make urine from body waste and water.'*
Genetics	Autosomal dominant is most common.
Features	Asymptomatic or there may be pain or haematuria.
Complications	Recurrent infections, stones, hypertension, renal failure and need for dialysis.
Investigations	U&E, BP, ACR and USS and seek renal advice.
Monitoring	USS and U&E.
Immunisations	*Pneumococcus* and influenza vaccine.

HNPCC (hereditary non-polyposis colon cancer)

Associations	Other cancers, e.g. ovary, prostate and stomach.
Screening	Colonoscopy, endoscopy, cystoscopy and pelvic screening.

Thrombophilias, e.g. Factor V Leyden

Explanation for patients	*'The blood has an increased tendency to form clots so you are more likely to get a blood clot in the large veins in the legs or the lungs – called a pulmonary embolism.'*
Genetics	Autosomal dominant BUT if homozygous (faulty gene inherited from BOTH parents) significantly increased risk of blood clots.
Features	DVT, increased risk of clot dislodging to form PE.
Complications	Increased risk of miscarriage – consider if multiple miscarriages in 2nd or 3rd trimester. Possible increased risk of pre-eclampsia, slow fetal growth, placental abruption.
Investigations	Screening test for APC (activated protein C) resistance, then genetic tests.

Genomic Medicine

Others which are or can be autosomal dominant

- Ehlers–Danlos syndrome
- Gilbert's disease
- Hereditary haemorrhagic telangiectasia
- Marfan's syndrome
- Neurofibromatosis
- Von Willebrand's disease
- Prader–Willi syndrome
- HOCM

There are more!

Autosomal-recessive disorders

Cystic fibrosis	*'An inherited condition in which the lungs and digestive system can become clogged with thick, sticky mucus.'*
Hereditary haemochromatosis	*'Hereditary means that it runs in families. The body absorbs too much iron from food that you eat, so levels build up in the body and, untreated, can affect the liver, joints, pancreas and heart.'*
Wilson's disease	*'The body stores too much of an element called copper and, if not treated, this can build up and cause problems in the body, particularly the liver, brain and eyes.'*
Sickle cell disease	*'The red blood cells are an unusual shape and do not live as long as healthy red blood cells. They can't carry as much oxygen and can block blood vessels causing problems such as pain, infections and anaemia.'*
Thalassaemia	*'People with thalassaemia don't produce enough haemoglobin, which carries oxygen around the body in the red blood cells. This means they can become short of breath and anaemic.'*

X-linked recessive

Haemophilia A (factor VIII) and Haemophilia B (factor IX)	*'A rare condition that means the blood can't clot normally so people tend to bleed for longer than usual if they have a cut. It usually affects boys rather than girls. It can't be cured but can be treated with injections of man-made clotting medicines when needed.'*
Becker muscular dystrophy	*'An inherited condition which affects boys rather than girls. Over time, it causes weakness in the muscles of the legs and pelvis. It can cause problems with walking and may also affect the heart.'*
Duchenne muscular dystrophy	*'An inherited condition which affects boys rather than girls. Over time, muscles become weak. It can affect all muscles in the body including those in the heart and lungs.'*

X-linked dominant

Fragile X syndrome (FRAX)	*'An inherited condition that affects both boys and girls, but is usually worse in boys. It causes problems with development such as delay in learning to crawl and walk and learning disabilities. It can also cause problems with speech.'*

Genomic Medicine

Chromosomal disorders

Turner's syndrome	*'An inherited condition that only affects girls. Girls tend to be shorter than average and their ovaries don't develop properly so they may not have periods and usually can't get pregnant without help.'*
Klinefelter's syndrome	*'An inherited condition that only affects boys. Babies may take longer to learn to crawl or walk, children may have trouble concentrating and teenagers grow taller than expected for the family. Most men with Klinefelter's will need help if they want to father a child.'*
Down syndrome (Trisomy 21)	*'People with Down syndrome have an extra copy of a chromosome. They are likely to have some degree of learning disability and may take longer to learn to crawl and walk. When they grow up, they may be shorter than average height. They may have other problems for example with their heart, and may get more infections.'*
Edwards' syndrome (Trisomy 18)	*'A rare but very serious condition which affects how long a baby may live and very sadly most babies will die before or just after being born. A few babies will live to become children, but may have learning disabilities and problems with their heart, chest, kidneys and digestive systems.'*
Patau's syndrome (Trisomy 13)	*'A rare but very serious condition that severely affects the baby's normal development and very sadly often causes miscarriage, stillbirth or the baby dies soon after birth or in the first year of life.'*

A useful analogy to explain genetics is that of an instruction manual: the words are genes, the chapters the chromosomes. Put all together and you have a plan to build a body and make it work.

Genomic Medicine

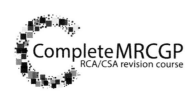

CHAPTER 9 OVERVIEW

Gynaecology and Breast

	Cases in this chapter	Within the RCGP 2020 curriculum: Gynaecology and Breast	Learning points in this chapter include:
1	Heavy Menstrual Bleeding	'Menstrual problems including heavy menstrual bleeding, dysmenorrhoea (primary and secondary), dysfunctional uterine bleeding'	NICE Guideline NG88. Heavy menstrual bleeding: assessment and management. May 2021
2	Polycystic Ovary Syndrome	'PCOS – gynaecological aspects and associated metabolic disorders such as insulin resistance and obesity and symptoms such as acne and hirsutism'	PCOS Metformin
3	Post-Menopausal Bleeding	'Post-menopausal bleeding'	CA125 test NICE Guideline NG12. Suspected cancer: recognition and referral. January 2021
4	Cervical Cancer – End of Life. Discussion with a Relative	'Cervical cancer, CIN, dysplasia'	How to discuss end-of-life care with relatives
5	Gynaecomastia	'Gynaecomastia' 'Breast lumps (men and women)'	Causes of gynaecomastia Examination, investigation, management.
Extra Notes	Menopause and HRT	'Menopause – treatment options including hormone replacement therapy – systemic and local methods'	Different preparations (oestrogen only/cyclical combined/continuous combined)
	HRT Risks	'The risks and benefits of hormone replacement therapy'	Vascular risks Breast cancer risk Side effects Stopping HRT
	Endometriosis	'Common and important conditions – endometriosis' 'Diagnosis of endometriosis' 'Endometriosis need(s) to be managed as long-term conditions…in primary care'	Endometriosis
	Ovarian Cysts	'Benign ovarian swellings including ovarian cysts, dermoid' 'Ovarian cancer including adenocarcinoma and teratoma'	Oxfordshire Guidance – Management of Ovarian Cysts

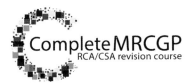

CompleteMRCGP
RCA/CSA revision course

CHAPTER 9 REFERENCES

Heavy Menstrual Bleeding

1. NICE Guideline NG88. Heavy menstrual bleeding: assessment and management. May 2021.
2. NICE Guideline NG12. Suspected cancer: recognition and referral. Jan 2021.
3. Mansour D. Safer prescribing of therapeutic norethisterone for women at risk of venous thromboembolism. *J Fam Plann Reprod Health Care* 2012; 38: 148–9.

Polycystic Ovary Syndrome

1. NICE CKS. http://cks.nice.org.uk/polycystic-ovary-syndrome#!scenariorecommendation. Sep 2018.
2. http://www.advancedfertility.com/progesterone-withdrawal-test.htm

Useful Resources

https://patient.info/womens-health/polycystic-ovary-syndrome-leaflet
https://patient.info/sexual-health/hormone-pills-patches-and-rings/progestogen-only-contraceptive-pill-pop

Post-Menopausal Bleeding

1. NICE Guideline NG12. Suspected cancer: recognition and referral. Jan 2021.
2. Postmenopausal Bleeding – Patient Care Pathway. https://www.oxfordshireccg.nhs.uk/professional-resources/documents/clinical-guidelines/gynaecology/post-menopausal-bleeding-pathway.pdf

Cervical Cancer – End of Life. Discussion with a Relative

1. https://www.gmc-uk.org/ethical-guidance/ethical-guidance-for-doctors/confidentiality

Useful Resources

http://patient.info/doctor/cervical-screening-cervical-smear-test-pro. May 2021.
HPV and cervical cancer. Fact sheet. http://www.who.int/mediacentre/factsheets/fs380/en/. Nov 2020.
NICE CKS. http://cks.nice.org.uk/cervical-screening#!scenario:1. Sep 2020.
https://www.mariecurie.org.uk/professionals/palliative-care-knowledge-zone/individual-needs/talking-approaching-end-life

Gynaecomastia

1. Porter K. GP management of gynaecomastia. http://www.gponline.com/gp-managementgynaecomastia/cancer/womens/article/1118276. Feb 2012.

Menopause and HRT/HRT Risks

1. NICE Guideline NG23. Menopause: diagnosis and management. Dec 2019.
2. FSRH Guideline: Contraception For Women Over 40. https://www.fsrh.org/standards-and-guidance/fsrh-guidelines-and-statements/contraception-for-specific-populations/aged-over-40/. Sep 2019.
3. https://bnf.nice.org.uk/drug/estradiol.html
4. NICE CKS. https://cks.nice.org.uk/topics/menopause/management/management-of-menopause-perimenopause-or-premature-ovarian-insufficiency/ Nov 2020.
5. Jones M.E., Schoemaker M.J., Wright L., et al. Menopausal hormone therapy and breast cancer: what is the true size of the increased risk? *Br J Cancer* 2016; 115: 607–15.
6. NICE CKS. https://cks.nice.org.uk/topics/incontinence-urinary-in-women/prescribing-information/intravaginal-oestrogen/ Oct 2019.

Endometriosis

1. https://www.nhs.uk/conditions/endometriosis/treatment/
2. NICE Guideline NG73. Endometriosis: diagnosis and management. Sep 2017.

Ovarian Cysts

1. RCOG Guideline. Green-Top Guideline No. 34. Ovarian Cysts in Post-Menopausal Women. Jul 2016.
2. RCOG Guideline. Green-Top Guideline No. 62. Management of Suspected Ovarian Masses in Premenopausal Women. Nov 2011.
3. Oxford Guidance. Price N., Traill Z., Goldstein M., et al. Management of Ovarian Cysts. Joint PCT/Radiology/Gynaecology/Gynae Oncology Guidelines. Version 4. Dec 2012.

Information taken from NICE guidelines with kind permission. Please note the guidelines change frequently and you should ALWAYS check for the latest updated guidance. Remember that NICE guidance is only applicable to patients in the UK.

Gynaecology and Breast

Doctor's Notes

Patient	Jacqui Mason 24 years F
PMH	No information
Medications	No current medications
Allergies	No information
Consultations	No recent consultations
Investigations	No recent investigations
Household	No household members registered
Previous consultation	6 months ago
	Attended with heavy periods.
	Normal abdominal and PV examination.
	Try tranexamic acid.

Example Consultation   Heavy Menstrual Bleeding

Open ☐	Oh dear, tell me more about them. What pain do you experience?
Impact ☐	How do your periods affect your life?
Flags ☐	Do you ever bleed between periods or after sex? Any pain during sex? Do you have pain at other times? Have your periods changed? When was your last period? Do you use contraception?
ICE ☐	Have you had thoughts as to what could be causing these heavy periods? Is there anything else that you have been wondering? Any other worries? Is there anything particular you were hoping for today?
History ☐	Tell me about your periods from when you first started them. I'm interested to know more about you… how is your general health? Any medical problems? Any other symptoms? Do you take any medicines? Do they help? Who are the important people in your life? Do you work? Any FH I should be aware of? Or of bleeding conditions?
O/E ☐	How do you feel about coming down for an examination? Your tummy and internally. This may be helpful; I may be able to feel a fibroid, a harmless lump in the womb which can cause heavy periods.
Sense ☐	I hear you feel strongly about seeing a gynaecologist.
Curious ☐	When did you start to think about endometriosis? Why did you think this may be endometriosis? Does anyone you know suffer with this?
Empathy ☐	Your periods are impacting on your life – especially at work, which is difficult and embarrassing for you.
SummarICE ☐	You are concerned about endometriosis and the possible complication of infertility. This is an understandable concern and you want tests to find the diagnosis.
Impression ☐	I agree, you are suffering from heavy menstrual bleeding. When there is no obvious cause for this, we call it dysfunctional uterine bleeding. Reassuringly, you do not have additional symptoms like pain during sex which may suggest endometriosis.
Experience ☐	Have you heard of any treatment options for heavy menstrual bleeding?
Explanation ☐	Everyone's periods are different. When women feel their periods are too heavy or they affect their life, we call this heavy menstrual bleeding. The clots you mention are blood which has grouped together.
InCludE ☐	There is always the possibility of endometriosis but the operation needed to diagnose endometriosis carries its own risk.
Recommend ☐	Therefore, without the additional symptoms, I would recommend trying treatment for heavy menstrual bleeding first.
Options ☐	We could do a blood test to check for anaemia. Meanwhile we can treat the bleeding with either a hormone treatment, the pill, which may reduce your periods, or a Mirena coil which can be helpful to reduce heavy painful periods. We could request an ultrasound to check for a fibroid. If we aren't winning, and we'll know soon, then we could think about endometriosis.
InCludE ☐	I appreciate this does not relieve your concern about blockages of the tubes. However, it is reassuring that you have regular periods and if you struggled to fall pregnant, we could have a low threshold for referring you to gynaecology? This way we have tried the least invasive route. What are your thoughts?
Empower ☐	Okay, I can see this is important to you. Okay.
Future ☐	Would you like to try a medication in the meantime? Can we arrange a blood test to check for anaemia? Would you like me to request an USS so the result is hopefully available for the gynaecologist?
Specifics ☐	Please book the blood test at reception. I will refer you and, if you do not receive an appointment within a month, please phone and speak to our secretary.
Safety net ☐	If your symptoms change – a change to your pain or bleeding pattern – let a GP know.

Gynaecology and Breast – 1

Patient's Story

Heavy Menstrual Bleeding

Doctor's notes	Jacqui Mason, 24 years. PMH: none. Medications: none.
How to act	A little pushy. Intelligent.
PC	*'It's my periods. They are very heavy.'*
History	Your periods started aged 14 years. They became heavy and painful a year ago.
	The pulling pain starts on the morning of your period in your lower stomach.
	The pain lasts 2 days. Your period cycle is 8/30 with 5 heavy days.
	You are changing a tampon every 2 hours. *'There are clots!'*
	During a period, you have to leave meetings, which is embarrassing.
	Paracetamol doesn't help.
	You saw another GP 6 months ago. You felt they didn't take you seriously and the tablet they gave you, tranexamic acid, didn't help.
	No IMB or PCB. You have no abnormal discharge.
	Jacob is your boyfriend of 2 years. No dyspareunia.
	You both had an STI check at the start of your relationship.
	You have never had an STI. You have never been pregnant.
	Your first smear was normal. For contraception you use condoms.
	You are otherwise well. No PMH, medicines or FH.
	No one you know suffers with it. Decline an examination. *'It will be normal.'*
Social	You are a graphic designer. You enjoy your job.
	You rent your home with your boyfriend and have a good relationship.
	You drink alcohol occasionally and do not smoke.
ICE	Two weeks ago you read an article in a magazine about endometriosis.
	It mentioned it causes heavy painful periods and can lead to blockages in the tubes.
	You believe you have endometriosis.
	You are concerned that this could make you infertile.
	You are hoping to get married next year and start a family.
	You do not want hormones as you want your body to be natural.
	You thought the GP may suggest the pill. You want a referral to a gynaecologist.
	Become angry if the doctor does not offer a gynaecology referral.
	You do not want to take medicines without knowing what is wrong.
	You demand to see a gynaecologist. You do not take no for an answer.

Learning Points

Heavy menstrual bleeding
: Excessive menstrual blood loss which interferes with the woman's physical, emotional, social and/or material quality of life … so ask about impact!

Cause
: DUB if no cause is found.

Iatrogenic (e.g. IUD), psychosomatic disturbance.

Fibroids, endometrial hyperplasia, cancer, endometriosis, PID.

Hypothyroidism, blood clotting disorders.

Red flags
: IMB, PCB, pelvic pain or pressure – possible structural or histological abnormality.

Examination
: If the history suggests heavy menstrual bleeding without a significant underlying cause then you may trial pharmacological treatment without examining the patient or performing any investigations unless treatment chosen is LNG-IUS. If other related symptoms, offer physical examination. Examine patient before any investigations or LNG-IUS fitting.[1]

Investigations
: FBC for all women with HMB. TFT and coagulation screen if other symptoms/signs present.

If PCB or IMB: view the cervix and refer for colposcopy if abnormal.

Infection (chlamydia) swab.

Imaging and biopsy
: Ultrasound or hysteroscopy are the first-line investigations.[1]

Pelvic USS if: uterus palpable abdominally, history or examination suggests pelvic mass, examination difficult or inconclusive (e.g. due to obesity).

TV USS if: significant dysmenorrhoea, or bulky tender uterus suggesting adenomyosis.

Hysteroscopy if: persistent IMB or risk factors for endometrial polyps, i.e. if considering submucosal fibroids, polyps or endometrial pathology.

2WW referral
: Consider if a 2WW referral is indicated – ensure you are up to date with all the 2WW criteria for gynaecological cancers in the NICE guidance for Suspected Cancer.[2]

Routine referral
: If investigations needed to diagnose cause of HMB and for consideration of alternative treatments including second generation endometrial ablation and hysterectomy.

Management options
: Consider LNG-IUS if no pathology or fibroids <3 cm, not distorting cavity or suspected or diagnosed adenomyosis.

If LNG-IUS declined or unsuitable, consider:

- Tranexamic acid (side effects include GI disturbance and headaches).
- Ibuprofen/mefenamic acid.
- Hormonal: IUS, COCP or cyclical norethisterone.
- Surgical, e.g. endometrial ablation or hysterectomy.

Norethisterone VTE risk
: Consider medroxyprogesterone acetate as an alternative to norethisterone to delay menses or in the treatment of menorrhagia in women with additional risk factors for VTE: >35 years and smokers or overweight or personal or FH of VTE.[3]

Doctor's Notes

Patient	Juliet Perkins	27 years	F
PMH	Acne		
Medications	Epiduo		
Allergies	No known allergies		
Consultations	Telephone call 6 months ago to repeat Epiduo treatment for acne.		
Investigations	No recent investigations		
Household	No household members registered		

Example Consultation   Polycystic Ovary Syndrome

Open ☐	Tell me more about your periods from when they first started.
Sense ☐	I can hear that you are worried.
Impact ☐	How has this been affecting you?
History ☐	When did your periods change? Have you noticed anything else that you don't think is right? I see you have acne in your medical history – how is that now? Have you noticed any hairs on the face or neck? Your general history – do you have any pain – generally or during intercourse? Have you ever been pregnant? Or had an STI? Have you had normal smear tests? Are you in a relationship? Do you live with anyone else? What work do you do? Do you smoke or drink much alcohol?
Flags ☐	Because you haven't had a period I need to double check – could you be pregnant?
Risk ☐	Has anyone in your family had trouble with their periods or other women's health problems?
ICE ☐	What has crossed your mind about what may be causing this? Is there anything else you have been wondering? Anything that you are worried about? What did you think I may suggest? Is there anything else you were hoping for?
Curious ☐	What conversations with others have you had about polycystic ovaries?
SummarICE ☐	To summarise, for several years your periods have been less than monthly which has made you question cysts in your ovaries. You came across this when your friend's sister needed IVF and her diagnosis of PCOS has made you worry about your own fertility.
O/E ☐	Do you know how tall you are and your current weight? Could you send me a photo of your skin?
Empathy ☐	I appreciate it may be worrying not having regular periods and a concern when you have heard that this may be linked to problems with fertility.
Impression ☐	I think you may be right. Polycystic ovaries are when we see cysts on your ovaries.
InCludE ☐	You have mentioned having a scan and I agree this would be helpful. If we see cysts on your ovaries, it is likely that you have PCOS because you have the associated problems, e.g. acne and infrequent periods. There are also some blood tests which help with the diagnosis such as checking your testosterone level.
Impact ☐	I appreciate this may be concerning; what is going through your mind?
Experience ☐	Do you know what doctors suggest if we see cysts on your ovaries?
Explanation ☐	The lining of the womb doesn't tend to get thicker and thicker but the alteration to your hormones can put you at increased risk of womb cancer in the long term.
Options ☐	To protect the womb, we should aim for four to five periods a year or protect your womb with the hormone progesterone. You have questioned whether metformin may be helpful. We should be guided by test results. Metformin is a tablet usually used for diabetes. The manufacturer did not intend it to be used for PCOS which means if prescribed it is off licence, but it has been shown to help with weight, the hair on the face and sugar levels which can creep up in PCOS. It can also help with fertility. However, I suggest waiting until we have your test results back and make the diagnosis.
Empower ☐	Because PCOS is linked with an increased risk of raised sugars and cholesterol, which in turn can increase the risks to the health of your heart and blood vessels, keeping active, which you already do with your sport, can protect you in the long term, as can eating a healthy diet. You may find significant lifestyle changes alone prevent the need for metformin. Would you like information leaflets on the hormone options we can use to ensure you have five periods a year and we can discuss this when we meet again?
Future ☐	Although it sounds like PCOS, I would like to arrange blood tests to check your testosterone and other hormone levels and make sure there is no other hormonal cause for this by checking your thyroid function and prolactin. I would like to check your general health bloods including your sugar and cholesterol. How does this sound? Are you happy for me to request an USS?
Specifics ☐	Please book a blood test with our healthcare assistant. Shall we catch up again, after your blood test, on the phone? We can then talk about the hormone options and also inducing a withdrawal bleed just before the ultrasound scan to get an accurate idea of the thickness of the lining of your womb.
Safety net ☐	I don't expect you to experience any new symptoms; however, occasionally cysts can cause pain so if you ever have stomach pain, please see a doctor.

Gynaecology and Breast – 2

Patient's Story

Polycystic Ovary Syndrome

Doctor's notes Juliet Perkins, 27 years. PMH: acne. Medication: Epiduo.

How to act Concerned.

PC *'I haven't had a period for 4 months.'*

History Your periods started aged 13 years and have always been every 4–8 weeks until about 3 years ago when they started to range from 1 to 5 months.

Your periods are not heavy. You have no IMB, PCB or dyspareunia.

You have no abdominal pain.

You have never had an STI.

You have never been pregnant.

Normal smear 2 years ago.

You have no other medical history apart from acne. You have no family history.

Social You are a teacher for children with learning disabilities.

You have a female partner of 2 years.

You drink occasionally <14 units a week and have never smoked.

You enjoy running and tennis.

ICE You have heard that you may have polycystic ovaries.

You are concerned that 4-monthly periods are not normal.

You worry that the lining of your womb is getting thicker and thicker; is this dangerous?

Your friend's sister, aged 33 years, has just started IVF treatment.

She mentioned that she has PCOS.

You would like a scan.

You have been reading and want to know if you can start metformin.

Height 165 cm. Weight 74 kg. BMI 27.

Examination Mild acne. Some long hairs below the chin.

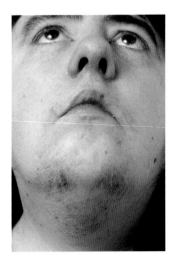

Credit: SPL/Science Source.

Learning Points

Diagnosis[1]	Two out of three of:
	Hyperandrogenism *Either* symptoms (e.g. hirsutism, acne, alopecia) *or* biochemical (abnormal blood tests).
	Cysts >12 in one ovary or ovarian volume >10 mL.
	Decreased ovulation Oligomenorrhoea or amenorrhoea.
Other symptoms	Weight gain or acanthosis nigricans.[1]
Investigations	Testosterone, SHBG, LH, FSH, TSH, prolactin, T4, HbA1c and lipids.[1]
Diagnostic	Hyperandrogenism – testosterone (increased) and SHBG (low/normal).[1]
Other causes	Premature ovarian failure – increased LH and FSH. [1]
	Hypogonadotropic hypogonadism – decreased LH and FSH. [1]
	Hypothyroidism – raised TSH and low T4.
	Hyperprolactinaemia – however, prolactin may also be mildly elevated in PCOS.[1]
Complications	Raised glucose and lipids.
USS	For diagnosis (ovaries) or if oligo/amenorrhoea induce a withdrawal bleed (see below) then refer for USS.
	If endometrial thickness >10 mm → endometrial sampling.[1]
Lifestyle	Decrease CV risk – exercise, weight loss and low GI diet.
Oligomenorrhoea	Prevent endometrial hyperplasia by inducing a withdrawal bleed every 3 months, with either cyclical progesterone or the COCP (unless protected by an IUS).[1]
For acne	Usual acne Rx or co-cyprindiol for acne and hirsutism.
For hirsutism	Bleach and electrolysis.
	Eflornithine cream but may cause skin irritation.
	Review and stop if no effect, e.g. at 4 months.
For weight	General advice and consider metformin and orlistat.
Complications	Weight gain, CVD, infertility due to anovulation, diabetes, high cholesterol.
	Endometrial hyperplasia and carcinoma.[1]
Pregnancy plans	GP – advice about lifestyle and weight loss.
	Specialists – metformin, clomiphene, gonadotrophins or fertility Rx.[1]
If pregnant	OGTT <20 weeks.[1] Increased risk of HTN, pre-eclampsia and premature birth.[1]
Metformin	Unlicensed for PCOS, initiated by a specialist[1], can improve insulin sensitivity, help to normalise menstrual cycle and it may help with weight loss or hirsutism.
Investigating secondary amenorrhoea	Consider a progesterone withdrawal test.[2]

Gynaecology and Breast – 2

Doctor's Notes

Patient	Hilda Rowland	53 years	F
PMH	Mirena coil inserted aged 48 years		
	Menorrhagia		
Medications	No current medications		
Allergies	No information		
Consultations	No recent consultations		
Investigations	No recent investigations		
Household	Brian Rowland	55 years	M

Example Consultation   Post-Menopausal Bleeding

Open ☐   What's led to this decision? Tell me more about the bleeding? Any pattern? And your periods prior to this?

History ☐   Is your general health good? Any other medical problems? Do you take any medicines? Tell me more about you? Are you active? Have you had any menopausal symptoms? Have you had children?

ICE ☐   You mentioned the bleeding is likely due to the coil. Why do you think that? Has anything else crossed your mind? Are you worried about anything? What did you think we may decide today?

Flags ☐   It is helpful to know if you are sexually active and if there is bleeding afterwards. I always check there is no risk of infection – any discharge? Other sexual partners? Any weight loss?

Risk ☐   Any family history you are aware of? When was your last smear? Have you had any abnormal smears?

Sense ☐   You seem relaxed about this bleeding.

Impact ☐   How has this bleeding affected you?

SummarICE ☐   To summarise, you were warned the coil may cause abnormal bleeding and is usually in for 5 years, therefore this bleeding has not come as a shock but has been irritating. You don't want the heavy periods to return but are hoping for a trial without the coil.

O/E ☐   I don't think we should remove the coil today as we don't yet know the cause of the problem. But may I examine you – feel your tummy, look with a speculum to see if the bleeding could be coming from the vagina or the neck of the womb called the cervix, and feel the womb? May I ask for a chaperone? Please go behind the curtain, undress from the waist down, get underneath the top sheet and tell me when you are ready… You have no sign of infection, but may I take swabs to be sure? May I check your weight and height?

Impression ☐   My concern is that you may have gone through the menopause. I say 'may have' because we don't know whether the absence of bleeding is due to your coil. Bleeding after the menopause can be common but needs investigation.

Explanation ☐   There are many possible reasons for the bleeding: a fibroid which is a harmless lump in the womb; a polyp which is originally harmless but may have the potential to become a cancer; it may be due to the coil, but the coil's hormone usually lasts for 7 years; the bleeding may also be coming from the cervix or vaginal walls which become more fragile as we age, but they look fine today. I will send the swabs to also rule out infection. The priority is ruling out a cancer, which can cause abnormal bleeding.

Options ☐   We refer all women who bleed after the menopause urgently for an USS, which is a jelly scan to check the womb shows no sign of a cancer. What are your thoughts?

Empathy ☐   I appreciate me mentioning the possibility of cancer may come as a shock, especially when the bleeding at the 5-year mark has made sense from what previous doctors have mentioned. As I say, in most cases nothing serious is found; however, I am sorry if this is upsetting and causes worry whilst we consider the possibility.

Future ☐   Let's now go through what you can expect in the next few weeks. At the USS they will insert the probe into the vagina to look at the womb. Depending on what this shows, you may need to see a specialist who will offer a camera test to have a closer look and take biopsies – little samples of the womb. If they do not remove the coil at the hospital, we can do this afterwards. Please make a follow-up appointment with me to go through what they have found, a few days after the ultrasound.

Safety net ☐   If your bleeding becomes heavier or you have pain let a GP know please.

Specifics ☐   You should be seen within 2 weeks from today. If you haven't received an appointment within 10 days let me know. If you have any questions just leave a message at reception and I'll phone you. Try not to worry – remember we are being thorough.

Gynaecology and Breast – 3

Patient's Story

Post-Menopausal Bleeding

Doctor's notes	Hilda Rowland, 53 years. PMH: menorrhagia. Mirena coil inserted aged 48 years. Medications: none.
How to act	Relaxed.
PC	*'I wondered if we could remove my coil now.'*
History	You had the coil inserted 5 years ago for heavy bleeding.
	You stopped being sexually active with your husband a few years ago.
	Over the last 3 months you have started bleeding.
	You have never been on HRT and take no other medication.
	Your last period was 3 years ago. Your smears are up to date.
	You have had no spotting until 3 months ago, with no pattern.
	You have no abdominal pain.
	You have not lost weight.
	You had hot flushes for a couple of years but these stopped a year ago.
	You have no urinary or bowel problems.
	You have been irritated by having to remember to take towels with you.
Social	A headmistress for the local primary school.
	You enjoy walking and you are a well-known member of the community.
	You lead a busy lifestyle with the school and church group charity events.
	You have never smoked and enjoy a sherry on weekends.
ICE	You believe your coil has started to run out which is why you would like it out.
	You are not worried, as you were told you may bleed at random times and it usually lasts for 5 years, so this makes sense to you.
	You expect the doctor will want to remove it today and then it will be sorted.
	Another possibility is that you could have another one. You just worry about the heavy bleeding coming back but wonder if you could try without it first.
	If the doctor mentions that this could be cancer react to this … *'You think I have cancer? You've got me worried now!'*
Examination	The vulva, vagina and cervix look healthy. The coil string is visible.
	No palpable pelvic masses.
	Abdomen soft, non-tender and no masses.
	BMI 25.

Gynaecology and Breast – 3

Learning Points Suspected Gynaecological Cancer

Always refer to the full text of NICE Guideline NG12: Suspected cancer: recognition and referral.

Cervical

When to examine the vagina and cervix with a speculum and palpate the uterus/ovaries:

- Every woman with abnormal or post-coital bleeding or pelvic pain.
- Do not rely on recent smear tests.
- Do not wait for the result of a smear test if there is any abnormality on the cervix. Refer 2WW.

Ovarian

When to request CA125 testing for possible ovarian cancer:

- Be suspicious in any woman, particularly those over 50 with symptoms of bloating, feeling full, loss of appetite, abdominal or pelvic pain or frequency/urgency in urination with symptoms occurring more than 12 times a month.[1]
- Consider also if 'unexplained weight loss, fatigue or changes in bowel habit'.[1]
- Be aware IBS rarely presents in women for the first time over the age of 50.

CA125 is ≥35 IU/mL:

- Urgently (within 2 weeks) 'arrange an ultrasound scan of the abdomen and pelvis'. [1] If this suggested a cancer the patient would then require a 2WW gynaecology referral.

CA125 is <35 IU/mL OR ≥35 IU/mL and the USS is normal:

- Reassess for other conditions then safety net for more frequent/persistent or new symptoms.[1]

Endometrial

2WW gynaecology ≥55 years with PMB.

Consider if <55 years with PMB.[1]

However, many GPs have direct access (2WW) to ultrasound (85% sensitivity) as a first-line investigation for PMB. If women also have a normal speculum examination, up-to-date smear, endometrial thickness of <4 mm and no risk factors (BMI >35, DM, Tamoxifen or previous hyperplasia) then, if the bleeding settles, no hysteroscopy is required.[2] If, however, bleeding persists then the GP should consider referral for a hysteroscopy which may detect a mass not seen on the ultrasound, for example an endocervical tumour.

Consider a direct access ultrasound scan for women >55 years with unexplained vaginal discharge if first presentation of this or have thrombocytosis or have macro/microscopic haematuria and: low Hb or high platelets or raised blood glucose. [1]

Reasons to send a 2WW gynaecology referral:

- Ascites and/or pelvic or abdominal mass.[1]
- If an ultrasound suggests cancer.
- Women with PMB – see above and your local guidelines.
- Consider if abnormal appearance of the cervix, vagina or vulva (e.g. lump, ulceration or bleeding).[1]

Doctor's Notes

Patient	Louise Barker	33 years	F

PMH Metastatic cervical cancer diagnosed 5 months ago.

Last hospital letter – TAH followed by chemotherapy. Now palliative care.

Normal vaginal delivery 2 years ago

Ex-smoker

Medications Cyclizine

Ibuprofen

Paracetamol

Codeine phosphate

Metoclopramide

Allergies No known drug allergies

Consultations 1 week ago with GP – abdominal pain. Codeine commenced.

Investigations No recent tests completed at the practice.

Household	James Barker	35 years	M
	Megan Barker	2 years	F

Husband has arranged an appointment to discuss his wife.

Example Consultation

Cervical Cancer – End of Life. Discussion with a Relative

Open ☐   Hello Mr Barker, my name is Dr X. What would you like to talk to me about today? What has been going through your mind?

History ☐   May I clarify what you understand about Louise's health? How is Louise physically? How is she coping emotionally? How are you coping? How is your mood at present? Who else is at home? Do you have any other support? Are you at work? Who is involved in Louise's care at present?

Sense ☐   I can hear that you are devastated and I hear that you have lots on your mind.

ICE ☐   When you are on your own, what thoughts do you have? Anything else that you have been wondering? All kinds of emotions occur at a time like this: sadness, fear, guilt, hopelessness. I'm interested to know what you have been feeling. Is there anything else that makes you feel anxious or worried? What would be helpful to you and your family? Is there anything else that you need or you are hoping for?

Impact ☐   Do you feel responsible for Louise's care day to day?

Curious ☐   When you say she will no longer be breathing… what else is going through your mind? What are your thoughts when you think of life without her? 'Back in time', what do you mean? What do you think is on Louise's mind? Have you shared how you feel with each other? Have you discussed going to a hospice?

Empathy ☐   You have many thoughts and emotions, whilst it sounds as if you are trying to be brave for your family.

SummarICE ☐   You have had fears of finding Louise no longer breathing and hope that when Louise is very poorly she will be in a hospice. You have had feelings of guilt and you can't imagine, at present, life with Megan without Louise, especially when you work and your family live 5 hours away. Have I understood you correctly?

Explanation ☐   You are correct that the virus that causes this infection can be sexually transmitted, but this virus is so common. Over a third of people your age will have this virus, which is far higher than other STIs. Louise has been extremely unlucky. Most women with the virus will remain healthy.

Options ☐   You mentioned that you would like someone to talk to, about how to talk to Megan. Would it be okay if I spoke to the palliative care nurses? They could talk to you and Louise about options for the future, the benefits of a hospice as well as how they can help within your own home, and also about talking to Megan.

InCludE ☐   You mentioned you fear finding Louise not breathing in the morning and how you will cope without her. I also wonder if speaking to a counsellor may be helpful to talk through your fears. How would you feel about that?

Empower ☐   Could you talk to any friends or family about who may be able to help you with Megan? If we were to think about how might they help you, what comes to mind? Have you thought about creating a memory box for Megan for when she is older? Some families find this helpful.

Future ☐   I'm just wondering about when we should speak again. What are your thoughts? Can we arrange for Louise and you to come into the surgery together?

Safety net ☐   If, in the meantime, you or Louise ever need help day or night, do you know who to call?

Specifics ☐   If we are open, please contact us or Louise's palliative care nurse. During the night you can call 111 for a doctor. Do you have all the telephone numbers to hand?

Patient's Story

Doctor's notes   Mr Barker has arranged a telephone appointment to discuss his wife. Louise Barker, 33 years. PMH: metastatic cervical cancer diagnosed 5 months ago. Last hospital letter; TAH followed by chemotherapy and now palliative care. NVD 2 years ago.

Medications: Cyclizine, ibuprofen, paracetamol, codeine and metoclopramide.

How to act   Quiet and polite.

PC   *'I just thought I should talk to you, Doctor.'*

Be slow to give information.

'There's so much in my mind I can't concentrate sometimes.'

History   You understand your wife was diagnosed with metastatic cervical cancer 5 months ago. She has had a TAH and the last scan showed the chemotherapy was not successful. Originally, she had bleeding and pain for months but put this down to her POP and IBS. She missed her smear because of the baby and then she forgot. Currently Louise is able to manage at home on pain relief but you worry about how you will look after her and Megan, who is now 2 years old, as Louise's disease progresses. The palliative care team has not visited as currently Louise's symptoms are controlled. Louise is strong emotionally with family but cries at night.

Social   Louise's family live locally and are around most days. Your family is 5 hours away. You are signed off work for 3 months. You are a surveyor. You met Louise 3 years ago and within a year you were married. Prior to life with Louise, life was centred around work and friends but once Megan arrived, life dramatically changed. You have no medical or psychiatric history. You do not feel depressed but incredibly sad. You eat and sleep but have many upsetting thoughts which are distracting. You have no thoughts of harming yourself or another.

ICE   *'I can't stop thinking that she won't be breathing.'* You mean you are frightened about finding Louise dead. Every morning you wait until you can feel her breathe before you turn to look at her.

'How will I cope without her?' By this you mean how you will care for Megan alone. You feel full of sadness when thinking about your future life. No one has brought up the subject of life after Louise as they don't want to upset you but you think it would be a relief to discuss this and will talk to the family.

'You know, if life could go back in time.' You feel guilty with your thoughts. You sometimes wish you had never met Louise, then you wouldn't be going through this. You also believe this is your fault. You read that the virus that leads to the cancer is sexually transmitted and you fear this was passed on from you. Louise told you 'not to be silly'. You cry with Louise if ever you talk about your feelings but you don't tell her things that you fear may upset her. You think Louise feels guilty that she will leave you and Megan alone.

You hope the doctor will visit Louise and talk to her about a hospice so she will be around nurses *'when it happens'*. You feel you need someone to talk to about how to talk to Megan about her mother. You need someone to help you with Megan after she has gone.

Learning Points

Confidentiality[1] Unless the patient has given consent, no information can be given to the NOK. However, you can speak in general terms about a condition or likely outcome, e.g. 'often in similar situations the hospice can offer support'.

You cannot give new information to the relative but can discuss what they already know. Again be general to avoid any confidentiality issues, e.g. in this case you can discuss cervical cancer in general (such as links to HPV) but not the specifics of Louise's case.

Do not Do not presume you understand their concerns. Explore their thoughts.

Do Ensure the relative feels understood – summarise their ICE!

Reassure they will receive the help they need specifically related to their concerns.

Example consultation structure when discussing end-of-life care with a relative

Allow the person to do the majority of the talking, be flexible with what they hope to discuss. The following structure may be helpful:

1. Silences, exploring thoughts or stating what you sense can help initiate a sensitive consultation.
2. Check their understanding of the situation.
3. Collect all thoughts, concerns, fears, anxieties and expectations.
4. Be curious. Explore any cues they may have hinted. Silences or repeating words to encourage further discussion may be useful here.
5. Understand the relative; are they well? Their mood, their responsibilities as a carer, other stressors in their life, the impact of the situation.
6. Summarise the ICE. A powerful way to help the relative feel understood and also focuses the management plan.
7. Empathise. The immensity of the situation and its potential impact on the person.
8. Enquire about communication between the relatives and patient.
9. Provide options/suggestions to manage each concern in turn.
10. Consider if other professionals or support groups may be helpful.
11. Empower with regard to their concerns.
12. Plan future meetings. Is anything required in the meantime?
11. Safety net: rescue treatment and contact numbers in the event of sudden deterioration.

If appropriate – in the event of death, do they know who to call? Usually, the GP or OOH GP to certify death, followed by the undertaker.

Doctor's Notes

Patient	Craig Mason	46 years	M
PMH	No medical history		
Medications	No medications		
Allergies	No information		
Consultations	No recent consultations		
Investigations	No recent investigations		
Household	Carolyn Mason	45 years	F
	Julianne Mason	15 years	F
	Thomas Mason	13 years	M

Sense ☐   I can sense you are worried.

ICE ☐   What has gone through your mind regarding what may have caused this? Is there anything you fear this could be? Is there anything in particular you thought I might suggest?

Open ☐   Anything else that you have noticed? Or are concerned about?

Flags ☐   Have you felt any lumps in the breast? Or elsewhere, for example the testicles? Any other symptoms elsewhere? For example, are your bowels normal? Any symptoms in the chest or tummy?

Risk ☐   Is it painful? Do you have a cough or any breathing problems? Any pain in the chest? Or weight loss? Do you smoke?

History ☐   You are otherwise well? Have you taken any medications or any supplements? What is in this supplement? How much alcohol do you drink? I'm interested to know more about you. Do you work? Do you live with anyone?

Impact ☐   Has this affected you or your relationship?

Curious ☐   What led you to start taking supplements?

SummarICE ☐   So to summarise, you have noticed your breasts have enlarged and this started after the addition of a body-building supplement. You are otherwise well with no symptoms. In the back of your mind, you fear this could be a cancer, or that I may suggest you need to go to a breast team. Have I understood correctly?

Empathy ☐   I can hear this has been a fright.

Impression ☐   I think you have developed breast tissue, which in men is called gynaecomastia.

Experience ☐   Have you come across this?

Explanation ☐   It has many different causes. In your case I believe it has been caused by the supplement. I think it is unlikely this will be cancer.

Examination ☐   However, I would like to examine you. Would you be able to come down to the surgery? I would check your height and weight, examine your chest to rule out any worrying breast lumps, and check your liver and neck looking for signs of any other underlying cause. It would be helpful to check your testicles are normal too as sometimes abnormal hormone release from testicles can cause gynaecomastia. If you were happy for me to do this, I would ask a chaperone to be present. Presuming your examination confirms my suspicion, I would expect your breasts to go back to normal a month or two after stopping the supplement.

Recommend ☐   I appreciate you wanted to increase your muscle tone but taking a supplement has risks, especially if from the internet and we do not know what is in the product. If I find any abnormal lump, you may need to see a specialist or we may need to do some blood tests.

Empower ☐   Do you think you will talk to your wife about our consultation today? Can you think of other ways to improve your fitness? Eating a varied diet that contains natural proteins and gradually improving your fitness is healthy.

Future ☐   You seem interested in your general health; would this be something you would like to talk more about? Is there anything specific that worries you about your general health? What tests did you have in mind? When you come down, ask reception to make you an appointment with the nurse for a cholesterol and blood pressure check.

Specifics ☐   I have booked you in at 3 p.m. Presuming all is well we can catch up in a month to see if there has been improvement and discuss your general health. Sometimes it takes up to 12 months to settle completely. Do you think reducing the amount of fat in your diet and increasing exercise is something you could do?

Safety net ☐   If you notice anything new, symptoms or lumps, then tell me straight away please.

Patient's Story

Gynaecomastia

Doctor's notes	Craig Mason, 46 years. PMH: none. Medications: none.
How to act	Concerned.
PC	*'I'm worried that my chest has grown. It's like I have breasts.'*
History	Your breasts have started to appear in the last few months.
	They are not painful. You have no PMH.
Social	You live with your wife and two children. Estate agent. Minimal alcohol. No stress.
	You started using a body-building treatment 6 months ago.
	Your wife encouraged you to go to the gym and tone up.
	You do not know what is in the supplement, you get it from the internet.
ICE	You think it may be fat as you have put on weight.
	At the back of your mind, you hope it's not breast cancer.
	Your fear would be being sent to a clinic full of women.
	You have no idea what the doctor may suggest.
	Late in the consultation, say you were worried about a decline in your health.
	You hope the GP offers a check-up including blood pressure and cholesterol.
	You are happy to come to the surgery for an examination.
Examination	Bilateral gynaecomastia, no lymphadenopathy.
	No hepatomegaly and no palpable thyroid.
	BMI 26.

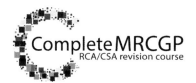
CompleteMRCGP
RCA/CSA revision course

Causes of gynaecomastia[1]

Idiopathic

Physiological	In teens and elderly.
Infection	Mumps.
Tumours	Lung (there may be an increased β-hCG) and testicular.
Systemic disease	Liver, thyrotoxicosis.
Iatrogenic	Drugs, steroids, PPIs, TCAs.
Hormonal	Hyperprolactinaemia, hypogonadism.
Alcohol	

Examination[1]

Breast examination and lymphadenopathy.

Signs of hyperthyroidism or goitre.

Chronic liver disease.

BMI.

Testicular examination.

Investigation

Not required in:	teens, if typical senile changes or if obvious iatrogenic cause.[1]
Consider	TFT, LFT, GGT, U&E, testosterone, prolactin, LH, β-hCG, oestradiol, DHEA, SHBG.[1]
If lung cancer suspected	CXR.
Testicular pain or mass	USS testes.
Mammography	Only if cancer is suspected.
Genetic cause suspected	Chromosomal karyotyping.

Management

Treat the cause, stop the drug and follow-up in 1/12.

Prognosis

Usually 1–12/12 to resolve after treating the cause.

In adolescent boys, physiological gynaecomastia is common and usually transitory. Reassurance can be given that most cases (90%) resolve within 3 years.[1]

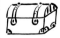 See the **Link Hub** at **CompleteMRCGP.co.uk** for a useful article on Gynaecomastia

---

Symptoms	Flushes, vaginal dryness, mood changes, low libido and urinary symptoms. Also sleep disturbance and often joint and muscle pains, headaches and fatigue.[1]

FSH testing

Measurement of FSH is unreliable whilst taking HRT.[2] Similarly FSH shouldn't be used to diagnose menopause in women using COCP, POP or high-dose progestogens.[1]

Consider using FSH to diagnose menopause in women aged 40–45 with changes in their cycle or vasomotor symptoms, or women <40 in whom POI is suspected.[1]

FSH testing may be helpful in women aged 50–55 taking POP or using IMP or LNG-IUS. If FSH is >30 IU/L, contraception can be stopped after 1 more year for any woman over 50 years. If FSH is <30 IU/L, contraception should be continued and FSH measured again after 1 year.[2]

General advice	Exercise, cotton clothing. Avoid: caffeine, spicy foods, smoking and alcohol.
	CBT may be helpful.[1]

Premature menopause

POI is confirmed if FSH is raised on two samples 4–6 weeks apart in women aged under <40.

Offer women a choice of HRT or a CHC unless contraindicated (e.g. hormone sensitive cancer).[1] NICE advises explaining to patients the importance of starting and continuing hormonal treatment until the age of the natural menopause and that this will offer bone protection and may benefit BP. The risk of cardiovascular disease and breast cancer is low in this age group.[1]

Ensure sufficient dietary calcium intake (blood tests and dietary calcium calculators) and encourage weight-bearing exercises to prevent the risk of osteoporosis and fragility fractures.

Contraception	Do not rely on HRT for contraception.[2]
Options:	Mirena (change every 5 years if used for endometrial protection)[2] + oestrogen-only HRT.
	The combination of Mirena with oestrogen-only patches provides both contraception with reduced VTE risk.
	POP + sequential HRT. 'All progestogen-only methods of contraception are safe to use as contraception alongside sequential HRT.'[2]
	'A woman who is under 50 years and free of all risk factors for venous and arterial disease can use a low-oestrogen combined oral contraceptive pill to provide both relief of menopausal symptoms and contraception; it is recommended that the oral contraceptive be stopped at 50 years of age since there are more suitable alternatives.'[3]
SSRIs/SNRIs[4]	For vasomotor symptoms consider a trial of SSRIs (off label) or SNRIs (off label) for 2 weeks in the first place. For mood disorders, consider self-help resources and a trial of CBT (low mood/anxiety). Use antidepressants if confirmed diagnosis of anxiety/depression. Beware that SSRIs paroxetine and fluoxetine should not be offered to women with breast cancer who are taking tamoxifen as they may inhibit its effect.

VTE risk	Transdermal is safer for menopausal women who are at increased risk of this, including those with a BMI >30 kg/m². Consider asking for advice from haematology when considering HRT in women at high risk of VTE.[1]
CVD risk	Cardiovascular risk factors are not a contraindication to HRT as long as they are optimally managed. Oestrogen-alone HRT is associated with no, or reduced, risk of coronary heart disease. HRT with oestrogen and progestogen does not increase in the risk of coronary heart disease in women under 60 years.[1]
Stroke risk	HRT involving oral oestrogen (but not transdermal) is associated with a small increase in the risk of stroke.[1]
T2DM risk	HRT does not increase the risk of diabetes or affect glucose control.
Breast risk	When using oestrogen-only HRT, there is little or no change in the risk of breast cancer, but HRT with oestrogen and progestogen can be associated with an increased risk. Any increase in risk reduces after stopping HRT and is related to the duration of treatment.[1]
	Note a recent study suggested the risk of breast cancer from combined HRT has been underestimated.[5]
Dementia risk	Unknown.[1]
How given	HRT is available as tablets, skin patches, gels, nasal spray or a vaginal ring.
Preparations	If the woman has had a hysterectomy – oestrogen only.
	If still having periods – a cyclical combined HRT to avoid random spotting.
	If periods have stopped – a continuous combined HRT product.
Safety net	If leg swelling/pain, or any sign of stroke, seek immediate help.
	Inform of the importance of BP monitoring and provide breast awareness advice.
Follow-up	3 months, then 6-monthly.
Side effects	Nausea, breast pain, leg cramps. Skin irritation from patches. See the BNF.
Stopping HRT	Can be either immediate or gradual. Tip – patches can be cut down in size gradually.
	Gradually reducing HRT may reduce the risk of recurrence of symptoms.[1]
Vaginal dryness	Oestrogen pessary for vaginal atrophy combined with Replens for dryness.
	You may consider vaginal oestrogen for women who cannot take HRT (contraindication) after seeking advice.[4]
Contraindications to use of topical oestrogens	Active breast cancer and undiagnosed vaginal or uterine bleeding.
	Current or previous thromboembolic event or thrombophilic disorder. Acute liver disease or history of this, if still have abnormal LFTs. Porphyria. See reference for full list.[6] The BNF advises that endometrial safety is unknown if long-term or repeated use, so patients should have 'annual break' to reassess continuing need. Any bleeding or spotting during treatment should be investigated including endometrial biopsy.[6]

 See the **Link Hub** at **CompleteMRCGP.co.uk** for useful PILs in gynaecology

Gynaecology and Breast

Extra Notes

Symptoms	Cyclical or chronic pelvic or ovulation pain. Pelvic or elsewhere.
	Dysmenorrhoea, menorrhagia and deep dyspareunia.
	Pre-menstrual or post-menstrual spotting.
	Cyclical or peri-menstrual bladder or bowel symptoms.
	Infertility in association with 1 or more of the above.
O/E	Likely to be normal. There may be a fixed retroverted uterus or tenderness.
Investigations	USS is likely to be normal. Endometriosis may be identified on MRI but patients are usually offered a laparoscopy for the diagnosis.
GP treatment[1]	NSAID – mefenamic acid or paracetamol – 3 month trial.
	OCP – may back-to-back (off licence).
	Progestogen – Mirena or implant.
	See NICE guidelines for a very useful flowchart about hormonal treatment.
Complications	Infertility.

 See the **Link Hub at CompleteMRCGP.co.uk** for helpful links to organisations for women with endometriosis

Due to difficulty making the diagnosis, consider referring all women with suspected endometriosis to a gynaecologist to confirm the diagnosis (laparoscopy).

In particular, offer referral for women with unconfirmed endometriosis if:[2]

- Symptoms are severe, persistent or recurrent.
- Pelvic signs of endometriosis.
- Initial management is not effective, not tolerated or is contraindicated.

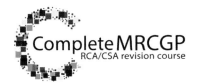
CompleteMRCGP
RCA/CSA revision course

Gynaecology and Breast

Ovarian cyst management

Post-menopausal women

In all post-menopausal women with an ovarian cyst, suggest measurement of serum CA125 in the report	
Simple cysts Simple cyst ≤5 cm	Recommend rescan with CA125 measurements every 4 months for 1 year
	If no change after 1 year (3 scans) consider cessation of scanning if there is no clinical concern
Simple cyst >5 cm	Recommend an urgent 2-week wait referral to gynaecological oncology. MRI assessment should be considered
Complex cysts Any complex cyst	Recommend an urgent 2-week referral to gynaecological oncology, fax report to GP/referring clinician

Pre-menopausal women

Simple cysts Simple cyst ≤5 cm	No follow-up required unless there is clinical concern. A statement to this effect should be included in the report
Simple cyst 5–7 cm	Rescan in 6–8 weeks If resolved or decreased in size, no follow-up required If persisting or increased in size suggest gynaecology referral
Simple cyst >7 cm	Suggest gynaecological referral. MRI assessment should be considered by gynaecologist
Complex cysts	
Any typical dermoid cyst	Suggest gynaecology referral
Haemorrhagic cyst	Rescan in 6–8 weeks to ensure resolution. If not resolved, likely to be endometrioma (follow recommendations for endometriotic cysts)

Endometriotic cysts:
  Symptomatic, any size
  Asymptomatic
  • <5 cm
  • >5 cm
	Suggest gynaecology referral
	
	Rescan in 6 weeks, if it persists, suggest gynaecology referral
	Suggest gynaecology referral

Complex cysts with features suspicious for ovarian malignancy	Recommend an urgent 2WW referral to gynaecological oncology Fax report to GP/referring clinician Recommend measurement of CA125 (Also LDH, α-FP and Beta-hCG if patient <40 years of age) Any woman/girl before the 19th birthday should be managed jointly by paediatric and gynaecological oncology MDT

With thanks to Miss Natalia Price for permission to include this Oxford University Hospitals NHS Foundation Trust guidance. Price N., Traill Z., Goldstein M., et al. Management of ovarian cysts. Joint PCT/Radiology/Gynaecology/Gynae Oncology guidelines. As guidance updates, the link can be found at the **Link Hub at CompleteMRCGP.co.uk**

CHAPTER 10 OVERVIEW

Haematology

	Cases in this chapter	Within the RCGP 2020 curriculum: Haematology	Learning points in this chapter include:
1	Suspected DVT	'Symptoms and signs of haematological disorders…DVT or PE' 'Evolving new agents for anticoagulation treatment and prophylaxis in primary care. Their appropriate use as an alternative to warfarin and the assessment of their potential benefit and risk' 'Anticoagulants: indications, initiation, management and reversal/withdrawal including heparin, warfarin, direct oral anticoagulants such as dabigatran, drug interactions and contra-indications'	Diagnosis and treatment of DVT Wells' score Treating DVT Capacity
2	Myeloma	'Common and important conditions…multiple myeloma' 'Relevant primary care investigations (e.g. X-rays, paraprotein urine testing in myeloma)' 'Disorders of calcium metabolism, e.g. myeloma'[1]	Diagnosis and management of myeloma
3	Splenectomy	'Common and important conditions… splenectomy' 'Health advice for travellers'	Splenectomy – indications, consequences, risks Advice for patients after splenectomy Travel risks after splenectomy
4	Anaemia	'Common and important conditions – anaemia and its causes including iron, folate and vitamin B12 deficiency, sideroblastic, haemolytic, chronic disease' 'Identify symptoms that are within the range of normal or self-limiting illness and differentiate them from underlying pathology, e.g. anaemia'	Differential diagnosis of tiredness in children Management of anaemia in children
5	Henoch–Schönlein Purpura	'Purpura: recognition and causes such as drug-induced, Henoch–Schönlein'	Diagnosis and management of HSP
Extra Notes	Capacity DOACs		Assessing capacity Apixaban for DVT/PE

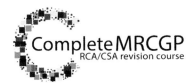

CompleteMRCGP
RCA/CSA revision course

CHAPTER 10 REFERENCES

Suspected DVT

1. NICE guideline NG158. Venous thromboembolic diseases: diagnosis, management and thrombophilia testing. Mar 2020.
2. NICE CKS. Anticoagulation – oral. https://cks.nice.org.uk/topics/anticoagulation-oral/ Jan 2021.
3. NICE CKS. Deep vein thrombosis. (Includes Wells' score.) https://cks.nice.org.uk/topics/deep-vein-thrombosis/management/management/ Nov 2020.

Myeloma

1. https://www.myeloma.org.uk/understanding-myeloma/what-is-myeloma/
2. NICE CKS. Multiple myeloma. https://cks.nice.org.uk/multiple-myeloma. Jan 2021.

Splenectomy

1. https://patient.info/doctor/splenectomy-and-hyposplenism. Aug 2020.
2. https://assets.publishing.service.gov.uk/government/uploads/system/uploads/attachment_data/file/399191/Splenectomy_DL_Leaflet_06_WEB__2_.pdf
3. Immunisation against infectious disease – the Green Book (latest edition); Public Health England. https://www.gov.uk/government/collections/immunisation-against-infectious-disease-the-green-book#the-green-book

Anaemia

1. Haemoglobin concentrations for the diagnosis of anaemia and assessment of severity: WHO/NMH/NHD/MNM/11.1 . World Health Organization 2011. https://www.who.int/vmnis/indicators/haemoglobin.pdf
2. British National Formulary for Children.

Henoch–Schönlein Purpura

1. https://patient.info/doctor/henoch-schonlein-purpura-pro. Jun 2019.

Haematology

1. https://bnf.nice.org.uk/drug/apixaban.html

Information taken from NICE guidelines with kind permission. Please note the guidelines change frequently and you should ALWAYS check for the latest updated guidance. Remember that NICE guidance is only applicable to patients in the UK.

Haematology

Doctor's Notes

Patient	Raymond Styles	86 years	M
PMH	Ankle fracture placed in cast 3 weeks ago.		
	Prostate cancer		
Medications	No current medications		
Allergies	No known drug allergies		
Consultations	No recent consultations		
Investigations	Recent U&E, LFT normal		
Household	No household contacts registered		

Example Consultation

Open ☐	I'm pleased your carer called. Tell me more about this pain and swelling. Is there anything else you have noticed?
ICE ☐	What do you think has caused the pain and swelling in your leg? Is there anything you fear it may be? What do you think we should do?
Flags ☐	Do you feel breathless? Are you coughing up anything? Any blood? Do you have any pain in your chest? Have you had a temperature?
Sense ☐	You don't seem worried.
History ☐	How are you in general? Do you have any other family?
Curious ☐	Tell me more about your experience of hospital.
Impact ☐	Things must have been hard since you lost Maggie. How do you spend your days?
O/E ☐	Your carer kindly sent me a photo, I can see your lower right leg looks swollen and is red all over. Could you squeeze the back of your leg and tell me if it hurts? If you press on your skin does it leave a dimple? How far up your leg does that happen?
Empathy ☐	I hear that you do not want to have the same experience as your wife and will not go to hospital.
Empower ☐	No one will force you. I must explain to you what I think so you can make an informed decision, but you are in charge.
SummarICE ☐	Although you suspect the pain and swelling may be serious, you are clear that you don't want to go into hospital but might be willing to have treatment at home, so long as it is straightforward and doesn't need blood tests.
Impression ☐	I believe you have a blood clot in your leg called a DVT. There is a real risk that this could travel to your lungs and make you very ill – you could even die from this. Your broken leg has made you less mobile and having prostate cancer puts you at increased risk, therefore I think this is most likely.
Recommend ☐	I would like to arrange for you to go to the hospital for a scan of your veins. At the hospital I would expect them to do a scan and a blood test so they could find out exactly what is wrong. If I were to explain to the medical staff your previous experience and tell them you would want to come home as soon as possible, would this be okay?
InCludE ☐	Can I check that we have understood each other correctly? You are aware that I believe you should go to hospital for tests, and not going to hospital may mean ongoing pain in your leg or serious breathing problems and you could die from this. Can you repeat to me what we have just talked about so I can check you understand? Thank you.
Options ☐	If you won't go to hospital, would you take some tablets at home that would thin your blood? They make it less likely that any blood clot goes to your lungs. The downside of this tablet is it can make you more likely to bleed and, rarely, they can cause serious bleeding. Okay good.
Explanation ☐	The tablet is called apixaban. You should take it twice a day and it's important to keep taking it and not stop it – otherwise your blood would soon start to clot again and this could cause serious problems. I will ask the nurse to call tomorrow to take a blood test from you to make sure your kidneys and liver are working well - but you won't need regular blood tests. Do you have any questions?
Future ☐	I suggest taking paracetamol, two tablets regularly for pain relief. Don't take ibuprofen as this interferes with apixaban. I will write to the DVT clinic to explain about your situation and get advice about how long you should take the apixaban but it is likely to be 3 months.
Safety net ☐	If you get short of breath, chest pain, cough up blood or your leg swelling or pain gets worse, please call the surgery, 111 if the surgery is closed or 999 if you have changed your mind about hospital. After starting the apixaban, if you notice any bleeding, please ring for advice straight away.

Patient's Story

Doctor's notes	Raymond Styles, 86 years.
	PMH: left ankle fracture placed in cast 3 weeks ago. Prostate cancer. Medications: none.
How to act	Respectful and apologetic. Dismissive of your symptoms.
	Under no circumstances are you going to hospital for any tests. You will accept tablets to thin your blood but want as little fuss as possible.
PC	*'Doctor, I'm sorry they called you. I'm fine now.'*
History	You have prostate cancer. You were offered but declined hormone treatment for this but are currently not troubled by it.
	Your carer called the doctor because she noticed that your right leg was swollen.
	You feel a little cross about this as you don't like to waste the doctor's time.
	You have no chest pain or breathlessness.
	You first noticed your leg swelling and pain yesterday. No fever. No confusion.
	You have never felt this pain before. *'I must have pulled a muscle.'*
Social	You live alone with four times daily care at present whilst your leg is in cast.
	You have no family.
ICE	You do not know what has caused the pain and swelling. You suspect it may be serious.
	If asked about any negative experiences: your wife, Maggie, died in the hospital and you do not want to have the same happen to you. Refuse to go to hospital whatever the doctor says. You will reluctantly accept tablets if the doctor persuades you but do not want injections or anything that needs frequent blood tests for monitoring, such as warfarin.
Examination if by phone	Clearly swollen lower right leg with generalised redness, left leg in cast. Patient states calf is painful and pitting oedema present to knee level.
Examination if F2F	Sats 95%. RR 18. HR 108 bpm. Chest exam normal. Apyrexial. Left leg in cast. Right leg red and swollen, with tenderness in the calf and pitting oedema to knee. Calf circumference cannot be compared because left leg is in a cast.

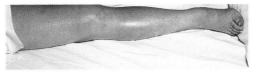

Reproduced from Browse's *Introduction to the Symptoms and Signs of Surgical Disease* (2021), CRC Press. With thanks to Kevin Burnand, Bijan Modarai and Ashish Patel.

Haematology – 1

Learning Points

Suspected DVT[1,2]

This case is testing your ability to clinically assess a patient, to prescribe appropriately but also tests your ability to assess capacity.

Assessing capacity – see Extra Notes, Chapter 16

Two-level DVT Wells' score[3]
NB – if suspect DVT in a woman who is pregnant or has given birth in the last 6 weeks – refer for same-day assessment and management. Otherwise use two-level DVT Wells' score: Score 1 point for:

- Active cancer (treatment ongoing, within the last 6 months, or palliative).
- Paralysis, paresis or recent plaster immobilisation of the legs.
- Bedbound for 3 days or more, or major surgery within the last 12 weeks requiring general or regional anaesthesia.
- Localised tenderness along the distribution of the deep venous system (such as the back of the calf).
- Entire leg is swollen.
- Calf swelling ≥3 cm compared with the asymptomatic leg.
- Pitting oedema present in symptomatic leg only.
- Collateral superficial veins (non-varicose).
- Previously documented DVT.

Subtract *two* points if an alternative cause is considered at least as likely as DVT.

Score ≥2 DVT is *likely*, <2 unlikely.

DVT pathway
For people who are *likely* to have DVT as assessed above:

- Follow local pathways (e.g. assessment on ambulatory medical unit) to arrange an urgent USS of the leg – ideally within 4 hours.
- If this is not possible, arrange D-dimer and start anticoagulation. The scan should be done within 24 hours.

For people who are *unlikely* to have DVT (based on the results of the two-level DVT Wells' score):

- Offer D-dimer test first. If results within 4 hours not possible then offer interim anticoagulation until result is available. In practice this is likely to involve referral to haematology through your local VTE pathway.
- If D-dimer positive arrange USS of leg.
- If D-dimer test is negative stop treatment and consider alternative diagnosis.

If interim therapeutic anticoagulation is required:

- First line: apixaban or rivaroxaban (follow local formulary).
- Second-line options: LMWH for 5 days followed by dabigatran, edoxaban or LMWH + warfarin.
- Consider comorbidities, contraindications and patient choice when selecting the anticoagulant.
- Check FBC, renal function, LFT, PT and APTT. Do not wait for result before treating. Ensure results reviewed within 24 hours.

Haematology – 1

Doctor's Notes

Patient	William Jefferies 65 years M
PMH	Nil
Medications	Paracetamol 1 g QDS
	Naproxen 500 mg TDS
Allergies	None
Consultations	Several consultations for back ache over the last 3 months. Prescribed paracetamol, codeine and NSAIDs. Had private physiotherapy.
	1 month ago – blood sugar, HbA1c and PSA – all normal.
	1 week ago – *'Continues to c/o low back pain. No neurological symptoms or signs. Full examination of back and neurology of legs – normal. Blood tests arranged.'*
Investigations	1 week ago:

FBC	Hb 110 g/L. Normochromic normocytic picture
ESR	90
U&E	Urea 11.3 mmol/LL (2.5–7.8)
	Creatinine 162 mol/L (59.0–104.0)
	Calcium – 2.8 mmol/L (normal range 2.1–2.6 mmol/L)
eGFR	54 mL/min/1.73 m^2

Lab comment 'CKD stage 3'

Total protein 120 g/L (60–80 g/L)

Lab comment – 'Sample sent for electrophoresis. Results to follow. Please send urine for Bence Jones protein'.

Household	Mary Jefferies 65 years F

Example Consultation

Open ☐	Hello Mr Jefferies. Yes, I do have your results. But as we haven't spoken before, it would help me to find out more about you first. Please tell me what symptoms led to the tests?
History ☐	Tell me more about the backache, e.g. where is it and when do you notice it most? Have you had any other symptoms such as tiredness or weight loss? Any constipation? How is your mood?
Impact ☐	You mentioned the backache interferes with gardening. Does it stop you doing anything else that you want to do?
Curious ☐	What does Mary think? What has made her think you are muddled? You mentioned you are retired. What was your work? How do you spend your days in retirement?
Flags ☐	Any weakness or numbness in your legs? An odd question, this, but are you always aware when your bladder is full? Any dribbling of urine? Any numbness around the back passage? That's good to hear, thank you.
Risk ☐	Has any relative had similar symptoms?
ICE ☐	What's gone through your mind? You sound worried – what's your worst fear? Is there anything in your mind you were hoping I might be able to do, as well as giving you the results?
SummarICE ☐	So, for the last 6 months or so you have been having troublesome low back pain, not getting better with either physiotherapy or painkillers and interfering with your ability to look after your garden, play golf and drive your car to see your grandchildren. You are worried it might be from prostate cancer. You had some blood tests last week and are here for the results.
Empathy ☐	This has been a worrying time for you and you can't spend your retirement how you wish.
InCludE ☐	Thankfully, I don't think this is prostate cancer as you had a normal PSA test and the symptoms don't fit. I think it's likely that the muddled thinking that your wife has noticed will improve with treatment and I'm also very hopeful you will be able to get back to gardening very soon.
Explanation ☐	Your blood test results appear to explain many of your symptoms. You are slightly anaemic, which will tend to make you tired. Your kidneys are not working as well as usual. We have also found more protein in your bloodstream than is usual and it is possible that you may have a condition called myeloma. Your calcium is also a little high which would fit with this.
Experience ☐	Have you heard of myeloma or known anyone with this?
Explanation ☐	Myeloma is a condition where some of the cells in your bone marrow, called plasma cells, start to be more active than they should be and produce too much of a particular protein called immunoglobulin. The cells start to crowd out other cells in the bone marrow, so the body can't make its normal red and white cells, making you anaemic. These excess proteins can also block up small tubes in the kidneys so they can't work as well.
Options ☐	I would like to get an urgent urine test done to measure how much protein is passing through the kidneys. This and a further blood test may confirm the diagnosis. If so, I would then suggest you see a blood specialist called a haematologist who will be able to start treatment. We would arrange this within 2 weeks. Do you have any questions at this stage?
Explanation ☐	No, this isn't leukaemia, although it is a type of blood cancer. At the hospital I expect the doctors will examine you and take more blood tests. They may want to take a sample of your bone marrow, look at this under the microscope and do a scan to look at all your bones. This will guide treatment, which may be chemotherapy, steroids or other drugs to bring this under control.
Empower ☐	There are some things you can do. Please stop the naproxen as this may affect your kidneys. Paracetamol and codeine are safe. Drink plenty of fluids so you are well hydrated and to help your kidneys. Exercise will help – perhaps a daily walk and build up the distance slowly.
Future ☐	May I book you an appointment for next week so we can talk through the rest of your results and I will answer any questions you have? We will also need to discuss immunising you against pneumonia and what to do if you get any infection.
Safety net ☐	If you get numbness around the back passage, lose that feeling of your bladder being full, or get weakness of the legs, you must contact a doctor at once, even at night or the weekend.
Specifics ☐	If you begin to feel very thirsty, sick, tired or have increased aches and pains, please telephone reception to speak to me or another doctor the same day as this could be a sign that your calcium levels have become too high.

Haematology – 2

Doctor's notes	William Jefferies, 65 years.
How to act	In discomfort with your back – it hurts when you walk. Worried.
PC	*'I've phoned for my blood test results – does it explain why I've been getting back pain?'*
History	For the last 3 months you have had troublesome back pain. Initially you thought you had done too much in the allotment. You took some paracetamol and ibuprofen, which did not help, and then went to a private physiotherapist. He gave you some exercises and you have been following these but no real improvement. The back pain is getting worse and you can no longer play golf. You are now in pain all the time and it's keeping you awake. You have lost a little weight without trying. You have been more tired than usual, and your muscles seem weak (e.g. when gardening). You have also been constipated and drinking more. The doctor thought you might have diabetes but a fasting blood sugar and HbA1c were completely normal. A week ago, you saw a different doctor who did a full examination of your back and legs (normal) and arranged some more blood tests. You are here for the results.
Social	You are a retired businessman and enjoy gardening as a hobby. You have always been fit and well and played sport including golf. You live with your wife who is also retired and have two grown-up children who live about 100 miles away and four grandchildren. Driving to see the grandchildren is really uncomfortable so you are going less often and miss these visits.

ICE	**Ideas**	Your good friend had back ache which turned out to be secondaries from prostate cancer.
		Your wife has noticed you are muddled at times – but you don't think so. It's just there's a lot on your mind.
		The blood test may have shown something to explain the back pain.
	Concerns	Could this be cancer?
		Is it going to get better?
		What can you do to help me get back to my gardening?
	Expectations	You hope the doctor will have found out what is wrong and you hope it's nothing serious like cancer.
		You have never heard of myeloma and will ask the doctor what it is if this is mentioned. If 'blood cancer' is mentioned, ask *'Is it leukaemia?'* A friend's son had this and died when he was 6.

Blood results	Mild anaemia, normochromic, normocytic.
	ESR raised.
	U&E show CKD stage 3.
	Total protein is raised.

Learning Points

What is it? A blood cancer arising from plasma cells. Represents 2% of all cancers. Mainly aged >65 years although can be much younger.

When to suspect Adults, especially if > 60 years with

- Unexplained back pain, especially thoracic or lower back.
- Fatigue (30%).
- Symptoms of hypercalcaemia (30%), e.g. pain (bone, abdominal), low mood, confusion, muscle weakness, constipation, thirst, polyuria.
- Weight loss (25%).
- Hyperviscosity symptoms, e.g. headache, cognitive impairment, visual disturbance, mucosal bleeding (7%).
- Cord compression symptoms.
- Fever (1%).
- Onset often gradual may be picked up following pathological fracture or recurrent infection.

Examination Normal or hepatomegaly (4%), splenomegaly (1%), lymphadenopathy (1%).

Blood tests FBC – normochromic, normocytic anaemia.

U&E – renal impairment (50%).

Bone profile – hypercalcaemia (15%).

Raised ESR, serum protein or globulin.

Management Blood tests – FBC, serum calcium, PV or ESR, U&E.

Consider X-rays of painful areas to rule out pathological fractures.

Arrange urgent plasma and urine protein electrophoresis (ideally within 48 hours) – be aware negative in 1–2% people with myeloma.

Urgent admission if suspected cord compression, corrected calcium >2.9 or AKI.

Otherwise – haematology 2WW referral.

Secondary care Bone marrow aspiration and trephine biopsy (monoclonal plasma cells).

MRI to detect extent of bone disease. Low-dose CT scan if MRI unsuitable or declined. Plain X-ray of spine, skull, chest, pelvis and upper limbs if MRI and CT unsuitable or declined.

Treatment – chemotherapy, steroids, anaemia treatments, bisphosphonates for pain, immunomodulatory therapy. Stem cell transplant.

Ongoing primary care Treat infections promptly.

Manage pain, e.g. paracetamol +/– codeine (avoid NSAIDs).

Offer flu and pneumococcal vaccination.

Monitor mental health and offer help where needed.

Support and advise family and carers, e.g. advise exercise and adequate hydration.

Discuss role of palliative care, when appropriate.

Advise re DLA, PIP payments.

Doctor's Notes

Patient	William Ashfield	19 years	M
PMH	Splenectomy – 3 months ago		
Medications	None		
Allergies	None		
Consultations	None		
Investigations	None		
Household	Jennifer Ashfield	45 years	F
	Peter Ashfield	44 years	M
	Fiona Ashfield	12 years	F

Example Consultation

Open ☐   Hello William, yes – let's talk about that. I'm sorry to hear you had to have your spleen removed. What led to that?

History ☐   Were you knocked out by the accident? Did you have any other injuries, for example broken bones or cuts? Did you need a blood transfusion?

Impact ☐   And tell me about you. You mentioned a gap year? What were your plans for the year? And when the year is over, what are you hoping to do next?

ICE ☐   Do you have questions in your mind about what happened in Thailand? How are you hoping I can help today? Your mum sounds worried – if she were here now, what would she say?

Curious ☐   Do you know what your spleen does? Have you read up about it? What did the doctors in Thailand tell you about life after splenectomy?

Experience ☐   Have you known anyone who has had their spleen removed? I'm sorry to hear about your gran.

Risk ☐   Where do you plan to travel next?

Flags ☐   In the past, have you ever had any serious infections, such as pneumonia?

Sense ☐   I sense you are keen to move on and get back to life as normal, and that's very understandable.

Empathy ☐   It must have been very frustrating to have to come home and continue to hear about all the adventures your friends are having.

SummarICE ☐   You had your spleen removed in Thailand after an accident and would really like to resume your gap year, travelling to India and around the Far East. You're not sure what it means to have no spleen, but your mum thinks you should take antibiotics.

Impression ☐   You feel almost back to full fitness and would ideally like the all-clear from me.

Explanation ☐   William – it's great that you are feeling better but there are some things we need to talk about. The spleen is important for fighting infection and you are now more at risk of getting infections – including significant ones, such as pneumonia or malaria, and these may affect your health. We need to do everything we can to avoid you getting a serious infection like your gran.

InCludE ☐   Let's think about whether you also need to take antibiotics every day, to prevent infection, as your mother thought. As you are aged over 16 and under 50, and have been healthy in the past, I don't think you need to, but you should definitely have a supply to keep at home in case you get a fever. Are you okay taking penicillin – not allergic to it? Good. I will give you a prescription for an antibiotic called amoxicillin which is effective against many bacteria. If you need to take it to treat an infection, you take it three times a day. We should also make sure you are immunised against common illnesses, including flu and pneumonia. Would you like to have these jabs?

Options ☐   Going to India is now riskier for you. Malaria is common and this infection, often serious and potentially fatal for anyone, could be very risky indeed. If you do go, please take all precautions against mosquito bites: protection in the evening – long sleeves and long trousers, tuck in your socks, use strong DEET repellent and mosquito nets overnight. Malarial mosquitoes are most active between dusk and dawn. Dog bites would also be risky for you because dog saliva contains an unpleasant infection that could overwhelm your immune system.

Empower ☐   You said your plans were flexible: have you thought about travelling to a country that will be just as interesting but safer for you because it's non-malarial? Most countries that are further from the equator are safe – check the WHO map online.

Recommend ☐   You could protect your health by choosing to travel somewhere else and still have an interesting gap year. Whatever you do, you must ensure you have travel health insurance and tell your insurers about the splenectomy.

Future ☐   You should carry a card with you at all times to let doctors know that you have had your spleen removed – you can download this from the NHS website. Getting an alert bracelet, so it's easy for anyone to see in an emergency, is a good idea too.

Specifics ☐   Always remind any doctor, dentist or other health professional that you have no spleen – you might need antibiotics earlier in an illness than normal. Keep a supply of antibiotics at home and carry them with you when you travel. Always check the expiry date as they do have a limited shelf life. Please make an appointment with our nurse for flu and pneumonia jabs.

Safety net ☐   If you develop a fever, sore throat or bad cough, start the antibiotics and see a doctor ASAP.

Patient's Story

Splenectomy

Doctor's notes	William Ashfield, 19 years.
How to act	Confident and cheerful.
PC	*'So I had my spleen removed after an accident in Thailand. I just want the all-clear to fly back and carry on with my gap year.'*
History	You had been abroad for 1 month at the start of your gap year before university and were travelling in Thailand where you went quad biking with friends. The quad bike slipped on a muddy track and you rolled down a bank with the bike on top of you. Thankfully you were rescued and taken to the local hospital but were very ill, and had an operation. You were not really aware of what went on but you had a big scar up and down your abdomen. You don't think you broke anything; no serious cuts and you are not sure if you had a transfusion. You were 'out of it' for a few days. When you were well enough to be discharged, the doctors told you they had removed your spleen and that you should talk to your doctor at home about this. Your travel insurance arranged a flight back to the UK and you have been convalescing for the last month. Your friends are still abroad, now in India, sending you daily WhatsApp messages and photos that make you jealous and you want to go out to join them. Your parents are very much against this, so you have come to the doctor to get the all-clear. You have no firm plans for the year – just to have a good time travelling.
Social	Lives with parents and younger sister. Due to start Edinburgh University next year to read history.
ICE	You have no real idea what your spleen does.
	You regard this as an unfortunate incident that could have happened to anyone and you want to get on with your gap year and your life. You think your parents are being overprotective.
	You want to know if there is anything you need to do or know about your spleen.
	Your maternal grandmother had her spleen removed because of cancer and had to take an antibiotic every day. She died of sepsis 2 years ago. You mother thinks you should be on an antibiotic too and has asked you to raise this. *'My mum thinks I need to be on antibiotics all the time, like gran.'* If asked, gran got very sick with an infection – you think it was her chest.

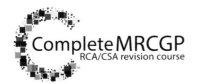

CompleteMRCGP
RCA/CSA revision course

Haematology – 3

Why splenectomy? Planned – e.g. hypersplenism, lymphoma or as part of total gastrectomy.

Traumatic – due to an accident, or trauma during surgery (25% of all splenectomies).

Autosplenectomy – loss of spleen function (hyposplenism) due to:
- Sickle cell anaemia
- Coeliac disease
- Dermatitis herpetiformis
- Essential thrombocythemia (ETP)
- Ulcerative colitis.

Management of patients after splenectomy

Risks Overwhelming infection: major long-term risk, but largely preventable.

Most common are: pneumococcal, Hib, *Neisseria meningitidis*:
- Occurs in 4% patients, if no antibiotic prophylaxis.
- Mortality risk 50%.

E. coli, malaria and babesiosis (tick-borne malaria-like infection, common in USA and parts of Europe).

Increased risk of severe falciparum malaria – use all possible antimalarial precautions and preferably avoid travel to malarial areas.

Immunisations All routine immunisations for children and adults can be safely given.

Live vaccines okay before travel (e.g. yellow fever, live oral typhoid).

Give all vaccines at least 2 weeks before splenectomy, but delay for 3 months if patient has been immunosuppressed, e.g. on steroids, chemotherapy, radiotherapy, methotrexate. See Green Book.[3]

If non-immunised, give at the first opportunity after splenectomy.

Re-immunise every 5 years as levels of antibodies decline.

Under 2's are at risk of vaccine failure – use PC7 where available as better response in this age group.

Prophylactic antibiotics – recommended if patients are at 'high risk'

High-risk patients generally <16 or >50.

Previous poor response to pneumococcal vaccine.

Previous invasive pneumococcal illness.

Underlying malignancy.

Use Pen V 250–500mg BD, or OD for compliance (or amoxicillin, or erythromycin).

Patients should take full therapeutic dose of antibiotic if pyrexia, malaise, shivering.

For all patients Carry a splenectomy card.

Wear an alert bracelet.

Be aware of risks of overseas travel – especially malaria and after animal bites.

Patient records should be alerted. Vaccine and revaccination status clearly documented.

Doctor's Notes

Patient	Connor McGowen	9 years	M
PMH	None		
Medications	None		
Allergies	None		

Consultations Four weeks ago by locum GP – mum noticed looks a little pale and seems lethargic. Connor reporting feeling tired. No other symptoms other than occasional abdominal cramps, usually when has been a little constipated. No red flags. Mum worried about coeliac disease due to family history (paternal cousin and grandfather). Agree bloods then review.

Investigations FBC: Hb 97 g/L

MCV 78 fl

WCC 7×10^9/L

Platelets 269×10^9/L

12, folate – normal. Ferritin low.

TFT normal

Coeliac screen normal

Household	Shona McGowen	42 years	F
	Patrick McGowen	43 years	M

Telephone consultation with mum – requests blood results.

Open ☐   How can I help? Yes, we do have the results. Could you tell me what led up to the blood tests being taken?

ICE ☐   Was there anything particular you thought might be going on? Have you been worrying about the results? How about Connor, is he concerned about anything? Other than going through the results, was there anything else you were hoping for today?

History ☐   You mentioned Connor had seemed tired and pale before. How is he now?

Impact ☐   How is the tiredness affecting him? Has it interfered with his hobbies or school work? Has it affected you as a family in any way?

Flags☐   Have any new symptoms developed since you saw my colleague? Any diarrhoea? Any blood loss from anywhere such as nosebleeds or blood from his bottom? Any weight loss? Or fever? Any bruising? Or lumps/bumps?

Risk ☐   What does Connor like to eat? Does he eat meat? What about green leafy vegetables? Do you find it a struggle to give him a balanced diet? Does this worry you? Is there any family history of anaemia or blood problems?

SummarICE ☐   So Connor has been more lethargic, just wanting to lie on the sofa after school and has appeared a little pale for the last couple of months. He hasn't had any bowel trouble, weight loss, fevers or any blood loss from anywhere. You try to encourage him to eat a balanced diet but he prefers chips and pizza to meat and vegetables and, as this is often quicker, you give in. You wondered about coeliac disease as two people on your husband's side have this. Shall we talk through the results?

Impression ☐   Most of Connor's bloods were reassuring and in particular his test for coeliac disease was negative. We did pick up one abnormality though. His blood count was a little low, something called anaemia.

Experience ☐   Have you heard of this? You're right it is common in pregnancy and yes Connor's anaemia appears to be due to low iron.

Explanation ☐   When we are short of iron, our red blood cells can't carry as much oxygen around and this can make us feel tired. The red blood cells have less of something called haemoglobin which carries the oxygen but this also makes the blood red so this is why some people with anaemia look pale. There are lots of reasons why someone can be short of iron. In Connor's case it is likely that he is not getting enough in his diet.

Empower ☐   There are things Connor can do to help. Eating foods rich in iron can boost his levels and give him more energy. Red meat, fish and green leafy vegetables all contain iron. Some cereals have iron added to them too. Increasing these foods will help Connor feel better and help reduce the chance of him becoming anaemic again. Do you think you could adjust the meals you make to increase iron rich foods?

Options ☐   You could try increasing dietary iron alone…

Recommend ☐   …but my suggestion would be to give Connor a course of iron to give his stores a boost and get him feeling better quicker. How does that sound? Is Connor able to swallow tablets?

Specifics ☐   I would suggest a 3-month course of iron called ferrous sulfate. He would need to take 1 × 200 mg tablet twice a day. These tablets can cause nausea and bowel upset – either constipation or diarrhoea, and do tend to turn poo black. However, most people tolerate them pretty well. Having vitamin C with the tablet, for example drinking a cup of orange juice, helps the iron absorb and can reduce any side effects. What are your thoughts?

Future ☐   Great, we will need to repeat his blood test in 4 weeks to check he is responding and will check the test again at the end of the 3-month course.

Safety Net ☐   If Connor has side effects from the tablets or develops new symptoms, particularly bleeding, bruising, weight loss, fever, sweats or bowel problems, please call me straight away.

Patient's Story

Doctor's notes Connor McGowen, 9 years. Telephone consultation with mum, Shona McGowen.

Previous consultation 4 weeks ago by locum GP – mum noticed looks a little pale and seems lethargic. Connor reporting feeling tired. No other symptoms other than occasional abdominal cramps, usually when has been a little constipated. No red flags. Mum worried about coeliac disease due to family history, (paternal cousin and grandfather) agree bloods then review.

Bloods show mild iron-deficiency anaemia. Normal coeliac screen, TFTs, B12 and folate.

How to act Relaxed.

PC *'Hi. I was hoping to discuss Connor's recent blood test results.'*

History Connor has been more lethargic and tired for the last couple of months. He has been lying on the sofa after school and doesn't feel like going out to play football. You think he looks pale but is otherwise okay. He does get occasional abdominal pain but this usually coincides with when he becomes a little constipated. He doesn't eat a lot of fruit and vegetables. He prefers to eat chips and pizza if he has a choice. He has not suffered any weight loss, sweats, fevers, bruising, diarrhoea or significant abdominal pain. No blood loss from anywhere. You were anaemic during pregnancy but no other family history of blood problems.

Social Connor generally enjoys school and plays for a football team. He has had less energy and has been less enthusiastic about going to football training. Connor's dad is a builder and works long hours. You work in a supermarket, long hours too, so it is often tempting to make quick meals like pizza rather than cooking lots of meat and vegetable meals. You feel you should make more of an effort with the family's diet. You could pick up some healthier ingredients at work. Perhaps you could encourage Connor to cook with you.

ICE You aren't sure why Connor has been so tired but wonder about coeliac disease as his paternal grandfather and cousin have this. You just wish to discuss the results though aren't impatient regarding this and are happy to discuss the background with the doctor.

You have heard of anaemia – you had this whilst you were pregnant with Connor and took iron tablets for a month or two. You are happy for Connor to try tablets. You didn't have any problems with them when you took them and you'd like him to be back to normal as soon as possible.

Learning Points

Haemoglobin concentration cut offs can vary between areas and laboratories but WHO suggest the following as cut offs for anaemia in children:[1]

- 6 months – 5 years: <110 g/L
- 5–12 years: <115 g/L
- 12–14 years: <120 g/L

Iron deficiency is most commonly due to inadequate dietary intake. Consider coeliac disease.

B12 and folate deficiency tend to cause megaloblastic anaemia. Again, usually dietary; rarely pernicious anaemia can occur.

Consider inherited anaemias, particularly in certain ethnic groups, e.g. sickle cell, thalassaemia.

Other genetic causes, e.g. sideroblastic anaemia, hereditary spherocytosis, G6PD.

Where there are other abnormalities on the FBC consider conditions affecting the bone marrow such as leukaemia, secondary cancers or fibrosis.

Acquired haemolytic anaemias can be caused by infections, e.g. malaria, hypersplenism, toxins and auto-immune conditions.

Treatment

Depends on cause.

For deficiencies consult BNF for children as doses vary with age and also whether medication is for prophylaxis or treatment. Both tablets and liquid forms available. Sytron (sodium feredetate) is a commonly used oral solution for children unable to swallow tablets.

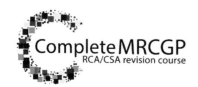

Doctor's Notes

Patient	Holly Forsyth	5 years	F
PMH	None		
Medications	None		
Allergies	None		
Consultations	None		
Investigations	None		
Household	Anne Forsyth	35 years	F
	Paul Forsyth	35 years	M
	Henry Forsyth	7 years	M

Example Consultation   Henoch–Schönlein Purpura

Open ☐   Meningitis – that must have been very worrying. Please tell me what you noticed this morning.

History ☐   How is Holly in herself right now? Please take me back to the beginning. How did this start? Have you noticed anything else, for example a temperature? And her appetite?

Impact ☐   How has she been in herself over the last few days? Has she been able to go to school and play with her friends?

ICE ☐   You were concerned about meningitis – did you have any other worries about what this might be?

Curious ☐   Have you known anyone with meningitis? Yes – I agree it is a worry, meningitis can be very serious.

Risk ☐   Did Holly have a viral infection, for example a bad sore throat, in the last couple of weeks?

Flags ☐   Has Holly had any tummy pains or sickness in the last few days? Any diarrhoea? Any blood in the diarrhoea? Has she had swollen ankles or a puffy face?

O/E ☐   May I examine Holly please? Check her temperature and pulse, feel her tummy and both look at and feel the rash on her legs and arms, examine her knees and test a urine sample. Thank you.

SummarICE ☐   To summarise, Holly had a sore throat 2 weeks ago and got better and has been well since then, going to school and playing as normal, but this morning you noticed this rash, which is on her legs, buttocks and arms. Her temperature and pulse are both normal and her tummy is fine. Both her knees seem a little swollen and her face is a little puffy. Her urine test shows a little protein but is otherwise normal.

Explanation ☐   I think that Holly has had a reaction to a recent infection, possibly the sore throat, and her body's defence system has gone over the top in responding to this, causing inflammation of the blood vessels, which we call vasculitis.

Empathy ☐   This is a lot to take in and not something you were expecting.

InCludE ☐   Thankfully it is much less worrying than meningitis and I am able to tell you what I think it is and get Holly on the right treatment.

Impression ☐   This condition is called Henoch–Schönlein purpura, or HSP. It's named after the two children's doctors who first described it and purpura means purple, so describes the colour of the rash.

Experience ☐   Have you heard of this condition before or known anyone with anything similar? It is fairly rare, affecting about 1 in 10,000 people each year.

Empower ☐   Thankfully most children make a complete recovery. Occasionally, children have a problem with their kidneys for a few weeks or months but this is usually mild and normally gets better on its own. I will print you a leaflet from patient.info that tells you all about HSP.

Options ☐   Holly should stay off school and rest for the next few days, with her feet up, for example on the sofa. This will help the rash on her legs to get better more quickly. Calpol will help if she is feeling achy or has pain anywhere. Use Calpol rather than ibuprofen, as ibuprofen can affect the kidneys in HSP.

Future ☐   I would like to arrange for Holly to see a children's doctor today for a blood test and to confirm that this is HSP. I don't think Holly will need to stay in. Please contact me again after this appointment if you have any questions and so we can discuss what has been said.

Specifics ☐   I will speak to the on-call doctor straight after this consultation and will phone you on your mobile with a time to go up to the children's assessment unit.

Safety net ☐   If, over the next few days, Holly becomes unwell, for example develops a fever, or if her legs or face swell more, or you notice blood in her poo please contact a doctor straight away.

Haematology – 5

Patient's Story   Henoch–Schönlein Purpura

Doctor's notes	Holly Forsyth, 5 years, accompanied by mum. PMH: none. Medication: none.
How to act	Concerned.
PC	*'Holly's been a bit off it for a few days and now she's come out in this rash on her legs. I did the glass test and I'm worried it's meningitis.'*
History	Holly had a sore throat 2 weeks ago which cleared up. A few days ago, she seemed slightly under the weather and then this morning, when you were helping her dress, you noticed the rash. The rash was on the backs of her legs and her buttocks and on her forearms – symmetrical. You checked her temperature, which was normal. In fact, Holly has seemed absolutely fine in herself today, playing happily with her brother, although you wondered if her face was a bit puffy.
Social	You work as a shop assistant at the local Spar, part time. You live with Holly's dad who is a refuse collector. Holly has an older brother, Henry. Both children have always been fit and well and attend the local primary school. Holly was at school yesterday and was fine.
ICE	You thought the rash looked like a bruise so did the glass test and it did not blanch.
	This has made you worried about meningitis. You have seen pictures of children who have lost limbs as a result of this. But Holly is well and you thought children with meningitis were really poorly.
	You hope the doctor will tell you what is wrong and act promptly to give Holly the best care.
	You have brought a urine sample, just in case.
Examination findings	Temperature 37.0 °C. HR 80 bpm regular. Cap refill <2 seconds. Abdomen soft, non-tender NAD. Knee joints slightly swollen. Urine dipstick – Protein +, Blood +. Otherwise NAD.

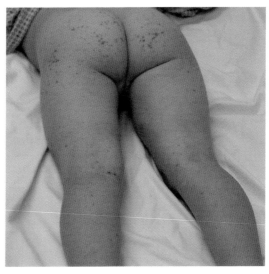

Reproduced from *Pediatric Emergency Medicine*, Second Edition (2019), CRC Press. With thanks to Emily Obringer.

Learning Points

Henoch–Schönlein Purpura[1]

What is it?
A systemic vasculitis mainly affecting children <10, especially ages 4–6 years.

Rare in infants and young children. Caucasians more affected than other ethnic groups.

May occur in adolescence and adults – generally more severe and renal problems more likely.

Affects 10–20 children/100,000 population. (GP practice of 10,000 patients would expect to see 1–2 cases per year.)

Aetiology
Cause unknown – ?mixture of genetic, immune and environmental factors.

Appears seasonal – mainly autumn and winter. May be preceded by infections such as group A streptococci, *Mycoplasma*, EBV, Coxsackie virus, hepatitis A and B, parvovirus B19, *Campylobacter*, varicella and adenoviruses.

May be triggered by vaccination.

May be associated with solid tumours, especially in adult men.

Presentation
Mild illness, low-grade fever.

Symmetrical, erythematous macular rash especially back of legs, buttocks, ulnar side of arms.

Macules become purpuric, spreading and coalescing to look like bruises. Often raised and just palpable.

10–40% patients have abdominal pain and vomiting.

Boys may develop scrotal pain or swelling.

Investigations
Diagnosis may be made on symptoms and typical appearance of rash.

Investigations: U&E, FBC to look for platelet levels + rule out leukaemia, tests for recent streptococcal infection, IgA levels (usually high in HSP).

Urine dipstick to look for protein, blood.

BP (may be raised).

Stool test for blood in stools.

Skin biopsy if diagnosis uncertain.

Renal biopsy may be considered if renal involvement.

Management
Painkillers – paracetamol rather than ibuprofen (because of risks of bleeding from kidneys or gut). Ibuprofen can be used if no renal involvement.

Rest – with legs elevated. Purpura tends to develop in dependent areas.

Steroids – if renal involvement, specialist guidance.

If thought to have been triggered by medication – stop this.

Referral to renal specialist for ?renal biopsy.

Treat BP if raised.

Plasma exchange if very serious complications.

Complications
Renal involvement in 50% – some may develop nephritis. Can happen up to 6 months after rash.

GI bleeding – 30% → passing blood in stools. Rarely, can be severe and life threatening.

Orchitis – in 30% boys affected.

Rare but serious:

    Brain and nervous system – seizures.

    Heart – MI.

    Lungs – bleeding into lungs.

Prognosis
If no renal involvement, full recovery in 4 weeks with no sequelae.

1/10 have serious renal complications, may lead to renal failure.

HSP may recur within 6 months, especially if kidneys were involved.

Haematology – 5

Assessing capacity – see also Extra Notes, Chapter 16

To do this you need to ensure that the patient:

1. Understands the information.
2. Is able to remember the information long enough to make a decision.
3. Is able to weigh up the risks and repeat these to the doctor.
4. Is able to communicate his/her decision.

If a patient has capacity, is aware of risk to life and all the risks of not following advice and you cannot persuade them, you must respect the patient's autonomy. You should ask about involving family members and consider how else you can help the patient, including end-of-life and DNACPR discussions. However, you should not simply wash your hands of the patient because they have ignored your advice. Think about ways you can still help the patient, keep them safe and allow them the opportunity to change their mind.

Patients may refuse to go to hospital for many reasons. Their reason should be explored in detail and the doctor should give an explanation of what they expect will happen in the hospital.

Caring for others or even dogs/cats is a common reason to refuse hospital admission. Know your local emergency care team. There are also organisations that can help with pets, e.g. Dogs Trust.

Apixaban for DVT and PE[1]

DVT and PE: 10 mg BD for 7 days then 5 mg BD.

Prevention of recurrent VTE: 2.5 mg BD (after 6 months treatment).

For people with renal impairment:

- If creatinine clearance is 15 – 29 mL/min:
  - VTE – use apixaban with caution (as above).
  - Non-valvular AF – reduce dose to 2.5 mg twice daily. Same reduced dose if serum creatinine is ≥133 μmol/L and patient ≥80 years or weighs ≤60 kg.
- Do not prescribe apixaban if creatinine clearance (CrCl) <15 mL/minute.

Duration of treatment

Treatment of DVT and PE – assess presence of transient risk factors (for example recent surgery, trauma and immobilisation), but minimum of 3 months. Patients will usually be followed up in a VTE clinic who will advise regarding duration of treatment.

Advice for people taking apixaban

- No need for regular blood tests to monitor, e.g. INR, but still need monitoring, blood tests and review of treatment:
  - Renal function and LFT usually once a year, but more often if the person becomes ill or has renal problems.
  - Review every 3 months – assessment of compliance and adverse effects.
- Reiterate the importance of good compliance:
  - Effect reduces after 12–24 hours. Missed tablets means no cover!
- If surgery needed, may have to stop apixaban treatment temporarily.
- Don't stop treatment abruptly.
- Seek medical advice if spontaneous bleeding that does not stop or recurs.

Haematology

Adverse effects

Seek immediate medical advice if:

- Spontaneous bleeding occurs whilst on apixaban and the bleeding does not stop or recurs.
- Sudden severe back pain (which may indicate spontaneous retroperitoneal bleeding).

Drug interactions which can affect the plasma levels of apixaban: see https://cks.nice.org.uk/topics/anticoagulation-oral/management/apixaban/#drug-interactions

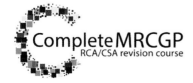

Haematology

CHAPTER 11 OVERVIEW

Infectious Disease and Travel Health

	Cases in this chapter	Within the RCGP 2020 curriculum: Infectious Disease and Travel Health	Learning points in this chapter include:
1	Recurrent UTI	'Renal diseases relevant to children – recurrent urinary tract infections'	NICE Guideline CG54. Urinary tract infection in under 16s: diagnosis and management. October 2018.
2	Lyme Disease	'Skin infections…Lyme disease' 'Tick-borne infections including Lyme disease'	NICE Guideline NG95. Lyme disease. October 2018.
3	Viral Illness	'Features of the acutely unwell child including rashes, irritability, breathing and circulatory signs'	NICE Guideline NG143. Fever in under 5s: assessment and initial management. November 2019.
4	Glandular Fever	'Multisystem infections – Epstein–Barr virus'	
5	Altitude Sickness	'You should be competent in diagnosing and managing common and important conditions related to travel and infectious disease, while at the same time knowing what services are available within your practice and locality' 'Travel-related conditions, e.g. altitude sickness' 'When prescribing, it is essential to follow the law and GMC guidance and to take account of licensing'	Prevention, diagnosis and management of altitude sickness HACE, HAPE Prescribing unlicensed medicines

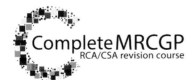
CompleteMRCGP
RCA/CSA revision course

CHAPTER 11 REFERENCES

Recurrent UTI
1. NICE Guideline CG54. Urinary tract infection in under 16s: diagnosis and management. Oct 2018.
2. NICE Guideline NG143. Fever in under 5s: assessment and initial management. Nov 2019.

Lyme Disease
1. https://patient.info/doctor/lyme-disease-pro. Aug 2016.
2. NICE Guideline NG95. Lyme disease. https://www.nice.org.uk/guidance/ng95. Oct 2018.

Useful Resource
https://www.lymediseaseaction.org.uk/about-ticks/tick-removal/

Viral Illness
1. NICE Guideline NG143. Fever in under 5s: assessment and initial management. Nov 2019.

Glandular Fever
1. NICE CKS. https://cks.nice.org.uk/glandular-fever-infectious-mononucleosis. May 2021.

Useful Resource
https://patient.info/ears-nose-throat-mouth/sore-throat-2/glandular-fever-infectious-mononucleosis#nav-5. Jan 2021.

Altitude Sickness
1. https://www.nhs.uk/conditions/altitude-sickness/ Mar 2020.
2. RCGP curriculum – Improving Quality, Safety and Prescribing.
3. GMC. Good Practice in Prescribing and Managing Medicines and Devices. Apr 2021.
4. Moore J.K., Ladbrook M., Goodyer L., Dallimore J. The provision of prescription-only medicines for use on UK-based overseas expeditions. *Wilderness Environ Med* 2017; 28: 219–24.

Information taken from NICE guidelines with kind permission. Please note the guidelines change frequently and you should ALWAYS check for the latest updated guidance. Remember that NICE guidance is only applicable to patients in the UK.

Infectious Disease and Travel Health

Doctor's Notes

Patient	Kalpesh Khan	6 years	M

PMH   Urinary tract infection 6 weeks ago – *E. coli*, fully sensitive

Urinary tract infection 6 months ago – *E. coli*, fully sensitive

Medications   No current medication.

Past medication – two courses of trimethoprim.

Allergies   No information.

Consultations   Last appointment 2 days ago:

Attended with mum. Temperature 37.9 °C, lower abdominal pain, dysuria, frequency and urgency.

Abdominal examination – suprapubic tenderness, abdomen soft, no masses. No loin pains.

Urine dip: protein +, blood +, leucocytes ++, nitrites ++.

MSU sent. Trimethoprim prescription given.

Weight 20 kg

Investigations   MSU result from 2 days ago – *E. coli*, resistant to amoxicillin and trimethoprim, sensitive to nitrofurantoin and cefalosporin.

Household

Asaf Khan	43 years	M
Yasmin Khan	41 years	F
Ayub Khan	7 years	M
Raja Khan	3 years	M
Sabeen Khan	2 years	F

Example Consultation

Open ☐   I'm sorry to hear that Kalpesh is no better. Could you tell me what has been happening over the last couple of days? How is he now? What is he doing at present?

History ☐   I see he has had two other urine infections in the past 6 months. In between his infections was he well? Has he had any other medical problems? Does he have any allergies? Is there any family history of kidney problems?

ICE ☐   What is going through your mind about this? Have you had any thoughts about what you would like to happen next? Is anything particularly worrying you?

Curious ☐   What is your experience of septicaemia? I'm sorry to hear that.

Empathy ☐   Infections must be worrying given your experience with your father.

Flags ☐   What is Kalpesh's temperature at present? Is he drinking well? When did he last pass urine? Do you know if his urine stream is normal? Have you seen any blood? Is he complaining of tummy or back pain? Has he vomited? Is he breathing normally? Is he drowsy or concentrating on the TV?

Risk ☐   Has he been growing and developing well? Were there any problems during your pregnancy? Does he ever struggle to open his bowels? Has he had any tests at the hospital?

InCludE ☐   So you believe Kalpesh has a urine infection but recognise that frequent urine infections in children aren't common. You are worried about septicaemia as this infection hasn't gone away.

Impression ☐   The laboratory sample confirms another urine infection, but unfortunately this one isn't sensitive to trimethoprim, which explains why he hasn't improved. The good news is that the laboratory has told us that another antibiotic should work.

InCludE ☐   From your description of Kalpesh it doesn't sound like he has septicaemia, but I agree this is a rare possibility if the infection isn't treated.

Experience ☐   Has another doctor talked to you about what tests we recommend with recurrent urine infections? Please tell me what you have read.

Explanation ☐   You are correct. Recurrent water infections in children aren't that common, and usually need investigation. However, they do usually respond to antibiotic medicines.

Options ☐   Today I could either see Kalpesh in the surgery, if you feel he needs review, or send you a prescription for nitrofurantoin antibiotic which should kill the bacteria. Which would you prefer? Okay, I will do a prescription for nitrofurantoin. Based on Monday's weight he will need 15 mg 4 times a day.

Future ☐   As Kalpesh has now had three confirmed infections, I would like to refer him to see a specialist, would that be okay? May I order an urgent ultrasound scan to look at his kidneys and bladder, which will be done within 6 weeks? It is likely the specialist will want to do some other tests such as a special test that checks that his bladder empties properly and that urine doesn't flow back up into the tubes towards the kidneys, because this is one cause of recurrent urine infection in children.

Safety net ☐   Keep an eye on how much urine he is passing. If he passes significantly less urine or you feel he is more unwell, don't hesitate to seek advice from a doctor straight away. I will get on with the referral to the specialist; you should receive an appointment letter within the next couple of weeks but please let the practice secretary know if this does not happen.

Specifics ☐   If Kalpesh gets any worse, please give us a ring straight away. I would expect him to improve within 48 hours, so if he is no better please let me know. Should you become worried in the evening, night or weekend you can phone 111 for advice. Are you happy with the plan? Thank you.

Doctor's notes	Kalpesh Khan, 6 years. PMH: two UTIs – *E. coli*, fully sensitive in past 6 months and further UTI confirmed on MSU, resistant to trimethoprim given.
How to act	Concerned.
PC	*'Hi Doctor, thanks for calling. I'm a bit worried about Kalpesh. He isn't responding to the antibiotics this time.'*
History	You attended the surgery 2 days ago when Kalpesh had symptoms of a urinary tract infection. You were given antibiotics by the doctor and told to phone back if he isn't improving. Unfortunately, this time he hasn't improved with trimethoprim. This is his third urinary tract infection in the last 6 months. Kalpesh was born at term following a normal pregnancy. He has been developing normally and is getting on well at school. He is otherwise fit and well (including since his last infection). He opens his bowels daily. Currently Kalpesh is lying on the sofa watching TV but is alert and concentrating. He is still having a low-grade fever intermittently, has lower tummy pain and dysuria. His fever is 37.2 °C at present after paracetamol and you plan to give him some ibuprofen. He is eating and drinking okay and passing urine every 2–3 hours. You have seen no blood and he has not complained of back pain. You have kept him off school for the last couple of days. There is no family history. He has no allergies.
Social	You are a married full-time mum and have three other children. They are all well. Kalpesh's father is a mechanic during the day and works as a taxi driver in the evenings, so works long hours.
ICE	You are worried that the antibiotics aren't working. You don't want Kalpesh to become really unwell. You are aware that infections can be serious – your father died of sepsis.

'I just don't want this to become a septicaemia.'

You have done some research and wonder if Kalpesh needs further tests. He has only had urine samples sent to date.

'I've read about tests he may need.' Reading included an ultrasound scan and a kidney scan but this is all you understand.

You would like to know what happens next. You are happy to accept antibiotics over the phone or an appointment at the surgery to check Kalpesh over. If given the option, and the doctor has clearly explained the problem and future plan, accept antibiotics over the phone. You would like Kalpesh to be referred.

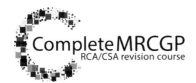
CompleteMRCGP
RCA/CSA revision course

Infectious Disease and Travel Health – 1

Most common signs and symptoms:

- Infants (0–3 months): fever, vomiting, lethargy, irritability.
  - Other: failure to thrive, poor feeding, jaundice, abdominal pain, haematuria and offensive urine.
- 3 months+ (pre-verbal): fever.
  - Other: abdominal pain, loin tenderness, vomiting, poor feeding, lethargy, irritability, haematuria, offensive urine, failure to thrive.
- 3 months+ (verbal): frequency, dysuria, dysfunctional voiding, changes in continence, abdominal pain, loin tenderness, fever, malaise, vomiting, haematuria, offensive urine, cloudy urine.

Management of children with urinary tract infections

Child's age	Testing	Management – refer to full guidance
		Also refer to NICE guideline N143 Fever in under 5s: assessment and initial management. November 2019
<3 months	Send urine for urgent MCS	Immediate admission to paediatrics for investigation and intravenous antibiotics in line with NICE Guideline N143
3 months-3 year	Dipstick testing	−ve nitrites and leucocytes – no antibiotic, no MCS +ve Leucocytes and/or nitrites – start antibiotics and send urine for microscopy
>3 years	'Dipstick testing for leucocyte esterase and nitrite is diagnostically as useful as microscopy and culture, and can safely be used.'[1]	+ve nitrite and leucocytes = treat +ve nitrite, −ve leucocytes = treat and send for culture −ve nitrite, +ve leucocytes = await MCS unless clinically UTI – may indicate infection outside urinary tract −ve nitrite and leucocytes = explore other causes of illness

Send an MSU if: suspected upper UTI (fever >38 °C or loin pain), child <3 years, recurrent UTI, single positive for leucocytes or nitrites, no improvement after 48 hours (if sample not sent already)[1], child with intermediate–high risk serious illness,[2] or 'when clinical symptoms and dipstick do not correlate.'[1]

For antibiotic choice see your local antibiotic guidance and BNF.

Which investigations and should I refer?[1] depends on the type of UTI and the child's age.

Typical UTI (UTI): *E. coli* responding to treatment/48 hours, no other features of AUTI or RUTI.

Atypical UTI (AUTI): seriously ill,[2] poor urine flow, abdominal or bladder mass, raised creatinine, non *E. Coli* species, not responding to treatment within 48 hours or septicaemia. Admission often required.

Recurrent UTI (RUTI): ≥2 UTIs (one must be upper) or ≥3 lower UTIs.

0–6 months: UTI: all require an USS within 6 weeks and if abnormal consider an MCUG.

AUTI: USS during acute infection UNLESS see * below. Also DMSA + MCUG.

RUTI: require urgent (during acute infection) USS,* DSMA + MCUG.

6 months–3 years: UTI: do not require investigation.

AUTI or RUTI: require USS (urgent for AUTI*, <6 weeks for RUTI) + DSMA ± MCUG.

Over 3 years: UTI: do not require investigation.

AUTI: urgent USS only UNLESS*.

RUTI: USS within 6 weeks and DSMA 4–6 months after the infection.

*UNLESS in non-*E. coli* UTI, responding to antibiotics + no other features of AUTI – USS/6 weeks.

Doctor's Notes

Patient	Paul Haydock	21 years	M
PMH	None		
Medications	None		
Allergies	None		
Consultations	None		
Investigations	None		
Household	Nicola Jones	21 years	F
	Tomash Komosa	24 years	M
	Gavin Thompson	22 years	M
	Tareeq Khan	23 years	M

Example Consultation

Lyme Disease

Open ☐	Yes of course. I'm sure we will be able to treat this. How did you first notice it?
ICE ☐	What's gone through your mind about the rash? What made your girlfriend think of ringworm? Did you have any other thoughts? Has anything worried you about this? I'll provide my recommendation but was there anything specific you were hoping for?
Curious ☐	Tell me about yourself – what are you doing in your life? And who do you live with?
History ☐	How has the rash changed since you first noticed it? Has it been itchy, sore or even painful?
Flags ☐	How have you felt in yourself? Any aches and pains or fatigue? Shortness of breath? Eye soreness or blurred vision?
Sense ☐	I sense you haven't been too worried yourself about this, but your girlfriend is concerned she might catch it from you.
Risk ☐	Have you been away from home in the last 3–6 weeks? Tell me about your trip to Scotland – in particular about any activities outdoors such as camping or hiking.
Examination ☐	I've had a look at the photo you sent, thank you. Are you able to check your own pulse and temperature? Thank you, that's really helpful.
Impression ☐	I don't think this is ringworm, although the rash is similar. I think it may be Lyme disease which is an infection that may be caused by tick bites.
Experience ☐	Have you heard of Lyme disease or known anyone who has had this? I'm sorry to hear about your friend's experience, but that isn't common. Most people get a rash like yours, rather than tiredness or other symptoms and the rash soon clears with antibiotics.
Explanation ☐	Lyme disease is caused when you are bitten by a tick that has already been infected with a bacterial bug. The bug is passed on in the tick saliva and infects the skin giving this rash which is called erythema migrans. Erythema means 'red' and migrans means 'spreading', so the name describes what the rash does if untreated.
Recommend ☐	There is no need to do a blood test because the appearance of the rash is so typical. Are there any antibiotics you can't take or are allergic to? Good – I suggest one called doxycycline. Please take one tablet twice a day for 3 weeks. You may get mild tummy symptoms such as loss of appetite, nausea or diarrhoea – these are common, ignore them if you can.
InCLudE ☐	You mentioned a cream, but that won't work for this rash – you need to have a course of antibiotics. I appreciate you were not expecting this? (Pause for response)
Empathy ☐	I agree that 3 weeks is a long time and I completely understand your hesitation about antibiotics but it's important that we completely get rid of the bug that's causing the rash, and this can take time. May I prescribe the antibiotics for you? Any other thoughts?
Empower ☐	If there were 100 people like you starting antibiotics for Lyme disease, about 16 would feel worse at first, for example fever, muscle aches and sweating. This shows that the immune system and the antibiotic are working and, if this happens, you should carry on with the treatment. Thankfully, you can't infect anyone else, so your girlfriend and others can't get the rash from you. Do you have any questions? Avoiding tick bites is the best way to prevent this from recurring. Although you've had the infection, you won't be immune and can catch it again if you get bitten. I would recommend that you wear long trousers when you are walking or working in any places where there may be deer, and always check your skin for ticks at the end of the day. Tuck your socks into your trousers so the ticks can't get in. You can safely remove ticks using fine-pointed tweezers and a steady pull. The UK-based Lyme Disease Action website has a video about how to do this.
Future ☐	Sometimes symptoms linger following treatment. If all clears up and you feel well when you complete the antibiotics, there is no need to see me again, however if you have concerns please let me know.
Safety net ☐	If you start to feel very unwell soon, or get a rash like nettle rash, or notice eye, breathing or nerve problems, please contact a doctor. Also see a doctor if you start to feel tired, weak or unwell in the next few weeks.

274

Patient's Story

Doctor's notes Paul Haydock, male, 21 years. No PMH, drugs or allergies. No recent consultations.

How to act Initially you are unconcerned. You become anxious if Lyme disease/3 weeks of antibiotics are mentioned

PC *'Can I have some cream for this rash on my leg?'* (Demonstrates the rash by showing the picture or state you have sent a photo.)

History Two weeks ago you noticed a red mark on your right leg. Since then, it has grown and seems to be spreading. The middle part has improved but it's growing in a ring. You do not feel unwell and the rash is not itchy or sore. Three weeks ago, you went on a field trip to Scotland when you were camping in an informal campsite. If asked, you did not notice a tick bite, nor remove a tick from your skin. You were wearing long trousers when outside but did not tuck them into your socks.

Social You are a geography student at Leeds University in your final year. You live with four other students in a shared house, including your girlfriend Nicola who is a medical student. *'Nicola thinks it's ringworm.'*

ICE Nicola has told you that she thinks this is ringworm and that you should get some cream to treat it. She is concerned she might catch a fungal infection from you. If the doctor suspects Lyme disease, you become alarmed. A fellow student got this and had to leave the course because they became so ill with fatigue. You ask for investigations and become concerned if the doctor prescribes antibiotics without doing tests. *'Can I have a blood test or something to be sure that's what it is?'* You are shocked at the length of antibiotic course *'3 weeks! That seems a long time. I thought antibiotics were bad for you.'*

O/E Temperature 37.0 °C. HR 68 bpm regular. No other skin rashes.

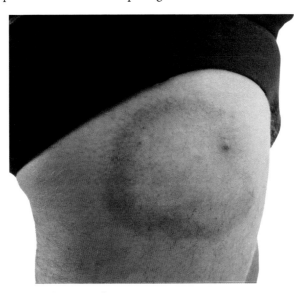

Credit: Shutterstock.

Learning Points

Cause	Body's response to infection with spirochaete *Borrelia burgdorferi*, transmitted from deer ticks.[1]
Pathophysiology	Once bitten by infected tick, there are several possible responses:

- Infection cleared by host defences (no symptoms but seropositive).
- Direct invasion of the skin causing typical rash, erythema migrans.
- Immune response with clinical symptoms, but no rash, e.g. neurological, MSK, etc.[1]

Epidemiology	More common in many areas of S. England, Thetford Forest, Lake District, N Yorks. moors and Scottish Highlands.[1] Grassy and wooded areas including gardens and parks.[2] Most tick bites do not transmit Lyme disease – prompt removal of tick reduces risk.[2]
Incidence	Estimated 3000 cases per year in the UK. All ages and genders. 15% acquired abroad.[1]
Presentation	*Erythema migrans*. Red rash, increase in size, not itchy, hot or painful. Usually appears 1–4 weeks (range 3 days to 3 months) after bite. May also get local reaction – usually develops and recedes within 48 hours of bite, more likely to be hot, itchy and/or painful. This is inflammation/infection with common skin pathogen, not *Borrelia*.[2]

Consider Lyme disease as possible cause of fever and sweats, swollen glands, malaise, fatigue, neck pain or stiffness, migratory joint or muscle aches and pain, cognitive impairment, such as memory problems and difficulty concentrating ('brain fog'), headache, paraesthesia.[2]

Lyme disease is an UNCOMMON cause of: neuro symptoms, e.g. facial palsy or unexplained cranial nerve palsy, mononeuritis multiplex, rarely encephalitis; inflammatory arthritis affecting one or more joints; cardiac problems, e.g. heart block, pericarditis; uveitis or keratitis; or skin rashes such as acrodermatitis chronica atrophicans or lymphocytoma.[2]

History	Ask about activities that might have exposed to ticks and travel to areas of high prevalence.[2] Consider possibility even with no clear history of tick exposure.
Investigations	Diagnose and treat erythema migrans without investigating further:

- If suspicious but no rash, offer ELISA test, treat with antibiotics until results.[2]
- If ELISA positive or equivocal, request immunoblot test and consider antibiotics.

Further details at https://www.nice.org.uk/guidance/ng95/chapter/Recommendations

Information for patients	Lab tests have limitations with false positives and false negatives. If symptoms persist and tests are negative, other diagnoses will be considered. Symptoms such as tiredness, headaches and muscle pain are common and a medical cause may not be found.[2]
Treatment	1. Emergency referral if CNS infection, uveitis, cardiac complications.

    2. Specialist advice if:

- <18, UNLESS single erythema migrans lesion only and no other symptoms.
- Adult with focal symptoms (e.g. to infectious diseases, rheumatology, neurology).

    3. Lyme disease without focal symptoms (i.e. typical rash only) – no investigations needed. Treat with antibiotics promptly:

- First choice: oral doxycycline – 100 mg BD or 200 mg OD for 21 days.
- Alternative: oral amoxicillin 1 g TDS for 21 days.
- Second alternative – oral azithromycin 500 mg daily for 17 days.

See https://cks.nice.org.uk/lyme-disease#!scenario for doses for children

Information for patients about treatment

- Symptoms may worsen in 15% of patients when they start treatment (e.g. fever, chills, muscle aches) – Jarisch–Herxheimer reaction due to cytokine release when antibiotics kill large numbers of bacteria. May last hours or 1–2 days. Unless there is evidence of allergy (e.g. urticaria) should continue the antibiotic.
- Use normal remedies for pain and fever, e.g. paracetamol.

If symptoms persist after treatment, review history and consider other possible causes. Also consider second course of antibiotics. Then discussion with national reference laboratory or specialist advice.

Infectious Disease and Travel Health – 2

Doctor's Notes

Patient	Jayden Hall	13 months	M
PMH	No information		
Medications	No current medications		
Allergies	No information		
Consultations	No recent consultations		
Investigations	No recent investigations		
Household	Donna Hall	29 years	F
	Liam Hall	6 years	M
	Carly Hall	4 years	F

Open ☐	Good morning, can I check who I am speaking to? Please could you confirm Jayden's date of birth and address? Great, how can I help? What is Jayden doing at the moment?
ICE ☐	Have you had any thoughts about what may be wrong with Jayden and what might need to be done? How worried are you about Jayden at this moment?
History ☐	What is he currently doing now? How long has Jayden been poorly? How high has his temperature been? Has it come down with paracetamol or ibuprofen? Has he been coughing? Does he have a runny nose? Any diarrhoea or vomiting? Does he seem in pain or distressed? Has Jayden had any medical problems? Any breathing problems in the past? Any problems in your pregnancy or around birth? And what support do you have with the children? Do you work? Is Jayden in contact with anyone who smokes?
Risk ☐	Has anyone he spends time with been poorly? Is he up to date with his vaccinations?
Flags ☐	Is he eating and drinking okay? Has he been having wet nappies? Have you noticed a rash? Does he seem to be breathing more quickly than usual? Is he moving around normally for him? Is he more drowsy?
Sense ☐	You seem to have a lot on your plate at the moment; is that right?
SummarICE ☐	So Jayden has been unwell for about 24 hours with a fever. You were hoping for a home visit so I could listen to his chest and prescribe some antibiotics.
Impression ☐	From listening to the description of Jayden's symptoms, it sounds as if he has a viral infection, but I agree we should have a look at him, especially his ears, and listen to his chest.
Explanation ☐	Usually when a child has a runny nose, cough and high temperature it is due to a viral infection, particularly if other people in the family have had similar symptoms.
InCludE ☐	In these situations, antibiotics don't help as they won't treat a viral infection and can actually make children more poorly by causing side effects like diarrhoea.
Empathy ☐	Having an unwell child, especially with a fever, is naturally a worry and it is very understandable you would like him checked. If ever you are unsure, calling the GP is the right thing to do. It must be really difficult having three poorly children at once.
Empower ☐	I can also provide you with a useful article called *When Should I Worry* that is helpful to parents. This provides some useful advice about fevers in children, common childhood illnesses, worrying symptoms and using medication at home.
Options ☐	But it would be really helpful if you could bring Jayden down to the surgery so I can examine him here and check that he is okay. We have to reserve home visits for housebound patients so we have time to see more patients, like Jayden, at the surgery. I would be happy to see him at whatever time you are able to get down, this morning or this afternoon.
Examination ☐	I would like to check his temperature, listen to his breathing and heart, have a look at his skin, check his ears and inside his mouth and have a feel of his neck and tummy. How does that sound?
Empower ☐	Could you ask a friend or relative to keep an eye on Liam and Carly while you bring Jayden to the surgery? Or get someone to come with you all to help? Thank you.
Recommend ☐	Meanwhile you can give ibuprofen as well as the paracetamol you have given. The two are safely used together and one option is to give them alternately, for example 3 hours after the paracetamol you give the ibuprofen, to avoid a fever coming on before the next dose is due. Do not give each more frequently than the instructions on the box.
Future ☐	We have a health visitor at the surgery who is a great resource for support, information and advice. They see all families with young children. May I ask the health visitor to contact you?
Safety net ☐	Please give me a call if Jayden gets any worse in the meantime. If the surgery is closed please call 111. If he becomes very unwell, for example, if he becomes floppy, his breathing changes or he develops new symptoms like a rash, you should phone 999. I don't expect this to happen. I will see you at the surgery later today.

Infectious Disease and Travel Health – 3

Doctor's notes	Jayden Hall, 13 months. PMH: no information.
How to act	Harassed.
	Push the doctor for a home visit. Be delighted if they agree to visit.
	If the doctor is insistent that you come to the surgery and suggests options, reluctantly agree to come down. You could call your mum and ask her to babysit.
PC	*'Morning Doctor, I was wondering if you could visit. Jayden has a high temperature and is not well.'*
History	Jayden has had a high temperature on and off for 24 hours. You have an ear thermometer which has shown temperatures up to 38.6 °C. You have given Jayden paracetamol which has brought his temperature down but it is creeping back up again and paracetamol isn't due for 2 hours. Jayden was coughing all night and kept you awake. You are tired and stressed this morning as Jayden's two older siblings (Liam 6 years and Carly 4 years) are off school with colds, which they have had for a few days. Thankfully they seem to be on the mend. Jayden has a runny nose and is pulling at his ears. His appetite has reduced but he is still drinking well. He has had plenty of wet nappies. He has not been sick and doesn't have diarrhoea. Jayden is currently playing with his sister in the lounge. You would like a home visit as you feel Jayden needs looking at, but you feel it will be too much to bring all three children down to the surgery. You live within walking distance of the surgery. Jayden is up to date with his vaccinations and there were no concerns during the pregnancy or neonatal period. He is growing and developing normally.
Social	You are a single mum. You have a part-time cleaning job. This is fairly flexible and you work when your mother can babysit Jayden whilst the others are at school. Your mother lives nearby and you have some supportive friends. Jayden's dad sees him at the weekends.
ICE	You feel Jayden probably needs antibiotics for a chest infection but aren't overly concerned about him. You expect the doctor to visit to examine his chest and give you a prescription for antibiotics.

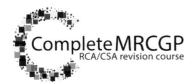

CompleteMRCGP
RCA/CSA revision course

Infectious Disease and Travel Health – 3

Management of children with urinary tract infections

This traffic light table should be used in conjunction with the recommendations in the NICE guideline on fever in under 5s.[1]

	Green – low risk	Amber – intermediate risk	Red – high risk
Colour (of skin, lips or tongue)	• Normal colour	• Pallor reported by parent/carer	• Pale/mottled/ashen/blue
Activity	• Responds normally to social cues • Content/smiles • Stays awake or awakens quickly • Strong normal cry/not crying	• Not responding normally to social cues • No smile • Wakes only with prolonged stimulation • Decreased activity	• No response to social cues • Appears ill to a healthcare professional • Does not wake or if roused does not stay awake • Weak, high-pitched or continuous cry
Respiratory		• Nasal flaring • Tachypnoea: RR >50 breaths/minute, age 6–12 months RR >40 breaths/minute, age >12 months • Oxygen saturation ≤95% in air • Crackles in the chest	• Grunting • Tachypnoea: RR >60 breaths/minute • Moderate or severe chest indrawing
Circulation and hydration	• Normal skin and eyes • Moist mucous membranes	• Tachycardia: >160 beats/minute, age <12 months >150 beats/minute, age 12–24 months >140 beats/minute, age 2–5 years • CRT ≥3 seconds • Dry mucous membranes • Poor feeding in infants • Reduced urine output	• Reduced skin turgor
Other	• None of the amber or red symptoms or signs	• Age 3–6 months, temperature ≥39°C • Fever for ≥5 days • Rigors • Swelling of a limb or joint • Non-weight-bearing limb/not using an extremity	• Age <3 months, temperature ≥38°C* • Non-blanching rash • Bulging fontanelle • Neck stiffness • Status epilepticus • Focal neurological signs • Focal seizures

CRT, capillary refill time; RR, respiratory rate.

*Some vaccinations have been found to induce fever in children aged under 3 months.

© NICE 2019. All rights reserved. Subject to Notice of rights. Table reproduced with kind permission from NICE.

Please remember that guidelines are constantly updated. Always refer to the latest guidance and remember that information from NICE is only applicable to patients in the UK.

Doctor's Notes

Patient	Daisy Atherton	18 years	F
PMH	None		
Medications	None		
Allergies	None		
Consultations	1 week ago 'Sore throat and tiredness for 2 weeks. O/E temperature 38.0 °C. Sats normal. RR normal. Throat – purulent tonsils. Some cervical glands. FeverPAIN 3: probable viral tonsillitis. Throat swab taken. Bloods for EBV. Use NSAIDs and paracetamol. See if not settling, treat with antibiotics if throat swab positive'.		
Investigations	Throat swab – no growth.		
	EBV – positive. Blood film done – many atypical lymphocytes. Confirms diagnosis of GF.		
Household	Henry Atherton	46 years	M
	Mary Atherton	44 years	F
	Jack Atherton	16 years	M

Daisy has given her written consent for you to discuss her health with her mother.

Example Consultation

Open ☐	Hello Mrs Atherton. I'm sorry to hear about Daisy. How is she now? I'm sorry to hear she's still tired and unwell.
ICE ☐	Please tell me what concerned you about the consultation with the practice nurse?
Empathy ☐	I'm sorry you felt disappointed and let down. Let's see if I can help address this and your concerns about Daisy's illness.
History ☐	Please could you tell me about the illness from the beginning.
Impact ☐	Tell me about Daisy – I gather she's at school. How is this affecting her studies? And what else does she do as well as her schoolwork, for example sports or hobbies? What about socially? And family life?
Risk ☐	Was Daisy in close physical contact with anyone who has, or has recently had, GF? For example, a boyfriend or girlfriend?
Flags ☐	And has she had any tummy pain?
Empathy ☐	She sounds very sporty. It must be very difficult for you seeing her so tired – and a worry.
Sense ☐	I sense you are very concerned about her.
Experience ☐	Have you known anyone else with GF?
Curious ☐	Tell me more about your friend's experience of GF.
ICE ☐	And what else, if anything, do you know about GF? You mentioned the nurse said it was a virus – what did this make you think? Now you know it's GF, what worries do you have? And as well as discussing Daisy's health, is there anything else you were hoping I might be able to do today?
SummarICE ☐	You are concerned that Daisy has GF which you think could have been diagnosed and treated earlier, and that the illness will affect her schoolwork, risk her not getting the grades she needs and her place at University.
Impression ☐	Mrs Atherton, you are right that the blood tests confirm GF. The test for the EBV, which causes GF, is positive – the virus is present.
Explanation ☐	A second blood test we did shows that some of her white blood cells have reacted to the virus – this means that they are actively working to fight the infection and kill the virus. So, the nurse was in fact right when she said that this was a viral illness – but it is a specific viral illness rather than a more general one that we can't name.
InCludE ☐	Our nurses are well trained to consult with patients with illnesses such as GF and if you had seen a GP, I'm sure the outcome of the consultation would have been no different. As with other viruses, there is no specific treatment.
Options ☐	There is probably no need to do any further tests, although if Daisy's skin tone becomes yellow, like jaundice, please arrange an appointment so we can examine her and arrange a blood test to check how her liver is doing because GF can cause a transient inflammation of the liver.
Specifics ☐	Taking paracetamol and ibuprofen will help Daisy's symptoms and her energy levels should start to improve gradually. There is no need for her to stay off school, but she should pace herself, resting when she is tired. There are no special precautions for home – her brother is not at risk. She should, however, avoid saliva contact or kissing as this could spread the virus to others. She should also avoid contact sports such as rugby for at least 4 weeks, if possible 8 weeks, from the start of the illness – this is because an organ in her tummy called the spleen may be enlarged and could be vulnerable in a tackle. She should be fine to be a bridesmaid but should avoid alcohol as this may affect her more than usual.
Future ☐	Daisy should be back to normal within a few weeks, but if you and the school feel that her exam performance is affected because of tiredness or because she can't revise properly, let me know and I would be happy to write a letter of support.
Safety net ☐	If Daisy's tiredness is not gradually improving over the next couple of weeks, please come back. It's not likely, but if she gets a bad tummy pain at any time, please contact a doctor straight away.

Infectious Disease and Travel Health – 4

Patient's Story

Doctor's notes Daisy Atherton, 18 years. Consultation with the nurse practitioner 1 week ago. 'Sore throat and tiredness for 2 weeks. Temperature 38.0 °C. Sats normal. RR normal. Throat – purulent tonsils. Some cervical glands. FeverPAIN 3: probable viral tonsillitis. Throat swab taken. Bloods for EBV and film. Use NSAIDs and paracetamol. See if not settling, treat with antibiotics if throat swab positive'.

Results Throat swab – no growth.

Monospot – positive. Blood film – many atypical lymphocytes. Confirms diagnosis of GF.

How to act You are Mary Atherton, the mother of Daisy Atherton. You are annoyed at not getting a GP appointment for Daisy last week and feel you have been fobbed off by the nurse. If the doctor today listens to you and appears to accept your concerns, you become more reasonable.

PC *'I brought Daisy to see the nurse practitioner last week and she told us she "just had a virus" I've had a phone call today to tell me it's glandular fever!'*

History Daisy had been feeling tired with a sore throat for the last 2 weeks. You wanted an appointment with the doctor but could not get one and had to see the nurse practitioner. She examined Daisy and took a blood test and throat swab and told you both it was probably just a virus. She suggested paracetamol, ibuprofen and fluids. You were not confident in her diagnosis. Now you have been told Daisy has GF.

Social Daisy and her brother attend the local comprehensive school. Daisy has her A-levels in a few weeks and her older brother has his GCSEs soon. Daisy is a keen member of the local girls' rugby team and plans to study sport and exercise medicine at University – she needs good grades to achieve her place.

You are an accountant and your husband is a lawyer.

It's your niece's wedding in 2 weeks' time and Daisy is looking forward to being a bridesmaid.

ICE Why couldn't I see a doctor?

We were told it was just a virus, but it's not, it's GF (false health belief).

Your friend's daughter had GF at a similar age and this was a lengthy and protracted illness that made her ill for months.

Will her A-level grades suffer – she's been too tired to revise.

Will her brother catch it?

Can she still do sport?

What about the wedding? Can she still be a bridesmaid?

What precautions should we take at home?

How long will this last?

If the doctor mentions 'atypical lymphocytes/white cells' you become concerned that it might be leukaemia. A friend's son had this and was very ill, although in remission at the moment.

When to suspect

- Fever.
- Lymphadenopathy – almost all, especially posterior cervical. Nodes mildly tender and mobile.
- Sore throat:
  - Usually severe.
  - Tonsillar enlargement – may meet in mid-line.
  - 'White wash' exudate.
  - Palatal petechiae – 1–2 mm diameter, crops last 3–4 days.
- Or sore throat that fails to improve or becomes worse. Can be difficult to distinguish from other types of sore throat especially streptococcal.
- Other features – prodromal malaise, splenomegaly, hepatomegaly, non-specific rash, jaundice.
- Most common 15–24 years.
- People >40 – rare. Atypical presentation, e.g. fever >2 weeks, jaundice (20%) but often no sore throat or lymphadenopathy.
- Children <3 – usually no symptoms, or symptoms of normal childhood viral illness.

Investigations

1. Children >12 and immunocompetent adults – FBC, white cell differential, monospot (week 2):
   - Likely to be GF if relative lymphocytosis or >20% reactive or atypical lymphocytes.
   - If monospot negative, repeat in 5–7 days if clinically indicated.
   - If rapid diagnosis needed, send blood for EBV serology.
2. Children <12 and immunocompromised of any age:
   - Serology for EBV if ill >7 days.
   - If two monospot negative and immunocompromised or pregnant, consider testing for CMV, toxoplasmosis and HIV – if at risk.
3. LFTs – AST and ALT may be 2–3 × normal.

Differential diagnosis

- Sore throat – streptococcal BUT less fatigue, no hepatosplenomegaly, anterior and submandibular lymphadenopathy.
- Other causes of lymphadenopathy:
  - Painful – local infection or inflammation.
  - Painless progressive – metastatic solid tumour or lymphoma.
  - Leukaemia – but rarely presents with lymphadenopathy.
- GF-like illness with atypical lymphocytes:
  - CMV – splenomegaly, hepatomegaly, negative monospot. Sore throat and lymph node enlargement rare.
  - Toxoplasmosis – hepatosplenomegaly but mild lymphocytosis.
  - Also consider: acute viral hepatitis, primary HIV, rubella, roseola, mumps, HSV-1.

Management (for most patients, but see NICE guidelines[1] for indications for hospital admission)

- Paracetamol, ibuprofen to reduce fever and pain. No evidence for steroids.
- Explain symptoms will last 2–4 weeks. Tiredness common – last symptom to go.
- School/work exclusion unnecessary but avoid kissing or saliva contact.
- Return to normal activities but tailor these to tiredness.
- Avoid contact/collision sports or heavy lifting for first month.

Doctor's Notes

Patient	Warren Edwards	56 years	M
PMH	None		
Medications	None		
Allergies	None		
Consultations	6 months ago – Well Man check with PN. Height 175 cm. Weight 110 kg. BMI 35.9. BP 152/83.		
	DNA blood test appointment and no consultation since then.		
Investigations	None		
Household	None		

Open ☐	A trek – that sounds exciting. Where are you going and when? And what's made you ask for Diamox? Are you able to tell me how high the trek goes? 5500 metres – that's really high.
History ☐	You are right to seek advice early – have you seen our practice nurse to see if you need any immunisations and for other health issues?
ICE ☐	Apart from altitude sickness, do you have any other concerns? You asked for a prescription for Diamox – is there anything else you were hoping for from me today?
Social ☐	Tell me about you. Which hobbies and what exercise do you enjoy? What do you do at work and who is at home? I'm sorry to hear about your marriage.
Flags ☐	What physical preparation have you done to get fit?
Sense ☐	You seem a little hesitant about your ability to do the trek – how are you feeling about the trek now?
Curious ☐	I'm curious about why you decided to go on this trek when you don't generally exercise.
Empathy ☐	I'm sorry to hear about your dad – it sounds like the hospice took good care of him, but you miss him a lot.
Experience ☐	Have you experienced altitude sickness in the past? That must have been very unpleasant – although it doesn't always follow that having had it once you will get it again.
Examination ☐	How has your weight been over the last 6 months? Do you happen to have a BP machine?
Impression ☐	My impression is that you are a bit less keen on the trek now than when you signed up and that you are more conscious about your health.
SummarICE ☐	To summarise, you came to ask for Diamox to take when trekking to Everest base camp. I have to tell you that this medication is not licensed for GPs in the UK to prescribe for altitude sickness and so unfortunately, I can't. You may, however, be able to get it at a local travel health clinic. There are some aspects of your health that concern me more than the risk of altitude sickness, particularly if you plan to go ahead with the trek. Your weight today is higher than it was 6 months ago, so your BMI is now >35. This is much higher than it should be and puts you at risk of diabetes, heart disease and other illnesses. Your BP was also raised at your last visit, so it may be that your BP is running a little high. These factors would put you at risk of developing problems on a trek and healthcare is not easy to come by in remote areas of Nepal, so this would be a risk.
Explanation ☐	Altitude sickness can affect anyone when they go above 2500 metres, particularly if the ascent is rapid. Having time to acclimatise as you gain height is important and you should check if your trek builds in rest days and days when you adjust to the height by climbing higher then sleeping at lower altitudes. Symptoms of altitude sickness include tiredness, headache, breathlessness and confusion. If you start to get symptoms, you must tell someone. The only real cure is to descend. Some people think that Diamox is useful, but others think that it masks the symptoms and may make things worse. As well as altitude, you also need to think about immunisations such as tetanus, diphtheria, polio, typhoid and Hep A. Dengue fever is also a problem at lower altitudes – this is transmitted by mosquitoes and there is no immunisation or cure. Ensure that your arms and legs are well covered between dusk and dawn and use a mosquito repellent containing DEET.
Options ☐	My suggestion would be that we arrange some blood tests to assess your general health and get your BP re-checked, how does that sound? Our nurse also runs a travel clinic and would be able to advise about immunisations for Nepal and other travel advice.
Empathy ☐	This has come as a surprise – you were hoping for a prescription rather than advice about your general health.
Empower ☐	You have many months before the trek – it's a really good chance to lose some weight and get fit – that way you would improve your general health as well as being able to raise money and help the hospice.
InCLudE ☐	How do you think you could improve your fitness? Regular walking and jogging sounds good and cycling to work would be excellent exercise and better for the planet.
Future ☐	If your BP continues to be raised, or there is a problem with any of the blood tests, we might need to see you soon to talk about blood pressure monitoring at home and consider medication.
Specifics ☐	Otherwise, shall we see you in 3 months to see how you are doing with your general fitness and weight?

Doctor's notes	Warren Edwards, 56 years. PMH: drugs, allergies. Household: none.
	6 months ago – Well Man check with PN. Height 175 cm. Weight 110 kg. BMI 35.9. BP 152/83.
	DNA blood test appointment and no consultation since then.
How to act	Initially you are confident and self-assured. If the doctor steers the consultation towards your general health, you keep coming back to the request for Diamox. You will come to see the practice nurse and will come to the travel clinic, if offered, but you do want to get an answer today about Diamox.
PC	*'I'm going on a trek next year. Will I be able to have some Diamox for altitude sickness?'*
History	You have signed up for a 2-week charity trek next year, going to Everest base camp to raise money for the local hospice, St Anne's. Your father died there last year. You miss him a lot and would like to do something to support the hospice. You have just received the preliminary trip notes from the organisers and it mentions the risk of altitude sickness and says to ask your GP if you will be able to have a prescription for this. When you were a student, you went to Peru on a trek and got sick with the altitude and had to be brought down by porters, which was embarrassing. You don't want this to happen again.
Social	You are divorced and live alone. You work in an office and are going on the trek with some friends at work, who are all younger than you and are keen runners and cyclists. At the time you were persuaded to join in, you thought it would be good fun and an amazing adventure – as well as raising money. You will fly to Kathmandu in Nepal first, then fly to the mountains. The trek goes as high as 5550 metres and the trip notes say that 7 nights are spent sleeping above 2500 metres (where altitude sickness may occur).
	At the Well Man check 6 months ago, you were told that you were obese and that you should lose some weight. You have not managed to do so. You put off coming back for blood tests and did not have your BP re-checked as suggested by the nurse.
	Since the divorce, you rely on takeaways and ready meals from the supermarket. You enjoy the TV in the evening and do not currently do any exercise at all. '*I don't have time for gyms and all that.*' You do not smoke and drink around 14 units per week.
ICE	Deep down you are anxious about the trek, as you are the oldest person in the group and the least fit by a long way, but you don't want to pull out now and lose face.
	You think you might be able to start regular walking and jogging and perhaps cycle to work.
Examination	Weight 112 kg. BP 160/110. BMI 36.5. If done remotely, able to tell the GP you are now 112 kg but you don't have your own BP machine.

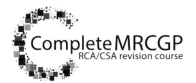

CompleteMRCGP
RCA/CSA revision course

Altitude sickness (also called acute mountain sickness – AMS)[1]

Symptoms	Headache, dizziness, tiredness, SOB, loss of appetite – usually worse at night. Judgement may be affected.
When?	6–24 hours after reaching heights >2500 m.
Who?	Anyone – regardless of age, gender, fitness.
	Previous history of altitude sickness is not a predictor of getting it again.
Prevention	Ascend slowly above 2500 m (300–500 m per day only). Have rest days.
	Eat light diet, high calories, plenty of fluids, avoid alcohol and smoking.
Plan ahead	Consider travelling with acetazolamide (unlicensed), paracetamol/ibuprofen for headaches, promcthazine for nausea.
Treatment	Stop and rest. Do not ascend for 24–48 hours. Treat symptoms with analgesia/ antisickness. If no better after 24 hours, descend – at least 500 m.
Complications	HACE (high altitude cerebral oedema). Above symptoms + confusion, disorientation, hallucinations. Lack of insight into being ill. Fatal if not treated. Rx descend, dexamethasone, bottled O_2.
	HAPE (high altitude pulmonary oedema). Cough, dyspnoea, chest tightness. Fatal if not treated. Rx descend, nifedipine, bottled O_2.

Prescribing unlicensed medicines

'When prescribing, it is essential to follow the law and GMC guidance and to take account of licensing and local prescribing guidance as well as other relevant regulations.'[2]

Unlicensed medicine = medicines that are used outside the terms of their UK licence or which have no licence for use in the UK.[3]

When can you prescribe unlicensed medicines?[3]

- No suitable licensed medicine available in the UK (e.g. child patient where only licensed medication is for an adult, or the licensed medicine would not meet the needs of a particular child but a medicine licensed for an adult would do so).
- The dosage specified for a licensed medicine would not meet the patient's needs.
- Patient needs a formulation not specified in the licence.
- Lack of availability of a suitably licensed medicine, e.g. temporary shortage.
- As part of a properly licensed research project.
- Due to a serious risk to public health, MHRA has temporarily authorised the sale/supply of a treatment or vaccine.

You must:[3]

- Be satisfied that there is enough evidence or experience to be sure it works and is safe.
- Take personal responsibility for prescribing, monitoring and follow-up OR ensure other suitable arrangements.
- Make clear, accurate, legible records of what you have prescribed and why.
- Explain to patients that you propose to prescribe off licence in a way that they can understand and so that they can make an informed choice.

Expedition medicines[4]

Some GPs may agree to prescribe medicines within their area of expertise, e.g. antibiotics and pain relief, to patients going on expeditions. If you do decide to do this it should be clearly documented on the prescriptions what the indications are and any follow-up/blood tests which would be required. The medicines should be prescribed as a private prescription. Be careful not to prescribe medications you are unfamiliar with, advise patients to see a travel/expedition clinic instead or take advice from an expert before prescribing.

Infectious Disease and Travel Health – 5

Kidney and Urology

	Cases in this chapter	Within the RCGP 2020 curriculum: Kidney and Urology	Learning points in this chapter include:
1	Acute Kidney Injury	'Identify and manage AKI, including taking early action, such as stopping medications, to reduce the risk of AKI' '.. a significant proportion of AKI starts in the community so GPs have a key role in its early identification and management'	NICE Guideline NG148. Acute kidney injury: prevention, detection and management. December 2019
2	Chronic Kidney Disease	'Common and important conditions… CKD including causes, classification, management, monitoring and indications for referral'	NICE Guideline CG182. Chronic kidney disease in adults: assessment and management. January 2015
3	PSA Test Result	'IPSS to assess LUTS' 'Prostatic carcinoma'	Bladder outflow obstruction PSA levels
4	Prostatitis	'Prostatic problems such as acute and chronic prostatitis'	Acute and chronic prostatitis
5	Overactive Bladder	'Overactive bladder syndrome'	Overactive bladder management
Extra Notes	UTI in Men and Haematuria Erectile Dysfunction Benign Prostatic Hypertrophy	'Urinary tract infections in children and in adults' 'Haematuria' 'Debate around the role of the PSA blood test as a screening test for prostate cancer'	UTI in men Haematuria Erectile dysfunction BPH PSA screening

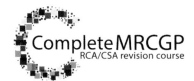

CompleteMRCGP
RCA/CSA revision course

CHAPTER 12 REFERENCES

Acute Kidney Injury
1. NICE Guideline NG148. Acute kidney injury: prevention, detection and management. Dec 2019.
2. https://ihub.scot/media/1401/20180424-web-medicine-sick-day-rules-patient-leaflet-web-v20.pdf. Apr 2018.

Chronic Kidney Disease
1. NICE Guideline CG182. Chronic kidney disease in adults: assessment and management. Jan 2015.
2. NICE Guideline CG181. Cardiovascular disease: risk assessment and reduction, including lipid modification. Sep 2016.

PSA Test Result
1. NICE CKS. https://cks.nice.org.uk/topics/prostate-cancer/diagnosis/psa-testing/. Jun 2021.
2. https://patient.info/doctor/prostate-specific-antigen-psa. Mar 2019.
3. http://www.uptodate.com/contents/screening-for-prostate-cancer

Prostatitis
1. NICE CKS. http://cks.nice.org.uk/prostatitis-acute. Nov 2020.
2. NICE CKS. http://cks.nice.org.uk/prostatitis-chronic. Sep 2019.

Overactive Bladder
1. NICE CKS. http://cks.nice.org.uk/luts-in-men. Mar 2019.
2. NICE Guidance. Lower urinary tract symptoms secondary to benign prostatic hyperplasia: tadalafil. Evidence summary ESNM 18. Oct 2013.

UTI in Men and Haematuria
1. NICE CKS. http://cks.nice.org.uk/urinary-tract-infection-lower-men#!scenario. Nov 2018.
2. NICE Guideline NG12. Suspected cancer: recognition and referral. Jan 2021.
3. NICE Guideline CG182. Chronic kidney disease in adults: assessment and management. Jan 2015.

Erectile Dysfunction
1. https://www.pcf.org/c/the-sexual-health-inventory-for-men-shim-questionnaire/
2. http://patient.info/doctor/erectile-dysfunction. Apr 2016.
3. https://www.relate.org.uk/
4. NICE Guideline NG12 Suspected cancer: recognition and referral. Jan 2021.

Benign Prostatic Hypertrophy
1. http://patient.info/doctor/benign-prostatic-hyperplasia. Oct 2015.
2. http://www.nhs.uk/Conditions/resectionoftheprostate/Pages/Risks.aspx
3. Cyproterone-acetate. http://www.cancerresearchuk.org/about-cancer/cancers-in-general/treatment/cancer-drugs/cyproterone-acetate. May 2020.

Information taken from NICE guidelines with kind permission. Please note the guidelines change frequently and you should ALWAYS check for the latest updated guidance. Remember that NICE guidance is only applicable to patients in the UK.

Doctor's Notes

Patient   Alexander Dickens   78 years   M

PMH   CKD, osteoarthritis and heart failure

Medications   Paracetamol

Furosemide 20 mg

Spironolactone 50 mg

Indapamide 2.5 mg

Ramipril 5 mg

Bisoprolol 5 mg

Allergies   No information

Consultations   Last week seen by GP. Pitting oedema to knees. Sats 95%.

Crepitations at lung bases. JVP 3 cm. Agreed to increase furosemide to two daily. BP 162/72. Ramipril increased from 2.5 mg to 5 mg.

Investigations   Blood test 1 week ago: eGFR 51 mL/min/1.73 m^2, creatinine 92 μmol/L, potassium 4.8 mmol/L and sodium 143 mmol/L.

Household   Dorothy Dickens   74 years   F

Message from biochemistry: eGFR 32 mL/min/1.73 m^2, creatinine 196 μmol/L, potassium 5.5 mmol/L and sodium 142 mmol/L.

Open ☐   Mr Dickens, I'm calling about your blood tests which show that your kidneys are struggling more than usual. I wanted to talk to you about what may be causing this so we can put them right again.

History ☐   Tell me the story about what led the doctor to see you last week. What medication changes did you both make? How have you been since the doctor last saw you? Do you feel more tired at all? Are you passing urine normally? Who is at home with you? Is Mrs Dickens well?

Risk ☐   It is likely that the cause is a combination of things: medicines and age, unfortunately. Do you have any problems with the flow of your urine or getting up at night? Good.

Flags ☐   Any fevers, any pain passing urine or going more frequently? Any loose stools or vomiting recently? You started taking furosemide last week. What dose are you taking each day? And can I check which other medicines you take?

Curious ☐   You mentioned your knee plays up. Do you ever take anything for that?

Impact ☐   How active are you generally?

ICE ☐   Is there anything that keeps worrying you? Anything else you have wondered? Is there anything else that you would like or would find helpful?

SummarICE ☐   To summarise, you have been very worried that your breathing is getting worse, as it did 6 months ago, when you needed to go into hospital. You have been well on 80 mg furosemide previously. Your main concern now is balancing the kidneys with the breathing.

Impression ☐   We call this acute kidney injury.

Experience ☐   Have you had problems with your kidney blood tests before?

Explanation ☐   I think what has caused it is a combination of factors that all impact on the kidney. The recent diarrhoea made the kidneys more dehydrated and increasing the ramipril and furosemide at the same time was just too much for the kidneys. The ibuprofen is also a contributor unfortunately.

Sense ☐   You sound very disappointed.

Empathy ☐   I appreciate it must be very disheartening going from one problem to another.

Options ☐   Have you taken your medicines this morning? I would suggest you hold off taking them until I've seen you. Can you come in to see me at the end of morning surgery?

Examination ☐   I would like to examine you. We can recheck the blood tests when you come. When you arrive, can you please do a urine sample. We can look at your medicines, take your BP, listen to your chest, look at your legs and knees and repeat your bloods. Does that sound okay? Your blood tests from today will be back in a few hours.

Recommend ☐   We can make a plan for your medicines based on if there is extra fluid in your legs or lungs, as well as your kidney result. I will call you again around 5.30 p.m. when the result will be back. We may have to reduce one of your water tablets and we should stop the ibuprofen. Do you have any thoughts or questions?

InCludE ☐   You aren't in the least a nuisance and I'm sure we can sort some treatment for your knees that won't affect your kidneys, for example physiotherapy.

Future ☐   I wonder whether, to help monitor your breathing, we could involve the heart failure nurses? It is likely I'll be suggesting a repeat blood test and discussion with me in the next few weeks so we can monitor the balance of fluid.

Empower ☐   You mentioned your weight has changed. Monitoring your weight is helpful to detect warning signs and guide your medications. I also have some information to give you which includes a card telling you what you can do when you feel unwell; it's called a medicines' sick day rule card. How will you get to the surgery? Great. See you at midday.

Doctor's notes	Alexander Dickens, 78 years. PMH: CKD, osteoarthritis and heart failure. Last week seen by GP. Pitting oedema to knees. Sats 95%. Crepitations at lung bases. JVP 3 cm. Agreed to increase furosemide to two daily. BP 162/72. Ramipril increased from 2.5 mg to 5 mg. Medications: paracetamol, furosemide 20 mg, spironolactone 50 mg, indapamide 2.5 mg, ramipril 5 mg, bisoprolol 5 mg. Blood test 1 week ago: eGFR 51 mL/min/1.73 m^2, creatinine 92 µmol/L, potassium 4.8 mmol/L and sodium 143 mmol/L.
	Message from biochemistry: eGFR 32 mL/min/1.73 m^2, creatinine 196 µmol/L, potassium 5.5 mmol/L and sodium 142 mmol/L.
How to act	You are surprised when the doctor calls.
PC	*'Hello Doctor, what can I do for you?... I'm very well thank you.'*
History	The doctor saw you last week. You were last in hospital 6 months ago when the fluid was on your lungs. This was frightening. Since then, you have been *'not too bad'* but you started to feel the fluid coming back last week so called the doctor. You had noticed you were not moving around the house as easily with your breathing. When the doctor suggested taking 40 mg furosemide, initially it didn't seem to help so you increased it to 80 mg. They have given you 120 mg in hospital before, so you thought 80 mg would be fine. You can tell your fluid is going as your breathing is better and you have lost a little weight. You feel fine. Last week, however, your grandchild came around and you had a day with diarrhoea. You feel fine now. You are passing urine normally. You have no symptoms of a UTI. You have no fever. Your knee arthritis does 'play up'. If asked, tell the doctor you buy ibuprofen OTC for this. Otherwise, you take only the prescribed medicines. You have not yet taken this morning's medication.
Social	You live with your wife. Your son lives around the corner with your grandchildren.
	You have a good circle of friends and don't let your medical conditions get you down.
	You have noticed a general decline in your health over the last few years.
ICE	You have never heard of the diagnosis 'acute kidney injury'.
	You become very apologetic that you have changed the dose yourself without consulting the doctor and apologise to the doctor for causing an inconvenience to them.
	'Oh dear Doctor, I am worried about my breathing… now my kidneys. I just can't win.'
	You are hoping the doctor will examine you again. Your son could bring you in.
	You would like reassurance that your chest is okay and to talk about your knees.

Definition[1]

Serum creatinine rise of ≥26 µmol/L within 48 hours.

≥50% rise in serum creatinine known or presumed to have occurred within the past 7 days.

A fall in UO to <0.5 mL/kg/hour for >6 hours in adults or >8 hours in children and young people.

25% or greater fall in eGFR in children and young people within the past 7 days.

Risk factors for development of AKI[1]

- Age over 65 years
- Nephrotoxic drugs
- Previous AKI
- CKD
- Neurological or cognitive impairment or disability, which may mean limited access to fluids because of reliance on a carer.
- Hypovolaemia
- Sepsis or infection (e.g. urine)
- Heart failure
- Diabetes
- Liver disease
- Severe diarrhoea (children and young people with bloody diarrhoea are particularly at risk)
- Oliguria (UO <0.5 mL/kg/hour)
- Iodinated contrast used in past week
- Urological obstruction
- Haematological malignancy
- Hypotension

Management Urinalysis, ± urgent USS, manage the cause, think about acute nephritis, refer (immediately if pyonephrosis, obstructed solitary kidney, bilateral obstruction, complications of AKI caused by obstruction) for relief of obstruction if present, review nephrotoxic drugs and repeat bloods and consider admission for renal replacement therapy.[1]

Complications Hyperkalaemia, metabolic acidosis, symptoms or complications of uraemia (pericarditis, encephalopathy), fluid overload and pulmonary oedema.[1]

Sick day rule card

The sick day rule card was originally developed by NHS Highland to advise patients which medicines to stop when they become unwell with either 'vomiting or diarrhoea (unless only minor), fever sweats or shaking unless only minor'.[2] Medicines to stop include ACEIs, ARBs, NSAIDs, diuretics and metformin.[2]

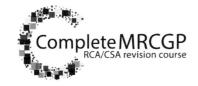

Doctor's Notes

Patient	Bob Riley	67 years	M
PMH	Hypertension		
Medications	Lisinopril 5 mg daily		
Allergies	No information		
Consultations	12 months ago – CKD G3bA2 diagnosed. Started on ACEI.		
Investigations			

Blood results:

12 months ago	**2 weeks ago**
eGFR 40 mL/min/1.73 m^2	eGFR 37 mL/min/1.73 m^2
ACR = 28 mg/mmol	ACR = 29 mg/mmol Hb 146 g/L
Na 137 mmol/L	
K 4.2 mmol/L	
ALT 12 IU/L	
ALP 60 IU/L	
PSA 0.8 ng/mL	
Cholesterol 3.1 mmol/L	
HbA1c 36.6 mmol/mol	

Household	Phoebe Riley	66 years	F

Sense ☐	Thanks for phoning back. I can hear you are worried and keen to know your results.
Curious ☐	To interpret the latest test in the context of your health, I'm interested to know how you have been feeling recently.
ICE ☐	Is there anything you are most concerned about today? And what did you think the blood tests may show?
Impression ☐	The latest kidney blood tests have shown that your kidneys are working pretty much the same as last year, which is good news.
Empathy ☐	I appreciate this is not what you had hoped to hear.
Experience ☐	Have you come across others with kidney problems like yours?
Explanation ☐	There is often no cause, but CKD can be caused by medical problems such as high BP, which is something you have had for a few years.
Risk ☐	Just to check other aspects of your health – in addition to hypertension, do you have any other medical problems? Are you taking any medicines including ibuprofen? Any family history of kidney problems? Have you ever smoked? Any problems passing urine, including needing to go at night, or again after you've just been or poor flow?
Flags ☐	May I just check – have you ever noticed any blood in your urine? Have you noticed any swelling around the ankles?
History ☐	Are you keeping active? Tell me about your work. And your family? How do you like to spend your time?
O/E ☐	Do you check your BP at home? Can you tell me the latest reading?
SummarICE ☐	So, to summarise, last year's diagnosis of CKD was a shock, but you've worked on your diet, reducing salt and processed foods, eating more fruit and veg and have felt well. You are surprised that the recent blood test is not back to normal and are worried about what this means. A friend is having dialysis and you hope you aren't also heading for this.
Options ☐	Your kidney function is pretty much the same as last year – this is good news. Over time, kidneys can become less efficient and so the numbers may get worse, but yours are stable. We wouldn't expect the kidney function to improve, but staying stable is very good. There is no suggestion that you are heading towards dialysis at the moment. One thing we could do is to protect your kidney blood vessels from the effects of raised cholesterol. I would like to recommend a cholesterol tablet. Although your cholesterol is good, research has shown that the tablet protects the vessels. The tablet is called atorvastatin 20 mg, which you take once a day. Have you heard of statins? There is the risk of side effects, e.g. muscle aches, but many people are fine on them. Rarely, there is a risk of muscle breakdown, so if your muscles did ache or you felt unwell then please tell your GP. This tablet can also affect the liver, but we will be monitoring your blood tests. If your kidney tests changed quickly or fell to below 30, we would ask the specialists to see you. The kidney test is currently at the level of 37. Normal is above 60. Do you have any thoughts or questions?
Empower ☐	To protect the health of the vessels, I suggest we monitor your BP; it is currently slightly high so we might need to alter your tablets if it stayed up. As much exercise as possible and decreasing your salt can be protective. If you decrease your salt by 6 g/day it can decrease your BP by 10. Might these be things you could do? You probably know this from before, but you need to avoid taking certain tablets from the chemist, such as ibuprofen, which can make kidney function worse. Check first before you buy anything.
Future ☐	Please can you check your BP twice a week for the next 4 weeks and then email me the results? Please then arrange a telephone consultation with me to see if we need to increase your BP medication. Regardless of this, we should repeat your blood test yearly to keep an eye on kidney function.
Safety net ☐	I'm happy with your kidney function at the moment but, if you ever do notice anything new, for example ankle swelling or blood in the urine, please let me know.

Patient's Story

Doctor's notes	Bob Riley, 67 years. PMH: hypertension. Medications: lisinopril 5 mg daily.
	Blood results 1 week ago: eGFR 37 mL/min/1.73 m^2, ACR = 29 mg/mmol
	Blood results 12 months ago: eGFR 40 mL/min/1.73 m^2, ACR = 28 mg/mmol
	Hb 146 g/L, Na 137 mmol/L, ALT 12 IU/L, ALP 60 IU/L, K 4.2 mmol/L, PSA 0.8 ng/mL, cholesterol 3.3 mmol/L, HbA1c 36.6 mmol/mol, ACR 28 mg/mmol
How to act	Concerned. You would like to know what the result means as soon as the GP tells you.
PC	*'You asked me to phone you to get my blood test results. What's wrong?'*
History	This is your first annual review following the diagnosis of CKD last year.
	This diagnosis came out of the blue – you had the blood tests a year ago for a routine health check. You have no family history.
	You have no outflow obstruction symptoms including no nocturia.
Social	You live with your wife. You walk the dogs twice a day. This is your only exercise.
	You enjoy the taste of your food but avoid sugary or fatty foods. You do add salt and think you could easily cut this down. You have never smoked. You drink alcohol occasionally. You take ramipril 5 mg, started 12 months ago.
ICE	You have been worried about your kidneys ever since the diagnosis last year. You thought that taking the tablets correctly would help your kidneys to return to near-normal (false health belief). A friend has recently had to start dialysis and you are worried this might happen to you.
	You want to know what has caused this CKD – the doctor didn't explain last year.
	You are keen to do anything you can to protect your kidneys *'Is there anything else I can do to help my kidneys?'* and willingly accept a statin if offered. If asked, you do check your own BP at home and the latest reading is 137/82.
Examination	BP is 137/82, urine dipstick is normal.

'People with markers of kidney damage and those with a glomerular filtration rate (GFR) of less than 60 mL/min/1.73 m^2 on at least two occasions separated by a period of at least 90 days (with or without markers of kidney damage).'[1]

Markers – kidney damage	Albuminuria (ACR >3 mg/mmol) or urine sediment abnormalities.[1]
	Electrolyte disorders, abnormal histology or renal imaging or history of renal transplantation.[1]
Offer testing for CKD using	eGFR creatinine and ACR to people with risk factors HTN, DM, CVD, AKI, structural renal tract disease, recurrent renal calculi or prostatic hypertrophy, multisystem diseases with potential kidney involvement – for example, SLE, FH of end-stage kidney disease (GFR category G5), opportunistic detection of haematuria.
	Do not use age, gender or ethnicity as risk markers to test people for CKD.
	Do not use obesity alone as a risk marker to test people for CKD.
CKD investigations	Repeat the test after 2 weeks to exclude AKI.
	To make a diagnosis of CKD another test is required in 3 months.
	ACR must be a first urine of the day.
	Avoid meat 12 hours before the blood test.
	eGFRcysC test – if available can differentiate borderline CKD.
	'African-Caribbean or African family origin… multiply eGFR by 1.159.'[1]
CKD diagnosis	eGFR <45 or ACR ≥3 (any eGFR) or eGFR <60 and eGFRcysC unavailable.
Progressive CKD	Change in CKD category/12 months or ↓eGFR 25% or 15 mL/min/1.73 m^2/year.[1]
Classification	eGFR 45–59 = G3a. 30–44 = G3b, 15–29 = G4, eGFR <15 = G5.
	ACR <3 = A1, ACR 3–30 = A2, ACR >30 = A3.[1]
Further investigations	FBC (?Anaemia) and if eGFR <30, calcium, phosphate, PTH and vitamin D.
	Urine dip for haematuria. Use ACR (not dipstick) for protein measurement.
	Renal USS if eGFR <30, progressive CKD, haematuria, FH PCKD or obstruction or may require a renal biopsy.[1]
Management	CVD lifestyle advice. No protein-free diet unless instructed by the renal team.
	If possible, stop nephrotoxic drugs.
	Offer antiplatelet drugs for CVD 2⁰ prevention but be aware ↑risk of bleeding.[1]
BP aim	<140/90 (target 120-139) or in diabetics <130/80 (target 120–129).[1]
Statins	See: NICE CG 181.[2] 'Offer atorvastatin 20 mg for the primary or secondary prevention of CVD to people with CKD.' See guidance for full details.
	ACE inhibitor. Start if ACR (mg/mmol): ≥70 or ≥ 30 + HTN or ≥3 + DM *and* K <5 mmol/L. Stop if change of eGFR ↓25% or creatinine ↑30% or K ≥6 mmol/L.
Monitoring frequency	See Table 2 within reference.[1]
Refer if	eGFR<30, ACR >70 (unless DM put on ACEI), ACR>30 + haematuria.
	Progressive CKD. Suspected renal artery stenosis or suspected inherited condition.
	≥4 antihypertensives.[1]
Discuss with medics if	AKI, severe uraemia, fluid overload or hyperkalaemia.
Type 4 tubular acidosis	In a diabetic with CKD and raised potassium… test for a low bicarbonate.
	Manage BP and discuss with a specialist whether the Rx of furosemide (if oedematous) and fludrocortisone is appropriate.

Doctor's Notes

Patient	Remigio Sanchez	48 years	M
PMH	No medical history		
Medications	No medications		
Allergies	No information		
Consultations	2 years ago for a soft tissue injury of the ankle		
Investigations	PSA 3.0 ng/mL		
Household	Perla Sanchez	48 years	F
	Sosimo Sanchez	16 years	M
	Manuela Sanchez	14 years	F
	Pilar Sanchez	10 years	M

Example Consultation

Open ☐ Thanks for talking to me on the phone. Can you tell me what led to this test being taken? I can see we haven't talked together for a long time.

Experience ☐ Tell me more about your father and brother's experience. What is your understanding of the PSA test? Has a doctor explained?

Sense ☐ I can tell you are keen to know the result.

Impression ☐ The result is slightly raised; however, activities such as running, cycling, ejaculating or intercourse can all increase this result. In the week prior to the test, did you do any of these activities? That is helpful to know. This result cannot be interpreted and I would expect your result to be raised if you have done those activities. I would like to repeat the test.

History ☐ Are you well? Any medical problems? Tell me more about you – your work and home. Do you notice any problems when passing urine? What is the flow like? Is it painful? Do you have to race to the toilet? Do you go frequently? Any fever? Any pain in the sides? How many times do you pass urine at night? Is the flow okay? Do you have to wait because it dribbles at the end? Afterwards do you feel your bladder isn't quite empty? Are you always thirsty? Any problems with erections?

ICE ☐ Is there anything else on your mind? What are you most fearful of? What did you think I might suggest today?

Flags ☐ Have you seen any blood in the urine? Have you noticed any new back pain? Have you lost weight? I'm pleased you have no symptoms.

Impact ☐ Getting a result can be worrying. How did you feel prior to phoning today?

Curious ☐ You mentioned 'I haven't got time to be ill.' Is this something that has been on your mind? If this result were raised, have you had thoughts about how it may affect you?

Empathy ☐ I appreciate that, with your family history and fear of the impact a diagnosis may have on your life, this result is very important to you.

SummarICE ☐ So to summarise, your brother and father have prostate cancer and you have arranged this test in the hope that if there was a cancer you are catching it early.

InCludE ☐ You fear how a diagnosis of prostate cancer would impact on your health and ability to provide for your family. This has been very stressful for you.

Future ☐ I would really like to see you for an appointment to examine your prostate if I may. It would involve lying on the couch behind the curtain, then I would insert one finger into the back passage as this is where we can feel the prostate. It is uncomfortable but not usually painful. I would also like to feel your abdomen. Would that be okay? I would ask for a nurse chaperone if that is okay with you? The reason for examining your prostate is to see if it feels normal, or if it is enlarged or feels lumpy. This would help us decide what to do – whether to repeat the blood test soon or refer you to see a urologist.

Explanation ☐ The PSA level can be raised in prostate cancer. But it can also be raised in harmless growth of the prostate. If the PSA level was raised, we would need a biopsy to diagnose or exclude a cancer. The biopsy is taken through the back passage; therefore, it can be an uncomfortable procedure with the risk of infection.

Future ☐ Please book an appointment to see me soon so I can examine the prostate. If it feels normal, we should repeat your blood test a week later. If this is raised, we would check your urine and kidney function before referring you to the urologist. If the prostate feels lumpy or abnormal, I would refer you to a urologist to be seen within 2 weeks.

Specifics ☐ If we do need to repeat the blood test, you should avoid sex, ejaculation and exercise for 48 hours before the test.

Safety net ☐ If in future you have any problems passing urine, or any new pain, let a GP know.

Doctor's notes	Remigio Sanchez, 48 years. PMH: PSA 3.0 ng/mL, nil else. Medications: none.
How to act	Eager to know what will happen to you.
PC	*'I've phoned for my PSA result.'*
PMH	You asked for the test as your brother has been diagnosed with prostate cancer.
	You made an appointment with the phlebotomist and told her you needed the test.
	You have never had any problems with your health.
	Your father also had a total prostatectomy for prostate cancer.
	You haven't noticed any symptoms.
	You attended the gym prior to the test being taken.
	You understand the PSA test will tell you if you have prostate cancer.
Social	*'I haven't got time to be ill.'*
	You moved from Argentina 6 years ago for work on oil rigs.
	You spend a lot of time away from home.
	Your work would not be sympathetic if you needed time off.
	They often make people redundant. You feel the pressure of finances at the moment with three children who want to go to university.
ICE	You assume you have prostate cancer too and want to catch it early.
	You are worried that you will need chemotherapy.
	You couldn't sleep last night because of fear of the result.
	You expect the doctor to send you for a biopsy. You have had no UTI symptoms.
Examination	Prostate and abdomen are normal.

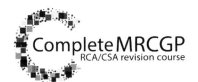

Kidney and Urology – 3

Consider a PSA test to check for prostate cancer in:

- Associated LUTS.[1]
- Visible haematuria.[1]
- Erectile dysfunction.[1]
- Unexplained symptoms (such as lower back ache, weight loss and bone pain) – might be due to secondaries.
- Men aged >50 after counselling (even if asymptomatic*).

*Prostate cells adjacent to urethra (transitional zone of the prostate) commonly change to become hyperplastic (BPH) whereas prostate cancer arises in the peripheral zone of the prostate – the part you can feel on DRE. Hence men with early prostate cancer are usually asymptomatic. Men who present with LUTS due to prostate cancer often have locally advanced disease. However, BPH and prostate cancer can coexist.

Occasionally tumours arise from the anterior portion of the gland, and are impalpable.

Symptoms from bladder outflow obstruction (from BPH or cancer of the prostate) may include:

- Urgency, frequency, incontinence or nocturia.
- Hesitancy, poor flow or post-micturition dribbling.

Symptoms of metastases may include back or bone pain, haematuria or weight loss.

Erectile dysfunction is not usually caused by prostate cancer but completes a Well Man history.

Men with low back pain: always consider a PSA test (as well as a myeloma screen and kidney/ureteric disease).

PSA counselling[2]

- Prostate cancer is not the only cause of a raised PSA.
- PSA cannot distinguish between aggressive and slow-growing cancers that would never have caused a problem.
- 15% of men with prostate cancer will have normal PSA.
- Prostate biopsies are negative in three out of four men with raised PSA.
- Prostate biopsy may cause infection and bleeding.
- Treatment of prostate cancer includes surgery, radiotherapy, hormones with side effects of incontinence, ED and fertility loss.
- NOT having test will avoid side effects of treatment – but may mean that early treatable cancers are missed.

2WW referral

1. Abnormal PSA levels. Normal is 0–4 but the PSA test is not diagnostic and the upper level varies according to race and age. NICE recommends 2WW referral for any man with PSA > age-specific range.[1]
2. Suspicious prostate on DRE.[1]

Significant rise in PSA whilst taking a 5-alpha reductase inhibitor.[3]

PSA rises in cancer, BPH, UTI, exercise (e.g. cycling), ejaculation, urinary retention or surgical intervention, e.g. flexible cystoscopy.

PSA is suppressed in men by up to 50% in the first year of taking finasteride or other 5-alpha reductase inhibitor.

Doctor's Notes

Patient	Arthur Smalling	49 years	M
PMH	Hypertension		
	Irritable bowel syndrome		
	Depression		
Medications	Amlodipine 5 mg OD		
	Mebeverine 135 mg TDS		
	Citalopram 20 mg OD		
Allergies	No information		
Consultations	No recent consultations		
Investigations	No recent investigations		
Household	Patricia Smalling	42 years	F

Open ☐	Please don't be embarrassed. Please tell me about the problem. How is going to the toilet?
History ☐	Some specific questions about your symptoms… Some of the questions are a little personal. How long have you had this pain? What sort of pain is it? Does anything bring it on or make it worse? How are your bowels? Have you passed any blood? Any mucus? How are your waterworks? Any pain passing urine? Going more often or in the night? Do you have to rush to the toilet? Does the urine flow start straight away or is there a pause? How is the stream? Does the flow stop and start? Do you get dribbling at the end when you think you have finished? Have you had a water infection before? Have you had any problems sexually?
ICE ☐	Have you had any thoughts about what could be causing your symptoms? Are you worried about anything in particular? Were you hoping I would do anything specific today?
Flags ☐	Have you ever seen blood in your urine? Or blood in your semen? Have you had a fever? Or any weight loss? Any new sexual partners?
Impact ☐	How have these symptoms been affecting you? How is your mental health?
Curious ☐	You mentioned being saddle sore. Have you been cycling a lot recently?
SummarICE ☐	So you have been experiencing pain in your back passage, pain between your privates and bottom, and discomfort passing urine. You have also noted that your stream isn't as fast as it used to be and have had some sexual issues and pain on ejaculation. You wondered if your symptoms were caused by cycling a lot, but the symptoms didn't improve with a month off cycling. You haven't had a fever or passed blood and your bowels are working normally.
O/E ☐	Do you have a thermometer at home? And are you able to check your pulse and BP? Good, thank you. It's reassuring that those are normal. It would also be really helpful if I could arrange to examine your tummy, testes and back passage. This will help me with the diagnosis. Would it be okay to see you later today? Would you mind if a chaperone was present? It would also be really helpful if you could provide a urine sample for testing; could you bring one with you?
Impression ☐	It is possible that you may have chronic prostatitis, which means inflammation of the prostate. A urine infection is less likely, given all your symptoms.
Experience ☐	Do you know much about the prostate?
InCludE ☐	You thought you might be saddle sore, but in fact I think this may be a prostate problem.
Explanation ☐	The prostate is a gland found in every man and is located in the pelvis. Prostatitis is a condition where the prostate becomes inflamed. Sometimes it's due to a bacterial infection but sometimes there is no obvious reason why the prostate becomes inflamed. It is not a form of cancer and isn't usually caused by sexually transmitted infections. Classic symptoms are pain in the region between your scrotum and anus – called the perineum – pain in the back passage and problems passing urine or with intercourse. Because the symptoms have been there for more than 3 months, we call the condition chronic. Unfortunately, it can be tricky to treat, but most men notice an improvement within 6 months. Any questions?
Future ☐	When I see you, I would also like to send a urine sample off to check for bacteria. It would be helpful if you could complete a couple of questionnaires before you come, to identify how the symptoms have been affecting you. One is called the International Prostate Symptom Score and the other is the National Health Institute – Chronic Prostatitis Symptom Index. I will email these to you. We would normally treat prostatitis with a month of antibiotics. Do you have any allergies?
Specifics ☐	If it is clear you do have prostatitis, I would like to start you on ciprofloxacin 500 mg BD (check local guidance), is that okay? We would review you in about 2 weeks to decide if you need any blood tests to check the kidney and prostate levels. If we are not making progress, we will ask a specialist to see you.
Safety net ☐	Should your symptoms worsen at any time or you develop a fever or pass blood, please let me know straight away. If the surgery is closed, call 111 for a doctor.

Doctor's notes	Arthur Smalling, 49 years. PMH: HTN, IBS, Depression. Medications: amlodipine, citalopram, mebeverine.
How to act	Embarrassed.
PC	*'Hello Doctor, I'm rather embarrassed, I've been getting a lot of pain in my bottom.'*
History	For the last 4 months you have been experiencing pain in your rectum. The pain can be sharp or a burning pain. You have been opening your bowels normally, passing a soft stool each day. No PR bleed or mucus. You have also had discomfort when passing urine for a number of weeks. You feel tender in the region between your *'privates'* and anus. Your stream isn't as good as it used to be but isn't too bad. You get up 1–2 times a night to pass urine. Until 4 months ago you hadn't noticed any frequency or urgency in the daytime. You have not seen blood in your urine. You don't suffer with hesitancy or terminal dribbling. You have had a couple of episodes of ED which you thought were due to your age (and possibly cycling), but you have also had pain during ejaculation which you thought was odd. No weight loss. No fever. No history of UTIs. You have been married for 25 years and have not had any other partners. You have been very well with your mental health.
ICE	You are a keen cyclist so initially thought cycling may be causing your symptoms. You have been training for a 100-mile bike ride for charity. You stopped cycling 4 weeks ago but unfortunately you haven't got any better so you thought you should get checked out.
	'I thought I'd got a little saddle sore!'
Examination	Temperature 36.3 °C. HR 68 bpm. BP 136/88.
	Abdomen soft and non-tender.
	Testicular examination normal.
	Tender perineum.
	Tender slightly enlarged smooth prostate on rectal examination.
	Urine dipstick: leuco ++, protein +, blood trace, nitrite negative.

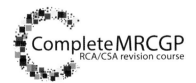

CompleteMRCGP
RCA/CSA revision course

Acute prostatitis[1]

Symptoms   Febrile illness, urinary symptoms + perineal/suprapubic pain.

Examination   Exquisitely tender prostate, leucocytes on urine dipstick.

Investigations   MSU and STI screening. Blood cultures.

Acutely unwell If severely ill, unable to take oral antibiotics or acute urinary retention admit to hospital.

Urgent referral Immunocompromised, diabetes, pre-existing urological condition or catheterised.

Chronic prostatitis (two types)[2]

1. Chronic bacterial prostatitis (10%).
2. Chronic prostatitis/chronic pelvic pain syndrome (CPPS = 90%).

Although prostatitis suggests infection and inflammation, the pathology is poorly understood. The histology does not always reflect the symptoms or treatment response. Chronic bacterial prostatitis is thought to be caused by recurrent UTIs, undertreated acute bacterial prostatitis, ascending urethral infection or lymphatic spread from the rectum. The cause of CPPS is unclear.

Symptoms:

Pain   Perineum, inguinal, suprapubic, penis, scrotum, testes, rectum, lower back or abdomen.

LUTS   Hesitancy, urgency, poor stream, terminal dribbling, frequency, nocturia or dysuria.

Sexual   ED, painful ejaculation, premature ejaculation or decreased libido.

History needs to identify/exclude: a UTI, acute prostatitis, haematospermia (may be prostatitis but also prostate cancer or STI), IBS (present in up to 30% of men with chronic prostatitis).

Duration of symptoms – minimum of 3 months.

Assess symptom severity using the National Institute of Health Chronic Prostatitis Symptom Index or IPSS.

Assess for depression/anxiety if cues to suggest this.

Examination: observations (rule out acute infection/sepsis), abdominal examination (tenderness, bladder distension or retention), external genitalia (urethral discharge, phimosis, meatal stenosis, penile cancer), DRE (prostate size, lumps? and tenderness).

Differential: acute prostatitis, prostatic abscess, UTI, urethritis, pyelonephritis, epididymitis, BPH, cancer of prostate/bladder/colon, urethral stricture, obstructive calculus in urinary tract or foreign body and pudendal neuralgia.

Investigations   Urine dip and MSU (try sending MSU after DRE to increase microbiology yield).

Consider full STI screen (esp. if <35 years or new partner).

Bloods: Consider PSA testing and routine bloods, e.g. FBC, U&E and CRP.

NB: MSU may be negative in chronic bacterial prostatitis so look for old MSUs.

Management   4–6 weeks antibiotic (check local guidance).

NICE – ciprofloxacin, ofloxacin or trimethoprim if quinolones not tolerated/allergy.

Trial alpha-blocker if LUTS present.

Paracetamol ± NSAID, laxatives if constipation also present.

Refer   If diagnosis in doubt.

Severe symptoms or if chronic bacterial prostatitis is suspected.

Doctor's Notes

Patient	Angus McLaughlin 72 years M
PMH	Chronic obstructive pulmonary disease
	Ischaemic heart disease
	Hypertension
Medications	Salbutamol PRN
	Tiotropium 18 mg OD
	Aspirin 75 mg OD
	Isosorbide mononitrate 20 mg BD
	Atorvastatin 80 mg nocte
	Bisoprolol 5 mg OD
	Ramipril 2.5 mg OD
Allergies	No information
Consultations	No recent consultations
Investigations	No recent investigations
Household	No household members registered

Example Consultation

Open ☐ Could you tell me a little more about your symptoms?

History ☐ How did it start? How often are you passing urine during the day/night? Do you have to rush? Do you have any episodes where you don't make it to the toilet in time, causing a leak of urine? What is the flow of urine like? Does the flow of urine ever take time to get going? Do you ever dribble urine after you think you have finished? How are your bowels? Do you drink much tea or coffee? How much alcohol do you drink? Have you avoided drinking fluids?

ICE ☐ You mentioned having to rush to the toilet; is there a particular concern you have? You also mentioned your prostate at the beginning; is that something you have been worrying about? Were you hoping that I'd do anything particular today?

Flags ☐ Is it painful to urinate? Any blood? Weight loss? Tummy or back pain? Recent angina?

Sense ☐ I sense these symptoms have become a real nuisance to you.

Impact ☐ Have you had to stop doing anything that you enjoy?
How is your mood? Have the symptoms been disrupting your sleep?

SummarICE ☐ So for several months you have been passing urine every hour during the day and every couple of hours at night. You find it difficult to rush to the toilet due to breathlessness and you fear bringing on an angina attack. Unfortunately, you have had to stop going to the pub as you worry about having an accident. You also worry about smelling of urine if you have an accident. You thought your symptoms may be due to your prostate and particularly fear prostate cancer.

InCludE ☐ I'm sorry to hear that this is stopping you getting out. Thankfully I don't think there is a problem with your prostate.

Impression ☐ I think you may have something called 'overactive bladder'. It would really help me assess your symptoms if I could examine you. Would you be able to come to the surgery this morning? Thank you. I would like to examine your abdomen, if possible your genitals and your prostate – this involves placing a finger into your rectum. Are you okay for me to do this examination? I would ask a chaperone to be present for the intimate examinations if that's okay with you? From what I've heard so far, I don't think it's cancer and you won't need an operation.

Experience ☐ Have you heard of overactive bladder?

Explanation ☐ Overactive bladder is a condition where the bladder is sensitive and empties suddenly, often when it's not even very full. It's not a harmful condition although it can cause troublesome symptoms. The main treatment is 'bladder training' but sometimes medications can help. What are you thinking at this point?

Empower ☐ There are some simple things you can do to help. Reducing caffeine and alcohol often improves symptoms as these both irritate the bladder and have a diuretic affect which means they make you pass more urine. Although reducing fluid intake may sound like a sensible thing to do, actually this can make the problem worse as concentrated urine can irritate the bladder. We can check the prostate blood test. If the level is raised, we would repeat the test. You may need a biopsy. I will give you information to read and we can discuss this next time. Any questions?

Future ☐ I would like to send a urine sample off to ensure that there is no water infection causing your symptoms. It would be really helpful if you could complete a 'frequency volume chart' for me. This simply means recording on a chart, which I will give you, each time you go to the toilet to pass urine and, if possible, measuring the volume of urine passed. Some people will buy a cheap plastic measuring jug to do this. Would it be possible for you to do this? Then we can have a look at the chart together and discuss the bladder training techniques. Would you like me to ask our district nurses to supply you with some pads you could use in the meantime – just in case?

InCludE ☐ I'm also mindful that your angina and breathlessness are causing problems and at your next appointment we should allow time to see if we can improve your symptoms perhaps by changing your medication.

Specifics ☐ I have an appointment free at 11 a.m. Would that suit? Great – I'll see you then.

Safety net ☐ When we meet up later this morning, we could also arrange a follow-up appointment in a couple of weeks to see how you are doing. If your symptoms worsen, you develop pain or see blood in your urine, please let me know straight away.

Doctor's notes	Angus McLaughlin, 72 years. PMH: COPD, IHD, HTN. Medications: salbutamol PRN, tiotropium 18 mg, aspirin 75 mg, ISMN 20 mg BD, atorvastatin 80 mg, bisoprolol 5 mg, ramipril 2.5 mg.
How to act	Concerned.
PC	*'Doctor, I'm having trouble getting to the toilet. Do you think it's my prostate?'*
History	For several months you have been having difficulty passing urine. You feel that you have to go every hour during the day and every couple of hours during the night. You suddenly get the urge to pass urine and if you don't find a toilet quickly you will often have an accident.
	You are often short of breath due to your COPD so find it difficult: *'I have to rush to the loo.'*
	As a result, you have started to avoid going out so that you can stay close to the toilet. You were fond of meeting friends in your local pub for a beer but now feel you can't do this.
	You worry that you'll have an accident and will smell of urine *'like an old man'*. You know some of your friends had difficulty with their waterworks and one needed an operation on his prostate. You drink two cups of tea in the morning and have another before bed.
	No dysuria. No hesitancy or terminal dribbling. Good stream. No intermittency. No ED. Normal bowel habit. No haematuria. No weight loss.
Social	You are a retired miner. Your wife passed away 3 years ago so you live alone now. You feel a bit lonely and isolated now you feel you can't go out.
	Ex-smoker.
	Drink 2 pints of ale a day.
ICE	You are worried you may have prostate cancer.
	You worry about getting angina attacks if you have to hurry but this has not happened.
	You have heard about prostate cancer and fear having an operation. You expect the doctor to examine your prostate. You hope the doctor will arrange some tests.
Examination	Abdominal examination normal.
	Prostate smooth and normal size.

NICE advice – Overactive bladder[1]

Take a full history of the symptoms as with other lower urinary tract symptoms. Look for drugs and lifestyle factors which may be exacerbating the symptoms. Ask about the impact on life.

Examination should include abdominal, genital and DRE.

Suggest patient completes a 'frequency volume chart'. The patient is asked to record the number of times they pass urine, the volume of urine passed each time and any other significant information such as episodes of incontinence, what they drink, how much and when. This helps to quantify the patient's symptoms and highlights problems such as nocturia.

Management

Conservative measures:

- Bladder training.
- Avoid caffeine and alcohol. Carbonated soft drinks and fruit juice may aggravate symptoms.
- Avoidance of dehydration (concentrated urine can exacerbate the problem).
- Weight loss may help.
- Pelvic floor exercises may help men, especially if history of stress incontinence as well.
- Offer containment devices, e.g. pads or external sheaths to help whilst problem is being investigated.

Drug treatment[1]

Offer antimuscarinic (anticholinergic) – oxybutynin (immediate release), tolterodine (immediate release), or darifenacin (once daily preparation) can be used first line. If first line fails, offer alternative. Common side effects of antimuscarinics: dizziness, drowsiness, dry mouth, blurred vision, constipation, headache, indigestion and abdominal pain. Do not offer oxybutynin (immediate release) to frail older men due to the risk of impairment of daily functioning, chronic confusion, or acute delirium (less common).

Second line (if antimuscarinic contraindicated or ineffective): mirabegron. Also consider this if the patient already has a high anticholinergic burden with the other medications they take, due to increased risk of Alzheimer's. (Even warfarin has anticholinergic effects.)

An antimuscarinic can be used alongside an alpha-blocker in patients with both voiding and storage symptoms.[2]

Refer if above measures are unsuccessful.

For assessment of LUTS in general use:

The International Prostate Symptom Score (IPSS) questionnaire to assess severity and impact on quality of life.
See below for more details about lower urinary tract symptoms and BPH.

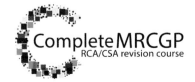

Differential diagnosis[1]	Urethritis, pyelonephritis, kidney cancer, calculi, epididymitis, bladder cancer, prostate cancer.
Investigations	Urine dipstick AND urine culture.
	If microscopic haematuria is detected in a man ≥60 years without dysuria and the MSU returns as negative → FBC and U&E.
Complications	Pyelonephritis, prostatitis and some bacteria increase the risk of stones.[1]
Treatment	1 week of treatment, e.g. trimethoprim/nitrofurantoin – see local guidance.[1]

When to refer to Urology for further investigations:

UTI fails to respond to antibiotics.[1]

Recurrent UTI – two or more in a 3-month period.[1]

'Even if >60 years – NICE advise this is a non-urgent referral.'[2]

'However, if recurrent UTI with haematuria present – see below.'

Genitourinary history suggests a cause or risk factor: e.g. stones, operations, bladder outflow obstruction.[1]

Persistent microscopic haematuria and normal renal function.[1]

If renal function impaired or proteinuria – refer to renal.[1]

Refer 2WW through the suspected cancer (for urological/renal cancer) pathway if:

>45 years	Unexplained visible haematuria (asymptomatic or negative MSU).[2]
	Visible haematuria which persists or recurs despite Rx for UTI.[2]
>60 years	Unexplained non-visible haematuria (negative MSU) AND EITHER dysuria OR ↑ serum WCC.[2]
Mass	Is identified (clinically or on imaging).[1]

Remember to use dipstick (not microscopy) to assess for haematuria and if one dipstick is positive → TWO more dipsticks are required. If EITHER of these shows a haematuria → refer (speed of referral depends on age as above).[3] 1+ on dipstick or more is significant. Routine referral if persistent non-visible haematuria which doesn't meet the above criteria for suspected cancer pathway referral.

Haematuria follow-up. 'Persistent invisible haematuria in the absence of proteinuria should be followed up annually with repeat testing for haematuria, proteinuria or albuminuria, GFR and BP monitoring as long as the haematuria persists.'[3]

Causes of ED

Vascular disease	Risk factors include: HTN, smoking, hypercholesterolaemia and DM.
Structural	Surgery within the pelvis. Peyronie's disease.
Skin disorders	Foreskin problems (lichen sclerosis, balanitis, xerotica obliterans).
Neurological	Tumour, spinal cord disease, MS, Parkinson's, stroke, peripheral neuropathy (DM).
Hormonal	Hypogonadism, Cushing's, thyroid, hyperprolactinaemia.
Drug induced	Diuretics, SSRIs, GnRH analogues and antagonists, antipsychotics.
Alcohol and recreational drugs	
Psychological causes	Stress, depression, anxiety, relationship difficulties, performance anxiety.
SHIM	Sexual health inventory for men[1] score may be useful.
	Tailor investigations to the likely cause depending on symptoms, age and risk factors.
	The patient may have their own terminology in a sexual health history. Use words they have chosen.
Make no assumptions	Ask about other sexual partners and confirm their partner's gender.

Management options

Sildenafil	CI include: already on a nitrate, unstable angina, recent MI or stroke, optic neuropathy.
	Side effects: headaches, flushing, N&V, dizziness and visual disturbances.
	Interactions: no alpha-blocker within 4 hours.
Other options	2nd line tadalafil (Cialis) with a longer duration of effect.
	Vacuum pumps. MUSE (alfraprostadil per urethra) and caverject.[2]
	Relationship counselling[3] or a referral to psychosexual medicine may be helpful.
	Show you have recognised the opportunity for health screening and promotion.
The Well Man check	CVD RFs, prostate and testicular screening, weight and bowel changes, stress/mood.
PSA screening	Offer all men with ED PSA screening.[4]

BPH management

Conservative   Reduce caffeine and alcohol. Bladder exercises.

Alpha-blocker[1]   E.g. tamsulosin

Explanation to patient: *'Acts by relaxing the prostate.'*

Side effects: drowsiness, light-headedness from low BP and retrograde ejaculation, which some men find very troublesome. Review after 4–6 weeks.

5-alpha reductase inhibitor[1]

E.g. finasteride

Explanation to patient: *'Acts by blocking the conversion of testosterone to a stronger hormone which increases the size of the prostate.'*

Side effects: loss of libido, ED, ejaculation problems and gynaecomastia.

Review in 3–6 months but can take up to 6 months to work.

Reduces PSA so avoid use if watchful waiting.

Transurethral resection of the prostate

90% risk of retrograde ejaculation. Other risks: incontinence, infection, retention, need for re-TURP, ED, strictures, bleeding, TURP syndrome and death.[2]

Tadalafil   Helps with ED and outflow symptoms.

Prostate cancer specialist management

Conservative   Watchful waiting (usually frail elderly) or active surveillance (regular MRIs ± biopsies) – usually in men with low-risk cancers.

Hormonal   Bicalutamide or cyproterone acetate prior to giving goserelin analogue.[3]

Goserelin – check LFTs 6 monthly.

Chemotherapy (increasing role of chemotherapy in metastatic prostate cancer) and radiotherapy.

Total/radical prostatectomy.

Counselling for PSA testing… an example

'The prostate is a gland that helps make semen. It is located near the bladder and rectum. As men get older it can become cancerous. Prostate cancer is the most common cancer in men, in fact 80% of men in their 80s have evidence of prostate cancer. Most prostate cancers are slow growing, especially in more elderly gentlemen and the cancer may be so slow growing that these men may never be affected by the cancer in their lifetime. Therefore, some men prefer not to know. However, in other men prostate cancer may be fast growing and spread to other areas like the bones in the back. There is a blood test called a PSA test which can be helpful in identifying prostate cancer in some patients. It checks for a chemical released from the prostate, called PSA. If this is high, it may be a sign of prostate cancer but may just be a sign of a large prostate, which is harmless. Because PSA can be raised when there isn't cancer, this can mean men having unnecessary tests done. Also, around 20% of prostate cancers have a normal PSA. To help find these cancers we also feel the prostate through the rectum to see if it feels abnormal. Any questions so far? If either PSA or examination are abnormal, we refer men to the urologists who would usually perform a biopsy. This biopsy, which means taking small pieces of the prostate, is taken through the back passage and is therefore an uncomfortable procedure and has a risk of causing an infection or bleeding in the prostate. You have/do not have symptoms of prostate problems but symptoms do not necessarily correlate with the cancer. You are welcome to take reading material home to think about it, or have you already made a decision?… If you would like the test, I suggest I examine your prostate, then we'll do the blood test in 1 week. I suggest waiting a week as examining the prostate can falsely increase the PSA level. So can exercise, cycling, sex and ejaculation. I will give you information on when to stop these activities prior to the test.'

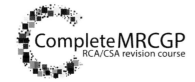

CompleteMRCGP
RCA/CSA revision course

Kidney and Urology

CHAPTER 13 OVERVIEW

Mental Health

Cases in this chapter		Within the RCGP 2020 curriculum: Mental Health	Learning points in this chapter include:
1	Anxiety	'Anxiety including generalised anxiety and panic disorders, phobias, obsessive–compulsive disorder, situational anxiety and adjustment reactions'	NICE Guideline CG113. Generalised anxiety disorder and panic disorder in adults: management. July 2019 CBT model
2	Depression Review	'Mood (affective) problems such as depression including features of a major depression such as psychotic and biological symptoms; bipolar disorder, assessment of suicidal risk; detection of masked depression'	NICE Guideline CG90. Depression in adults: recognition and management. October 2009
3	Personality Disorder	'Personality disorders including borderline, antisocial, narcissistic'	NICE Guideline CG78. Borderline personality disorder: recognition and management. January 2009
4	Postnatal Psychosis	'Pregnancy-associated disorders such as antenatal, perinatal and postnatal depression. Puerperal psychosis'	NICE Guideline CG192. Antenatal and postnatal mental health: clinical management and service guidance. February 2020
5	Eating Disorder	'Eating disorders including morbid obesity, anorexia and bulimia nervosa, body dysmorphia and Other Specified Feeding and Eating Disorders (OSFED)'	NICE Guideline NG69. Eating disorders: recognition and treatment. December 2020

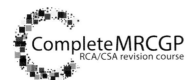

CompleteMRCGP
RCA/CSA revision course

CHAPTER 13 REFERENCES

Anxiety

1. NICE Guideline CG113. Generalised anxiety disorder and panic disorder in adults: management. Jul 2019.
2. Williams C.J. *Overcoming Depression: A Five Areas Approach.* London: Arnold. 2001.
3. Williams C., Garland A. A cognitive–behavioural therapy assessment model for use in everyday clinical practice. *Adv Psychiatr Treat* 2002; 8: 172-9.

Depression Review

1. NICE Guideline CG90. Depression in adults: recognition and management. Oct 2009.

Personality Disorder

1. http://patient.info/doctor/emotionally-unstable-personality-disorder. Jan 2016.
2. NICE Guideline CG78. Borderline personality disorder: recognition and management. Jan 2009.
3. https://www.nice.org.uk/news/article/new-standard-to-improve-the-care-of-people-with-personality-disorders. Jun 2015.
4. https://www.rcpsych.ac.uk/mental-health/problems-disorders/personality-disorder

Postnatal Psychosis

1. http://www.rcpsych.ac.uk/healthadvice/problemsdisorders/postnataldepression.aspx
2. NICE Guideline CG192. Antenatal and postnatal mental health: clinical management and service guidance. Feb 2020.
3. http://patient.info/doctor/postpartum-psychosis-pro. Mar 2015.

Eating Disorder

1. NICE Guideline NG69. Eating disorders: recognition and treatment. Dec 2020.

Information taken from NICE guidelines with kind permission. Please note the guidelines change frequently and you should ALWAYS check for the latest updated guidance. Remember that NICE guidance is only applicable to patients in the UK.

Doctor's Notes

Patient	Stephen Harper	42 years	M
PMH	Irritable bowel syndrome		
Medications	No current medications. Previous medications include mebeverine.		
Allergies	No information		
Consultations	GP consultation 5 weeks ago. Intermittent bloating. No red flags. Impression IBS.		
	A&E attendance with chest pain – discharge letter, tests all normal and reassured.		
Investigations	FBC, U&E, LFT, TFTs, GGT, CRP, HbA1c, ESR and coeliac screen all normal 1 month ago.		
Household	Judith Harper	43 years	F
	Bridget Harper	15 years	F
	Aidan Harper	14 years	M

Open ☐	Can you tell me more about your bowels? Anything else you have noticed? Do you feel well?
History ☐	Any other problems in the past? Have you taken any medication? Did it work? As it's the first time we've spoken, please tell me more about you. How are things at home? Work?
Flags ☐	Any change in your bowels? Any bleeding? Any weight loss? Any pain? What is your sleeping pattern? Your appetite? Are you able to enjoy activities? What comes to mind when you think about the future?
Sense ☐	You seem quiet today; is there anything else on your mind?
ICE ☐	What do you think is the main problem? Is there any other diagnosis that has crossed your mind? What were your thoughts regarding what we may decide today? Any other thoughts about this? What is your biggest fear?
Curious ☐	I'm interested to know what you mean by 'turning 40… a mid-life crisis'. Where do you think this has come from? Has a terminal illness happened to anyone you know?
Impact ☐	What triggers these thoughts? Does it make you feel unwell? Then what do you do?
Risk ☐	Any thoughts of hurting yourself or suicide? How much alcohol do you drink? Any other drugs?
SummarICE ☐	You are worrying about your health, in particular the risk of bowel cancer and the possibility of dying from this or from a heart attack.
Impression ☐	Thankfully, there are no worrying bowel symptoms. There is no weight loss, bleeding or change in your bowels and I see your blood tests were reassuring. I am a cautious doctor but I am confident that we do not need a colonoscopy. My feeling is that anxiety is driving your symptoms and fears, causing panic attacks. What are your thoughts about all this?
Experience ☐	Has anyone else you know suffered with anxiety? Do you know of ways to help?
Explanation ☐	Everyone has negative thoughts, but when these start to impact on your life we need to help you recognise the triggers and help you find ways to manage them. Panic attacks occur when normal hormones in the body get released inappropriately. These hormone reactions are normal when we are in dangerous situations but, when you have anxiety, they can occur in everyday situations when there isn't any danger.
InCludE ☐	Your symptoms of a racing heart, breathlessness, etc. are real but are triggered by a psychological process and thankfully aren't being caused by a heart problem.
Options ☐	There are things that you can do for anxiety, things I can help with and things others can help you with too. Relaxation exercises may help. You could contact MIND who will advise on local support groups. I can help with suggestions, monitoring and prescribing if needed, but help which doesn't involve medication can be just as powerful or more so. Others who can help may include family, friends or therapists for anxiety. There are useful resources, websites such as FearFighter.com and, on the Mindfulness website, a '3-minute breathing space' exercise. There are also books: do you enjoy reading? I recommend *Mindfulness: A Practical Guide to Finding Peace in a Frantic World*. What are your thoughts if I provide a list of all these suggestions for you to consider.
Empathy ☐	Anxiety can have a huge impact on one's life. Here is an explanation of the therapy called CBT. If anyone thinks they have terminal illness, we would expect the *emotional* and *physical* responses. These are natural. The *behaviour* response and initial *thought* is where the CBT can help, over time, gradually giving you tools to step out of the circle.
Empower ☐	Do any of these suggestion sound like they might work for you? Who else could help?
Future ☐	I would recommend that you have a look at the information. Recognising that your symptoms are anxiety can help you feel more in control but, if next time we meet we need more help, I would recommend calling Talking Space to arrange CBT.
Specifics ☐	I can give you their phone number and website details and you can refer yourself by ringing them or contacting them online. Shall we catch up again in a month to see how you are getting on? You can prebook an appointment online. Please phone me earlier if you need to.
Safety net ☐	If you feel your mood drops or you have new symptoms, for example your bowels change, you lose weight or see blood in the stool, please tell a doctor.

Doctor's notes	Stephen Harper, 42 years. PMH: irritable bowel syndrome. Medications: no current medication. Past medication: mebeverine.
	GP consultation 5 weeks ago. Intermittent bloating. No red flags. Impression IBS.
	A&E attendance with chest pain – discharge letter, tests all normal and reassured.
	FBC, U&E, LFT, TFTs, GGT, CRP, HbA1c, ESR and coeliac screen all normal 1 month ago.
How to act	Hesitant and quiet.
PC	*'It's my bowels again, Doctor.'*
History	You go to the toilet three times every morning.
	Your bowels are loose (not watery) but then they settle down. No other GI symptoms.
	No red flags – no weight loss, no bleeding and no change in bowels.
	You have seen previous doctors and *'they said it is irritable bowel'*.
	You have been struggling with financial pressures.
	Your children want to go to university.
	You have no thoughts of hurting yourself or anyone else.
	You have no features of depression, only worry. You eat and sleep okay.
Social	You work at an electronics store. At work, your concentration is good.
	You exercise to keep healthy. Your parents are elderly, which upsets you.
	Your relationship with your wife is good. She knows you worry.
	Children aged 15 and 14. You do not drink much alcohol. No drugs.
ICE	Deep down you think this must be due to stress.
	You often think when alone and especially on waking.
	Thoughts include financial worry and waiting to be told you have a life-limiting illness.
	Lots of things remind you of this: adverts and articles.
	You think about death a lot and it frightens you. It can make you cry.
	Your chest can become tight, you feel sweaty and can feel breathless. You recently had an episode of chest pain which frightened you, so you went to A&E and were told it was muscular.
	You had a mild pain in your lower chest which had no features of cardiac, gastric or respiratory disease. You accepted this but you fear you have bowel cancer, perhaps near the top of the tummy because of the recent chest pain.
	If the doctor senses you are quiet say: *'Well, you get to forty.'*
	If asked what you meant you say: *A mid-life crisis.'* If asked about it further tell the doctor – *'You hear of people going to the doctor and 6 weeks later they are dead.'*
	No one you know has had this happen. You don't know what to do.
	You wondered whether you should have a colonoscopy.
	You expect the doctor will restart your mebeverine. It doesn't help.
	You would follow any guidance from the doctor.
Examination	If the doctor examines you the abdomen is normal. Observations normal.

Open questions help the real problem to surface. Red flags steer diagnosis. Risk assessments guide management. 'Has anything else crossed your mind?' was useful here to avoid missing his multiple ICE. There were no red flags for lower GI symptoms, but this fear needed to be acknowledged and resolved.

NICE guidance – the stepped care model for the management of generalised anxiety.[1]

Step 1	'Identification and assessment; education about GAD and treatment options; active monitoring.'[1]
Step 2	'Low-intensity psychological interventions: individual non-facilitated self-help, individual guided self-help and psychoeducational groups.'[1]
Step 3	'High-intensity psychological intervention (CBT/applied relaxation) or a drug treatment.'[1]
	SSRIs. Side effects: upset stomach and may increase anxiety initially.
	Propranolol may be required in addition. Care of contraindications, e.g. asthma.
	Alternative drug treatments: SNRI and pregabalin.
	Benzodiazepines may be used for crisis management only.
Step 4	'Highly specialist treatment, such as complex drug and/or psychological treatment regimens; input from multi-agency teams, crisis services, day hospitals or inpatient care.'[1]

A simplified version of the CBT model adapted from Williams[2] and Williams and Garland[3] can be used in whole or in part even in a normal length consultation after excluding red flags for the physical causes. This model helps patients to visualise why their physical symptoms are linked to their anxiety and not a sign of something sinister. It is also a great way of summarising and demonstrating you have listened.

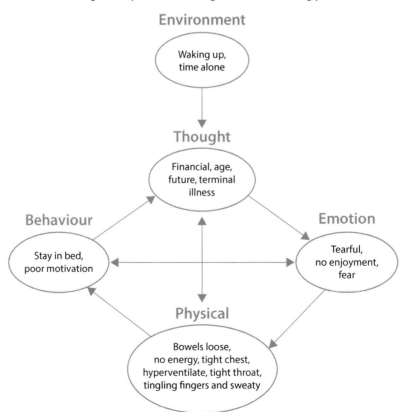

Environment
Waking up, time alone

Thought
Financial, age, future, terminal illness

Behaviour
Stay in bed, poor motivation

Emotion
Tearful, no enjoyment, fear

Physical
Bowels loose, no energy, tight chest, hyperventilate, tight throat, tingling fingers and sweaty

Doctor's Notes

Patient	Jessica Miller	24 years	F
PMH	Depression diagnosed 3 months ago		
Medications	Sertraline 50 mg daily		
Allergies	No information		
Consultations	No recent consultations		
Investigations	No recent investigation		
Household	No household members registered		

Example Consultation

Open ☐	Thank you for phoning. How have you been since starting the sertraline?
Sense ☐	You seem very quiet today.
ICE ☐	What has been going through your mind? Tell me what worries you? Is there anything particular you were hoping I might suggest or do today?
History ☐	Please take me back to the beginning. When do you think you started to feel this way? What was happening in your life at the time? How is the job going? I'm sorry to hear that. Please tell me about your family. Are you close to them? Can you confide in anyone? Do you live with anyone? Have you felt this way before? Tell me what happened then. What helped? Have you been able to take the sertraline regularly, each day? Any side effects?
Curious ☐	What does your mum think? What have you told her? What haven't you told her? Are people at work aware? Do you have any difficult thoughts? Or thoughts you can not explain?
Flags ☐	What is your sleeping pattern like? Do you wake with an alarm? Are you able to enjoy activities? How is your concentration? What comes to mind when you think about the future? Are you eating? Any thoughts of not wanting to be alive? Hurting yourself or suicide? Have you ever hurt yourself or tried to end your life? Have you made any plans to? Do you think you might? Could you tell someone about these thoughts if they became stronger? Any thoughts of hurting another person? How much alcohol do you drink? Do you take any drugs?
Impact ☐	How do you spend your days? And what about when you are not at work?
SummarICE ☐	So to summarise, you have been feeling this way for 6 months now, impacting on your energy levels. You have had upsetting thoughts of how you could end your life but have made no plans to do this as you do not want to upset your mum. You started sertraline 3 months ago and don't feel any different at all. You are wondering if they are working and whether we should change them. Work has been tough lately.
Impression ☐	I wonder if we should increase the dose of tablets? Sertraline is an effective drug for depression but takes time to work and often a higher dose than 50 mg is needed.
Experience ☐	Do you know anything about the causes of depression?
Explanation ☐	Causes can include new challenges in your life or a chemical imbalance in the brain. The sertraline helps with this but it does take time and you need to keep taking them: 50 mg is a good starting dose but I think we should now increase that to 100 mg daily.
Empathy ☐	It is very hard to move away from those you love for both you and your mum.
Options ☐	Depression can prevent you from looking after yourself and from performing well at work. It sounds as if your mum would like you to go home; have you considered this? That sounds sensible. Going home may provide time to decide together what to do in the longer term. What do you think? When it comes to depression there are things that you can do to help, such as getting more exercise and eating well, things I can help with, for example increasing the medication, and other people, such as your parents or counsellors, can give you support. You may find that returning to a happy and caring environment will help you feel better, but it may be that you need a little more help. It seems you are suffering significantly at the moment so we need to work out a plan which is best for you. What are your thoughts regarding increasing antidepressants or talking therapies? I suggest that I issue a work note for 4 weeks. Would you like the number of a counsellor? Would you be interested in some online help?
Empower ☐	What exercise could you do? Is there anyone else who could help you?
Future ☐	Can we catch up in a couple of weeks? Would you like me to talk with your mum? We need to make sure you are safe and so if your mum is aware of what thoughts you have had she can help you... would it be okay if I explained to her what you have told me?
Specifics ☐	If you decide to stay with your mum, can you book another telephone appointment to let me know and so we can discuss the ongoing plan? Avoid alcohol as it lowers mood.
Safety net ☐	If you feel your mood is dropping or you ever have thoughts of hurting yourself, call a GP, me if available, but there is always a GP on call here. If the surgery is closed there is 111 or the Samaritans. You could even go to A&E. Here are all the contact numbers.

Patient's Story

Doctor's notes	Jessica Miller, 24 years. PMH: depression diagnosed 3 months ago. Medications: sertraline 50 mg daily.
How to act	Quite short sentences. Your depression makes it hard work for the doctor to retrieve information from you. Often initially answering, 'I don't know.'
PC	After a pause… 'I don't know what's wrong with me. The tablets aren't working.'
History	You started to feel this way when you moved for your job about 6 months ago. No physical symptoms but you have no energy. No psychotic features. Anhedonia and hopelessness. You felt like this in the past, whilst doing your GCSEs, and were seen by the school counsellor – you found this helpful. You saw the GP 3 months ago and were started on sertraline. You have been taking the tablets regularly and not missed any. No side effects from the tablets. You are struggling at work and making mistakes. You have no features of psychosis.

> **Risk:** You have had occasional thoughts of not wanting to be alive. You sometimes think it would be good if you didn't wake up in the morning.
>
> You drink some alcohol. You take no drugs. No thoughts of hurting others.
>
> Never self-harmed.
>
> You have never made a plan to harm yourself.
>
> Thoughts have included jumping off a bridge or taking an overdose.
>
> If the doctor asks whether you intend to do this say, 'I don't know,' and if they ask if you would tell someone say, 'yes but I won't do that'.

> **Protective factor:** You are very close to your mum and you would hate to upset her by committing suicide.

Social	You work in marketing. You have been late for work as you struggle to get out of bed, despite being awake since 4–5 a.m. Your boss is nice and told you to come to the GP. You have fallen out with your flatmates over bills. You moved here for work 6 months ago.

You are eating less. You can't think about cooking.

You spend your days in your room watching TV.

You don't see your friends. You have no hobbies.

You do not exercise. You confide in your mum.

Your parents live 4 hours away. You miss them. They want you to go home.

Your mum is worried. She speaks to you on the phone every night.

ICE	You are not sure why you feel like this. You are not worried about anything.

You don't know what to expect today.

You accept a work note and a prescription for an increased dose of antidepressants.

You will go on walks with your mum. You will also see your local vicar.

If offered, accept a referral to counselling services.

You give consent for the GP to speak with your mum if the GP offers this.

Recommend a few suggestions tailored to their needs and capacity. Provide a list of the suggestions and contact numbers for organisations. You may have a collection of books you can lend. Structure your management plan: you can do, I (GP) can do, others can do and other resources. Depending on how much the patient can absorb.

'Things that you can do: a healthy sleep and meal regime to give you energy, avoid alcohol which lowers mood, and exercise every day should help to make you feel better. I can help with providing suggestions, monitoring and prescribing medication if needed. Other people who can help may include family, friends or professionals. You could contact MIND who will advise on local support groups. I suggest arranging counselling if you feel there are emotions or experiences you want to talk about. There are other useful resources, websites such as MoodGym or Mindfulness. There are helpful books also, such as Living in the Moment: with Mindfulness Meditations *by Anna Black. I have a list of all of these suggestions and here are the contact numbers.'*

NICE guidance–The stepped care model for the management of depression.[1]

Step 1 'Assessment, support, psychoeducation, active monitoring and referral for further assessment and interventions.'[1]

Step 2 'Low-intensity psychosocial interventions (self-help CBT or structured group physical activity programme), psychological interventions, medication and referral for further assessment and interventions.'[1]

Step 3 'Medication, high-intensity psychological interventions (e.g. CBT or behavioural couples therapy), combined treatments, collaborative care ('Only for depression where the person also has a chronic physical health problem and associated functional impairment'[1]) and referral for further assessment and interventions.'[1]

Step 4 'Medication, high-intensity psychological interventions, electroconvulsive therapy, crisis service, combined treatments, multiprofessional and inpatient care.'[1]

Duration of treatment of medication therapy

First episode of depression: continue for 6 months after the depression has improved.

Second episode: continue for at least 2 years.[1]

Combining drug medication in the patient resistant to first-line therapy needs careful consideration and 'should only normally be started in primary care in consultation with a consultant psychiatrist'.[1]

Be aware of:

Serotonin syndrome – see https://patient.info/doctor/Serotonin-Syndrome

Malignant neuroleptic syndrome – see https://patient.info/doctor/neuroleptic-malignant-syndrome

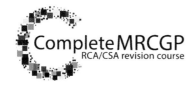
CompleteMRCGP
RCA/CSA revision course

Doctor's Notes

Patient   Andrea Lockwood   36 years   F

PMH   15 years old – under Child and Adolescent Mental Health Services for depression.

17–20 years old – under secondary care for major depression and self-harm. Discharged by mental health services for repeated failure to attend.

Mid-20s – managed by GP for moderate depression and superficial wrist cutting.

Overdose of paracetamol aged 27 years, seen by Crisis Team and discharged.

Termination of pregnancy 29 years old, referred to counselling team. Disclosed a history of sexual abuse as a child (by stepfather), declined to inform police.

Further episode of severe depression in early 30s, suicidal ideation but not attempts, wrist cutting, referred to secondary care but repeatedly failed to attend appointment. Discharged back to primary care.

Medications   Sertraline 50 mg daily.

Several courses of antidepressants in the past including fluoxetine, sertraline, mirtazapine.

Allergies   No information.

Consultations   GP appointment 4 weeks ago:

'Becoming depressed again, feeling low. Not sleeping or eating well. Got into trouble at work. Only had the job for 4 weeks when got into an argument with a colleague, resulting in her quitting the job on the spur of the moment. Feels colleague was out to get her. Worried about money. Lives alone, no local family. Finds it hard to keep friends, says no close friends. Has a nice neighbour who looks in on her occasionally. Having fleeting thoughts of suicide, no plans or attempts. Has been cutting wrists again, superficial wrist wounds seen.'

Plan: Restart sertraline, TCI 3–4 weeks for review. Crisis team number given to patient and worsening advice given.

Investigations   No information

Household   No household contacts

Example Consultation

Open ☐ Can you tell me a bit more about how you feel? Tell me your story. That sounds tough. (Pause) How have you been since you last saw the GP?

Impact ☐ Has the way you are feeling caused you any difficulties in life recently?

ICE ☐ Do you have any thoughts about what could be causing all these problems for you? Are you worried about anything specific? Was there anything specific you hoped we would achieve today or anything in particular that you wanted?

History ☐ I'm sorry you are feeling so low. Is your mood affecting how you sleep? Or eat? Are you able to go out and enjoy yourself? I can see from your records that you have had problems with your mood in the past; do you feel that you are always battling with low mood? Can you tell me more about what contact you have had with health professionals? Do you think your mood affects how you develop or keep relationships? Who is in your life? How do you get on? Has anyone in the family suffered with mood problems? Have you ever been in trouble with the police? Do you drink alcohol? Or smoke? Have you ever taken illegal drugs? Do you find that sometimes you act without thinking things through? Has this had any bad consequences for you? Do you ever feel paranoid, as if people are watching you or out to get you? Do you ever hear or see things which other people cannot?

Flags ☐ You told the GP last time that you had been harming yourself; is this still the case? How often? Is it possible to explain what drives you to cut yourself? Does it make you feel better afterwards? Have you ever felt so bad that you have wanted to end your life? Have you made plans to end your life? What would stop you from ending your life? Do you know where you can get help if you do feel suicidal?

Sense ☐ I sense that life can be very complex for you at times, would you agree?

SummarICE ☐ So you feel you have had problems with your mood since you were a teenager. This may have begun as a result of abuse you sadly suffered as a child. You have seen lots of different doctors and you have felt this has been without much success. You find it difficult to maintain relationships and can sometimes act on impulse without thinking of the consequences. You find cutting yourself releases tension and makes you feel better. You do have thoughts that it would be better if you weren't around but haven't recently made plans to end your life. You would like help and for a medical team to stick with you. Is there anything I have missed or you would like to add?

Explanation ☐ You're clearly suffering with an episode of depression at present, Andrea, but I do wonder if the problem runs a little deeper and if there may be another explanation as to why you have had such complex problems in your life. I wonder if you may have a personality disorder. Have you heard of this? Our personalities are quite complex but in general they are a set of qualities which control how we think, feel and behave. Our personalities develop in a particular way partly due to our genes but also due to our experiences and upbringing. In some people, their personality develops in such a way that it causes them great difficulties in life. These difficulties vary greatly but can be with their mood, their relationships or their behaviour, such as committing crimes. Do you think this could be the case for you?

Recommend ☐ I would like to refer you to our complex needs team who can assess you to see if they think you may have a personality disorder. If they do, they can help you by providing a community mental health nurse who will visit you. They can also put you in touch with a support worker and can help you access talking therapies. Sometimes medication, such as sertraline, can also help but I would like to be guided by their expertise. Is that okay?

Empathy ☐ I realise this is a lot to take in and may be a bit scary; how do you feel about it?

Future ☐ Let's continue the sertraline for now as it's helping and I will do the referral.

Specifics ☐ Can I talk to you again in 3 weeks? Please book an appointment online or by phoning reception.

Safety net ☐ If you are worsening in the meantime, please let me know. If you feel suicidal you can phone the Samaritans, but if you feel in danger call the crisis team. Thanks for talking to me today.

Doctor's notes	Andrea Lockwood, 36 years. PMH: see below. Medications: sertraline 50 mg daily. Past medication: fluoxetine, sertraline, mirtazapine.
	GP appointment 4 weeks ago: 'Becoming depressed again, feeling low. Not sleeping or eating well. Got into trouble at work. Only had job for 4 weeks when got into an argument with a colleague, resulting in her quitting the job on the spur of the moment. Feels colleague was out to get her. Worried about money. Lives alone, no local family. Finds it hard to keep friends, says no close friends. Has a nice neighbour who looks in on her occasionally. Having fleeting thoughts of suicide, no plans or attempts. Has been cutting wrists again, superficial wrist wounds seen. Plan: restart sertraline, TCI 3–4 weeks for review. Crisis team number given to patient and worsening advice given.'
How to act	Low.
PC	*'So, things aren't much better, Doctor.'*
History	You had a tough start in life as your natural father was an alcoholic so your home life was chaotic. Your father died following an accident related to alcohol. Your mother was devastated but over time came to terms with what had happened. Your mother suffered with anxiety and depression and was once hospitalised due to her depression. She met a new partner whom you did not like. You disclosed to a counsellor that your stepfather abused you when you were 13 years old but you do not want to go to the police about this now. He and your mother are separated and you do not see him anymore. Your relationship with your mother is variable. It's good at the moment. Over the years you have seen many health professionals about low mood. They never help you. You have repeatedly self-harmed and on one occasion took a paracetamol overdose, although you didn't really intend to die. You find that you can make friends easily but often the friendships fail due to arguments; you often feel that the friend doesn't really care about you. You can be impulsive. You have never had a job which lasted more than a few months. You will spend money that you don't have and react to situations without thinking of the consequences. You have once been in trouble with the police due to shoplifting, and you were let off with a caution. At present you feel low and worthless. You have been cutting your wrists as this gives you a sense of relief. You have had thoughts that it would be better if you weren't alive but haven't made plans to end your life. The sertraline has helped a little.
	You have no symptoms of psychosis. You want your life to get better and feel you need help from people who *'won't let me down'*. People always give you a tablet then pass you on to someone else. You would like continuity of care. You call the Samaritans regularly. This helps to release anger if you don't want to cut yourself.
Social	Currently unemployed, you were given a 'Med 3 fit note' by the GP in your last appointment. You drink alcohol occasionally. You smoke 15 cigarettes a day. No illicit drug use. You live alone in a rented flat.
ICE	You think you are depressed. You would like to continue sertraline. You are open to the idea of seeing a specialist if the doctor suggests this.

Personality disorders can be quite difficult to identify but be suspicious in patients with repeating patterns of behaviour, such as self-harm, emotional instability, criminal activity, problems maintaining relationships or difficulties functioning in day-to-day life (unable to keeps jobs, etc.). Personality disorders are thought to develop due to a combination of genetic factors and 'nurture' factors (early life experiences, abuse). Our personalities have normally formed between our mid-teens to early 20s. Although our personalities cannot be changed (hence personality disorders are often labelled untreatable), intervention can help patients cope with their difficulties and enable them to function better and have a more stable and fulfilling life. NICE recommends a structured approach to assessment and management. Psychotherapy can be effective and drug therapy may help in some cases (e.g. antidepressants to treat depressive symptoms). Antipsychotics or sedatives can be used for short-term crisis management but are not advised long term.[1-3]

Below is a summary of the different categories of personality disorder and their typical features. From http://www.rcpsych.ac.uk/healthadvice/problemsdisorders/personalitydisorder.aspx

Cluster A: ('Odd or Eccentric')	Features:
Paranoid	Suspicious, feelings of persecution, feel easily rejected, hold grudges[4]
Schizoid	Emotionally cold, prefer being alone, 'have a rich fantasy world'[4]
Schizotypal	'Eccentric behaviour, odd ideas, difficulties with thinking, lack of emotion or inappropriate reactions',[4] visual or auditory hallucinations, may have features of schizophrenia[4]
Cluster B ('Dramatic, Emotional and Erratic')	**Features:**
Antisocial or Dissocial	Lack of empathy, easily frustrated, aggressive, criminal activity, difficulty forming close relationships, impulsive, lack of guilt, do not learn from unpleasant experiences[4]
Borderline or Emotionally Unstable	Impulsive, hard to control emotions, features of depression/low mood/low self-worth, self-harm, difficulty maintaining relationships, may feel paranoid, can have auditory hallucinations[4]
Histrionic	Over-dramatic, self-centred, suggestible, worry about appearance, look for excitement and new things, and can be seductive[4]
Narcissistic	Strong sense of self-importance, desire success, power and intellectual greatness, crave attention but don't reciprocate, take advantage of others and don't return favours[4]
Cluster C ('Anxious and Fearful')	**Features:**
Obsessive–Compulsive (Anankastic)	Worry, doubt, perfectionists, rigid routines, cautious and preoccupied with detail, difficulty adapting, judgemental, sensitive to criticism, obsessional thoughts, high moral standards[4]
Avoidant (Anxious/Avoidant)	Very anxious/tense, insecure, feels inferior, extremely sensitive to criticism, have to be liked[4]
Dependent	Passive, can't make decisions, submissive, difficulty coping with daily tasks, feel hopeless and abandoned[4]

Doctor's Notes

Patient	Chloe Livingstone-Smith 28 years F
PMH	Failed forceps delivery and emergency lower segment caesarean section 2 weeks ago
Medications	No current medications
Allergies	No information
Consultations	Midwife visit at home yesterday.
	'Baby doing well, no jaundice, yellow stool nappies. Regained birth weight. Forceps mark fading. Breastfeeding. Up 2-hourly in the night. Mum tired. Not been out, says worried baby will pick up an infection, made an odd comment about the government, seems a little tearful, suggested talks to GP, asked husband to make her an appointment tomorrow.'
Investigations	No information
Household	Damian Smith 32 years M
	James Smith 2 weeks M

Open ☐	I see you had a baby 2 weeks ago, congratulations! Is James your baby's name? How has it been going? How are you? How is James? What has been the biggest challenge?
History ☐	How was your delivery? Is this your first child? How are you getting on with feeding? Is James sleeping well? Have you managed to get any rest? Who's at home? What support are you getting?
Sense ☐	You said that you couldn't talk for long on the phone; is there anything particular making you feel the need to rush?
Flags ☐	Have you been feeling particularly sad or worried since James was born? Why do you think he may be getting an infection? Is there anything that has happened to make you think the government wants to take him away? Do you believe that the government is speaking to you or sending you messages? Do you worry that the government can hear your thoughts or interfere with your thoughts? Do you ever hear or see things which other people cannot? Have you ever had thoughts about harming James? Or harming yourself? Have you done anything to protect James from the government?
Risk ☐	Do you know if any other woman in your family has had problems with their mood after having a baby? Have you ever had problems with your mood before?
ICE ☐	I see that your husband made the telephone appointment for you today, but had you any thoughts about what you would like to happen? You are clearly worried that James may become ill and that the government may take him away; would you like my help with this?
Experience ☐	Have you ever come across a situation where a mother has become unwell with mood problems after having a baby?
Curious ☐	What does your husband think? Is he worried about you or James?
SummarICE ☐	So you had your baby, James, 2 weeks ago. You had a tough time during the delivery but did recover well. Now, however, you feel unable to take James out of the house due to fear of him becoming unwell or that the government will take him off you as you believe it thinks you are a bad mother. You have been avoiding other people and have been keeping James clean by bathing him 3 times a day and changing his nappy every hour. You have unplugged the TV to stop the government sending you messages and to stop it spying on you. You would like help to protect yourself and James but aren't sure whom you can trust. Is there anything else you would like to tell me?
Explanation ☐	It seems to me, Chloe, that you may be suffering from a condition that can develop after having a baby and causes the mother to have severe mood problems. The condition is called postpartum psychosis. It sounds like your grandmother may have had the same problem.
InCludE ☐	Your feelings of being scared and anxious are very real but they are because you are unwell, not because anyone wants to take James away from you.
Recommend ☐	I would really like to get you some help with this today. To get the best help, I would like to speak to our specialist colleagues at the hospital and ask them to see you today.
Empathy ☐	I understand this is a scary prospect and it must seem that we are ganging up on you but I would really like to get you some help.
Future ☐	There is a special ward at the hospital where you and James can go until you are feeling better. James will stay with you so you don't need to worry that someone will take him away. How does that sound? Can I call your husband and ask him to come home to be with you? We can then arrange for you to go up to the hospital.
Safety net ☐	Is your friend able to stay with you until your husband arrives? If you feel worried or change your mind about seeing the hospital doctor, let us know and we can talk it through again.
Specifics ☐	When I phone your husband, may I explain to him what you have told me? When you are discharged, please let me know and I will come and visit you and James at home.

Patient's Story

Doctor's notes
Chloe Livingstone-Smith, 28 years. PMH: failed forceps delivery and ELSCS 2 weeks ago. Medications: none. Midwife visit yesterday: 'Baby doing well, no jaundice, yellow stool nappies. Regained birth weight. Forceps mark fading. Breastfeeding. Up 2-hourly in the night. Mum tired. Not been out, says worried baby will pick up an infection, made an odd comment about the government, seems a little tearful, suggested talks to GP, asked husband to make her an appointment tomorrow.'

How to act
Agitated. You want to reassure the doctor that all is well; however, you open up to the doctor when he/she explores your thoughts.

PC
'Can we make this quick, Doctor, I can't talk for long.'

History
You had your first baby, James, 2 weeks ago. You were induced due to being overdue and had a torrid time in hospital. The induction took a long time and resulted in a failed forceps delivery followed by an emergency caesarean section as James had become distressed in the womb. You were in hospital a couple of days recovering. James needed to be monitored as he had inhaled some meconium and the doctors were worried about infection. Since being discharged, you have become extremely anxious about James becoming unwell, especially that he will get an infection. You change his nappy hourly to keep him clean and bath him three times a day. You worry that the government is trying to take him away from you. You think that it sends messages through the television to you, telling you to give him up as you can't look after him properly and keep him safe and clean. You have unplugged the television and won't allow your husband to watch it. James is at home in another room and you have booked the phone consultation as you didn't want the government to snatch him if you went out. Your husband has told you that you need a telephone consultation check-up to see how you are getting on after the caesarean. He has booked the appointment for you. You remember your mother telling you that her mother went into an 'asylum' after giving birth to her. A friend is with you now, holding James whilst you phone the doctor. You have no thoughts of harming yourself or anyone else. You want to keep the baby safe. You trust your husband and friend.

Social
You are a designer for a large fashion company; previously you have travelled the world through your work. You married a photographer, whom you met whilst working on a fashion show. Your husband was keen to have children as he is a little older than you. You weren't sure at first as you didn't want to take a lot of time off work but were happy when you fell pregnant. Your parents live in Miami, so you don't see them often. You are an only child. Your in-laws live fairly locally and have been helping out.

ICE
You believe that your baby will be taken from you by the government as it thinks you are an unfit mother. You love your baby and have been doing everything you can to protect him, especially from infection. You do not want to go back to hospital. You think the doctor may be on the government's side but, if he/she explains kindly and empathetically, you agree to his/her plan. You are happy for the doctor to speak to your husband on the phone.

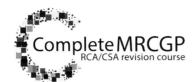
CompleteMRCGP
RCA/CSA revision course

Mood changes after delivery are common but we must all be on the lookout for women who may be struggling with a mental illness.

'Baby blues' – Very common (>50%). Low mood, irritability, anxiety and tearfulness are common symptoms. Usually occurs day 3–4 postnatally and has usually resolved by day 10. Be suspicious if symptoms persist beyond 2 weeks.

Postnatal depression – Occurs in 10–15% of women. Typically begins within the first 8 weeks but can occur several months later. Often there is a history of depression during pregnancy, although this isn't always picked up. More severe and longer lasting than 'baby blues'. Same symptoms as with non-pregnancy related depression, i.e. low mood, tearful, changes in sleep, changes in appetite, anxiety and anhedonia. May be some more specific symptoms related to having a new baby, e.g. difficulty bonding with the baby, lack of emotional connection to the baby, feeling guilty for not loving the baby enough, resenting the baby for the way they feel, thoughts of harming the baby. As with all patients with depression, it is essential to assess any risk posed by the patients to themselves or others. In postnatal depression, be especially alert to risk to the baby or other children in the household.

Screening questions – NICE recommends the following screening questions to help identify PND. '*During the past month, have you often been bothered by feeling down, depressed or hopeless? During the past month, have you often been bothered by having little interest or pleasure in doing things?*' Any positive response should lead to further assessment, possibly using a tool such as the Edinburgh Postnatal Depression Scale. NICE also recommends screening for anxiety with the following two questions (GAD-2):

Over the last 2 weeks, how often have you been bothered by feeling nervous, anxious or on edge?

Over the last 2 weeks, how often have you been bothered by not being able to stop or control worrying?[1]

Depending on the severity of the symptoms, the mother may be able to care for herself and her baby without much extra support, but in severe cases the mother may struggle to complete simple tasks. In milder cases, health visitors, community mental health teams, etc. can be called upon to help treat the patient in the community setting, with support from the family, partner or a carer. In more severe cases, involvement of the perinatal psychiatry team or even admission to a specialist mother and baby unit may be required. Where possible, the mother and baby should be kept together.

Postpartum psychosis (puerperal psychosis – Much rarer, occurring in 0.1%. Typically begins suddenly within the first 2 weeks following delivery. Symptoms vary but include severe depression, mania, hallucinations and delusions. It may occur in a woman with no history of mental illness, but the risk is increased if there is a personal or family history of mental illness (particularly of postpartum psychosis). There are frequently delusions about the baby: 'the baby is evil'. The patient may demonstrate typical features of psychotic illness, e.g. pressure of speech, knight's move thinking, delusions (e.g. paranoia, grandiose thoughts or ideas of persecution) or auditory/visual hallucinations.

Postpartum psychosis is a psychiatric emergency and NICE recommends referral for immediate assessment (within 4 hours) and, where possible, the mother should be treated in a specialist mother and baby unit. Thankfully the prognosis is good with the worst symptoms usually improving around 12 weeks and the majority of cases resolving between 6 and 12 months. However, there is a 50% chance of recurrence in future pregnancies.

Antipsychotic-induced hyperprolactinaemia
See the Link Hub at CompleteMRCGP.co.uk for helpful advice when commencing an antipsychotic.

Doctor's Notes

Patient	Eleanor Cartwright	15 years	F
PMH	Constipation aged 4 years		
	Lower respiratory tract infection 11 years		
Medications	No current medications		
Allergies	No known allergies		
Consultations	No recent consultations		
Investigations	No information		
Household	Brian Cartwright	55 years	M
	Faith Cartwright	54 years	F
	Attends with mother.		

Example Consultation

Open ☐ Hello Ellie. Please tell me what led you to book the appointment today? What have you talked about at home? How do you feel about this? How do you feel about your health? Faith, what are your thoughts please? Have you noticed anything else that has worried you?

Impact ☐ Ellie, have you noticed a change to your body? Have things at home changed? What about at school? Faith, have you noticed a change in Ellie? Have teachers?

History ☐ Ellie, have you had any medical problems? Do you take any medicines? Who is at home? Faith – may I speak to Ellie alone briefly? It is always helpful, thank you. Ellie – how are things at home? What is your mum worried about, do you think? What do you like to do when you are not at school? How is school? Have you noticed a change to any parts in your body? Going to the toilet, headaches or periods? Are you pleased or is that a worry?

Curious ☐ Ellie, your mum says you sometimes get angry. What makes you feel this way?

Risk ☐ Is anyone at school horrible? Because your periods have stopped, I have to make sure you are not pregnant: do you have a boyfriend? Have you had sex? Has anyone made you feel uncomfortable or hurt you? Do you take drugs or drink alcohol?

Flags ☐ Do you feel unhappy or tearful? Do you sleep okay? Can you concentrate? Do you ever wish you were not alive? Have you tried to hurt yourself? Do you ever see or hear things that others can't? Or receive instructions that others are not aware of? Are you happy for me to share with your mum your feelings and periods?

Sense ☐ Ellie and I have talked about her missed periods. I do sense you are very worried.

ICE ☐ Ellie, do you know why we are concerned? Is there anything you are worried about? When you were waiting for the call-back, what did you think I might say? Faith, what are your thoughts about what Ellie may be going through? What worries you most? Is there anything else? Is there anything specific you were hoping I would do today?

Examination ☐ Ellie – can you tell me what your height and weight are? Thank you. As your height is 165 cm and your weight is 40 kg, it means that your BMI is 14.6, so you are very underweight.

SummarICE ☐ To summarise, Ellie, you decided to change what foods you eat and exercise more over the past 5 months. Since then, your parents and school teacher have been concerned about you and especially after your mum heard you being sick.

Experience ☐ Ellie, do you know the risks of losing weight? Faith, can you tell me more about what you have read? Faith, have you come across this before?

Examination ☐ I would like to see you and your mum at the surgery later today please – to confirm your height and weight, check your blood pressure and pulse, and feel your tummy and your neck to make sure there is no other reason why you may have lost weight. Is that okay?

Recommend ☐ I would also like to do a full set of blood tests to check what may be out of balance including your hormones, thyroid, sugar, liver and kidneys and blood cells and also a heart tracing (ECG). Can you come in at 3.30 p.m. today?

Impression ☐ Ellie, it sounds as if you have decided that controlling your weight is really important to you. Sometimes, without realising it, a person can lose too much weight as they continue to focus on avoiding food and start to be sick to avoid absorbing food. This is called an eating disorder and your weight is now at a dangerous level. What is going through your mind?

Explanation ☐ The body needs nutrition to work. Periods stopping is a sign your body is not healthy.

InCludE ☐ Exercise is not safe at present as you may become extremely unwell if you lose more weight.

Recommend ☐ I would also like to write to the children's psychiatry team who can help you be in control again at a safe and healthy level.

Specifics ☐ I will call you with the blood results and the children's team should see you in the next week.

Safety net ☐ If either of you are concerned, don't hesitate to speak to a doctor. Call 111 if we are closed.

Patient's Story

Eating Disorder

Doctor's notes   Eleanor Cartwright, 15 years. PMH: constipation aged 4 years. LRTI aged 11 years. Medications: none.

How to act   Eleanor is quiet. Mother (Faith) is initially abrupt but then quiet also.

PC   **Faith**   *'I want to know what is wrong with Ellie. I'm very worried. She keeps to herself and is getting angry when we try to talk to her. We just want to help you, Ellie!'*

History   **Eleanor**   You don't know what's wrong and tell the doctor you don't know why your mother has made the telephone appointment. However, you are aware that your mum and dad are watching you eat and don't trust you. You sleep okay. You deny losing your appetite or decreasing your meal size. You just eat healthier food. You are annoyed that your parents have stopped you from exercising when you return home from school. You just want to be healthy. It started when you realised that the other girls at swimming looked 'better' than you. You felt 'fat' so just decided to eat better and exercise – that's what everyone tells you is good for you anyway so you don't see the problem. You eat with your parents but feel annoyed if they try to sneak extra food onto your plate. You hope to lose more weight as you don't think anything has changed since you started being healthier 5 months ago. You do not use laxatives. You do not disclose to the doctor that you have started vomiting. You have always been well and there is no family history. Your periods stopped 4 months ago. You have never had sex. You have no other symptoms.

Faith   You heard Ellie vomiting whilst the shower was running yesterday which is why you have made the appointment today. Ellie has lost a lot of weight. Originally you thought this was because her body was changing. When you were at college, a girl died from an eating disorder. Ellie has lost contact with her friends.

Social   **Eleanor**   You are in all the top sets at the local school. Your mother is a journalist and you don't know what your father does exactly but he is always very busy. You get on 'fine'. You play the piano and the clarinet and have your grade 6 piano exam next month. You have stopped liking school.

ICE   **Eleanor**   You don't know why your mother has made the appointment but, if pushed for an answer, your mum is watching what you are eating. You are not worried and expect the doctor will tell you to eat more. You don't like periods and you are thrilled they have stopped.

Faith   You believe Ellie is becoming very obsessed with her weight. You do not mention the words anorexia but you do admit to *'looking on the internet at problems with eating'.* However, you haven't yet come to terms with Ellie having this problem. You are concerned that Ellie has become a recluse and no longer goes out with her friends and her test results have dropped. The schoolteacher called you to say she was worried about Ellie's weight. Since this call last week, you have been watching Ellie. You feel very guilty and worry what the school will think. You would like the doctor to tell Ellie that she cannot exercise until she puts on more weight and to refer her for counselling. You are aware Ellie's periods have stopped and have talked about this.

Examination   BMI 14.6. BP 90/60. HR 58 bpm. Abdomen soft, non-tender with no masses or organomegaly. No lymphadenopathy. HS normal. No palpable thyroid.

Information taken from NICE Guideline NG69. Eating disorders: recognition and treatment. December 2020.[1] Please refer to full guidance.

As well as an unusually low or high BMI or body weight for their age, other factors should raise suspicion[1]

- Rapid weight loss
- Weight concerns and not overweight
- Menstrual disturbances

- Atypical dental wear (e.g. erosion)
- Gastrointestinal symptoms

Diagnosis

'Do not use single measures such as BMI or duration of illness to determine whether to offer treatment for an eating disorder.'

Assessment should include[1]	Physical
	Psychological
	Social
	Possibility of alcohol or substance abuse
	Risk to self and risk of abuse
	Need for emergency care in people whose physical health is compromised or who have a suicide risk
Observations/ Investigations	Heart rate, BP, weight.
	Be vigilant for refeeding syndrome, bradycardia and hypotension.
Management	Refer **immediately** to and be guided by your local community eating disorder team. Watchful waiting not considered appropriate for suspected eating disorders.
	Consider emergency admission if: 'severe electrolyte imbalance, severe malnutrition, severe dehydration or signs of incipient organ failure.'[1]
	For adults, consider psychological treatment such as:
	'Individual eating-disorder-focused cognitive behavioural therapy (CBT-ED)
	Maudsley Anorexia Nervosa TReatment for Adults (MANTRA)
	Specialist supportive clinical management (SSCM)'[1]
	Advise people with an eating disorder who are misusing laxatives or diuretics that laxatives and diuretics do not reduce calorie absorption and so do not help with weight loss [and] to gradually reduce and stop laxative or diuretic use.'[1]
	Regular medical and dental reviews if vomiting.[1]
	Osteoporosis risk – 'Advise people with anorexia nervosa and osteoporosis or related bone disorders to avoid high-impact physical activities and activities that significantly increase the chance of falls or fractures.'[1]
	'Advise people with an eating disorder who are exercising excessively to stop doing so.'[1]
	'Monitor growth and development in children and young people with anorexia nervosa who have not completed puberty (for example, not reached menarche or final height).'[1]
	At least annual review if stable/remission.
Respect confidentiality	Hold discussions in places where confidentiality, privacy and dignity can be respected but explain the limits of confidentiality, i.e. which professionals have access to information and when this may be shared. For children or young people <16, respect Gillick competence.

Metabolic Problems and Endocrinology

	Cases in this chapter	Within the RCGP 2020 curriculum: Metabolic Problems and Endocrinology	Learning points in this chapter include:
1	Hyperglycaemia	'Recognise and manage metabolic and endocrine emergencies' 'Systems of care for people with metabolic/endocrine conditions'	Case involves offering continuity of care and follow-up after the acute treatment of hyperglycaemia Ketones, HONK and lactic acidosis
2	Hyperparathyroidism	'Disorders of calcium metabolism, including hypoparathyroidism, hyperparathyroidism and osteomalacia; association with chronic kidney disease'	Hypercalcaemia differential Differential diagnosis of raised PTH
3	Tired All the Time	'Adrenal diseases including… Cushing's syndrome'	Cushing's syndrome
4	Hyperthyroidism	'Thyroid diseases including… hyperthyroidism'	Managing hyperthyroidism flow diagram
5	Diabetes in Pregnancy	'Gestational diabetes'	Counselling pre-conception and risks of diabetes in pregnancy
Extra Notes	Antihyperglycaemics	'Medication in diabetes management, including glucose and lipid lowering therapies, anti-platelets, ACE inhibitors and antihypertensives; recommended treatment targets; and insulin regimes, administration and dosages'	Antihyperglycaemics

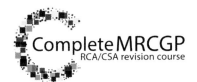

CompleteMRCGP
RCA/CSA revision course

CHAPTER 14 REFERENCES

Hyperglycaemia
1. https://www.nhs.uk/conditions/diabetic-ketoacidosis/. May 2020.

Hyperparathyroidism
1. http://patient.info/doctor/hyperparathyroidism-pro. Mar 2016.
2. NICE Guideline NG132. Hyperparathyroidism (primary): diagnosis, assessment and initial management. https://www.nice.org.uk/guidance/ng132. May 2019.

Tired All the Time
1. http://patient.info/doctor/cushings-syndrome-pro. Aug 2020.

Hyperthyroidism
1. NICE CKS. https://cks.nice.org.uk/topics/hyperthyroidism/. Jan 2021.
2. British Thyroid Foundation leaflet – 'Your guide to hyperthyroidism' and 'Your guide to antithyroid drug treatment to treat hyperthyroidism'.

Diabetes in Pregnancy
1. NICE guideline NG3. Diabetes in pregnancy: management from pre-conception to the postnatal period. https://www.nice.org.uk/guidance/ng3. Dec 2020.

Antihyperglycaemics
1. NICE Guideline NG28. Type 2 diabetes: management. Dec 2020.
2. NICE CKS. https://cks.nice.org.uk/topics/diabetes-type-2/prescribing-information/. May 2021.
3. https://patient.info/doctor/antihyperglycaemic-agents-used-for-type-2-diabetes
4. https://www.gov.uk/drug-safety-update/pioglitazone-risk-of-bladder-cancer
5. https://www.gov.uk/drug-safety-update/sglt2-inhibitors-updated-advice-on-increased-risk-of-lower-limb-amputation-mainly-toes
6. https://www.gov.uk/drug-safety-update/sglt2-inhibitors-updated-advice-on-the-risk-of-diabetic-ketoacidosis

Useful Resource

NICE Guideline NG28, Type 2 diabetes: management (Dec 2020) contains a very useful algorithm for blood glucose lowering therapy in adults with type 2 diabetes.

Information taken from NICE guidelines with kind permission. Please note the guidelines change frequently and you should ALWAYS check for the latest updated guidance. Remember that NICE guidance is only applicable to patients in the UK.

Metabolic Problems and Endocrinology

Doctor's Notes

Patient	Mary Owen 35 years F
PMH	Type 1 diabetes
	Anxiety
	IBS
Medications	Insulin glargine, NovoRapid, citalopram and buscopan
Allergies	No information
Consultations	DNA letter from hospital diabetes clinic
Investigations	No information
Household	No household members registered

Example Consultation

Open ☐ Oh dear. In what way unwell? When did you last feel your normal self? Okay, take it from that day and tell me what symptoms you noticed in sequence if you can. How is your general health usually?

Flags ☐ How are your blood sugars at the moment? Do you have a ketone meter?

Risk ☐ Any symptoms that may suggest infection, for example a cough, sore throat, diarrhoea, changes passing urine or tummy pain or abnormal vaginal discharge? Is it painful to pass urine? Are you racing to the toilet? Or passing a small or large amount each time? Any blood? Any rash, stiffness of the neck or discomfort looking at the light?

ICE ☐ What do you think may have caused this? What is worrying you? What did you think I might suggest today?

History ☐ Is the insulin regime appropriate for your lifestyle? Has everything been okay with taking your insulin recently? Do you have any other medical problems? How is your anxiety? How are your bowels at present? Do you work? Tell me more about work. Is anyone at home? Are you in a relationship? 'Not really?'

Curious ☐ You say you have been forgetting to take the insulin. Why might this be? Why are you missing meals? You say you haven't got time to worry about work: is everything okay? I'm sorry your mother is not well.

Impact ☐ Have you been struggling with your normal day? Are you feeling low?

O/E ☐ I would like to check your BP, pulse, temperature, listen to your chest, feel your tummy and do a finger prick test for sugar and ketones. I think we also need a urine specimen from you. Please could you pop to the toilet whilst I make a plan.

SummarICE ☐ To summarise, you have felt unwell for 2 days. You believe you have a urine infection, are frightened by your blood sugars being so high and thought I would suggest how to bring them down.

Empathy ☐ It sounds like you are under stress physically and emotionally with a busy career, whilst taking care of your mother to whom you are very close.

Impression ☐ Mary, I believe the raised blood sugar is likely due to a combination of stress and missing insulin doses.

InCludE ☐ And, I agree, a urine infection may have contributed to this. Urine infections are more likely after having sex and with raised sugars. I believe the diagnosis is a urine infection and diabetic ketoacidosis or DKA for short.

Experience ☐ Have you heard of this?

Explanation ☐ Because you do not have a good supply of insulin to move all that sugar into your muscles, your body breaks down fat to make ketones.

Options ☐ You need to go to hospital for treatment through the veins otherwise you will be extremely unwell.

InCludE ☐ Unfortunately, although I know this is what you hoped, we cannot give this care at home. Is your mother a patient with us? What does she need? I can call your mother and suggest arranging emergency care through the Single Point of Access Team whilst you are in hospital. I will phone the medical team at the hospital to let them know you need to come in. I will arrange for an ambulance to take you to hospital.

Future ☐ At the hospital, I expect you will be given fluids, insulin and antibiotics.

Empower ☐ When you are better, please return to see me to discuss your general health, support we could offer and changes to your insulin regime to suit your lifestyle better. I also recommend going to the toilet after sex to prevent water infections as this helps flush out the bacteria that may be pushed up to the bladder during sex. Does this make sense?

Specifics ☐ We can also prescribe a ketone meter and testing strips for you and book an appointment with our PN to demonstrate how to use this.

Safety net ☐ If you feel unwell again, please don't hesitate to speak to a doctor.

Metabolic Problems and Endocrinology–1

Patient's Story

Doctor's notes	Mary Owen, 35 years. PMH: type 1 diabetes, anxiety and IBS.
	Medications: Insulin glargine, NovoRapid, citalopram and Buscopan.
	Consultations: DNA letter from hospital diabetes clinic.
How to act	Slightly breathless and lacking in full concentration.
PC	*'I keep being sick. I feel really unwell.'*
History	Two days ago you started feeling unwell and tired and started to develop stomach pain.
	This morning you started vomiting with abdominal pain and a headache.
	You have no rash and no fever. You have no neck stiffness and no neurological symptoms.
	If the doctor asks you about your breathing, you do feel more breathless but have no other respiratory symptoms. Your blood sugar is 24.
	'I have been forgetting to take the insulin.'
	This is usually because you are *'always on the go'* and you have missed meals.
	You have no fever, but you have been passing urine more frequently over the past week.
	At first you thought you needed to go but then nothing came out and now you are passing much more urine, you have seen some blood and it is painful.
	Your bowels are currently normal. Your anxiety has been controlled recently.
	You have no other systemic symptoms. You do not have a ketone meter.
Social	You live alone. You are *'not really'* in a relationship. By this you mean you caught up with an old boyfriend and had sex 10 days ago. You used condoms.
	You work in advertising and have been successful in your career which can be stressful and you have suffered with the stress of meeting deadlines and presentations to clients in the past but *'I don't have time to worry about this now.'*
	You only drink minimal alcohol socially. You do not smoke.
	Your mother was diagnosed with leukaemia 3 months ago and she is currently having chemotherapy. You have been driving to see her after work and at the weekends, sometimes staying up with her through the night if she feels unwell.
	She isn't well at present but she made you come to the GP. You are very worried about your mum and will go back to see her after the consultation with the GP.
	You need to return to be with your mother. She has no one else. However, if the doctor explains why you need to go to hospital you will go. Your mother is a patient at the same GP practice. Can the doctors help? She needs someone to check in on her and make sure she has fluid and food tonight. She is very weak and in bed.
ICE	You are worried about your health and you are frightened that your blood sugars are so high. You believe you have a water infection after having sex.
	If the doctor mentions DKA, you have heard of it. You expect the doctor will tell you what to do with your insulin today to bring your sugars down.
Examination	HR 125 bpm. Sats 97%. BP 115/70. RR 19. Temperature 37.4 °C. Abdomen soft, generally tender, no peritonism. Urine dipstick: leucocytes ++, nitrite +++, protein +, blood ++, ketones ++++
	BM = 30 mmol/L. Blood ketones = 3.1 mmol/L. Clinically dehydrated.

Metabolic Problems and Endocrinology – 1

The consultation

When asking if a patient has been compliant with medication, avoid sounding confrontational by asking: 'Are you taking your medicines correctly?' Instead ask: 'Has everything been okay with taking your medication in the way the doctor prescribed?' This is a much softer question and more likely to yield a truthful answer. This case challenges your skills at managing an emergency, practising holistically and negotiation. Without a thorough social history and consideration of the patient's concerns, it is unlikely that the key information about the patient's mother will be uncovered. It is essential to address this concern and offer a solution to allow your patient to accept potentially life-saving treatment.

Most areas have a 'crisis team' who can put emergency care in place (either at home or within a care home) for short-term care issues. It is very important to invite the patient back to discuss ways in which she can access help with her mother (both practically and financially) or at the very least signpost her to local carers' support groups. It is likely she will need long-term support to prevent her own health suffering.

Ketones[1]	<0.6 mmol/L	A normal blood ketone value.
	0.6–1.5 mmol/L	Indicates that more ketones are being produced than normal. Test again in 2 hours.
	1.6–2.9 mmol/L	A high level of ketones and could present a risk of ketoacidosis. It is advisable to contact your diabetes team or GP for advice as soon as possible.
	≥3.0 mmol/L	A very high risk of DKA which will require immediate medical care.[1]
HONK		In type 2 diabetes: Hyperglycaemic Hyperosmolar Non-ketotic Coma.
		This may present with extreme thirst, frequency, confusion and nausea and may progress to coma if not treated promptly.
Lactic acidosis		Diabetic patients may become acidotic especially if they are taking metformin.

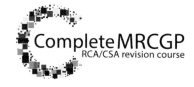

Metabolic Problems and Endocrinology – 1

Doctor's Notes

Patient	Avani Virdee	57 years	F
PMH	No medical history		
Medications	No current medications		
Allergies	No information		
Consultations	Bloods taken for routine health check		
Investigations			

3 weeks ago:

FBC	normal	
U&E/LFT/TFT	normal	
Lipids	normal	
HbA1c	normal	
eGFR	80 mL/min/1.73 m^2	
Corrected Ca	2.73 mmol/L	(2.2–2.6 mmol/L)
Vitamin D	51 nmol/L	(>50 nmol/L) = sufficient
		(30–50 nmol/L) = deficiency
		(<30 nmol/L) = severe deficiency

1 week ago:

PTH	7.9 pmol/L	(1.6–7.2 pmol/L)

Household   No household members registered

Example Consultation

Open ☐	Mrs Virdee, thank you for phoning. What led you to have these tests taken?
Sense ☐	I can hear you are worried and keen to know your result.
Impression ☐	The blood test has shown that a little gland in your neck may be releasing too much hormone which increases the body's calcium level. This is called hyperparathyroidism. The word 'hyper' means too much and the 'parathyroid' is a gland that sits in the neck. All your other blood tests are normal. This can be serious as high calcium levels can make you feel unwell. You are likely to have had it for many months but the good news is that we can often cure this problem.
Experience ☐	Any questions so far? Calcium is good for you in moderation, like most things! Too much calcium can cause you to feel unwell, but we don't usually advise calcium restriction in this condition.
History ☐	To help me work out the best course of action, can I ask a little more about you? Have you felt unwell? Do you have any medical problems? Do you take any medicines?
Flags ☐	Are you more thirsty recently? Passing more urine than normal? Any pain at all? Are your bowels okay? Have you ever had a kidney stone?
ICE ☐	Before you phoned today, did you have any thoughts about what may be wrong? Was there anything else you were hoping to talk about today?
Curious ☐	You mentioned you were tired; what might be causing that do you think?
SummarICE ☐	So to summarise, you were invited for a health check. We have detected a raised calcium level and raised parathyroid hormone level, which is likely to be due to a condition called hyperparathyroidism.
InCludE ☐	Apart from feeling tired, which may be due to your work and family commitments, you feel well. You are keen to know what happens next. Have I got it right so far?
Empathy ☐	I appreciate that any new diagnosis causes worry and apprehension.
O/E ☐	It would be helpful to examine you; to have a feel of your neck for lumps. Would you be able to book an appointment soon for this? Thank you.
Recommend ☐	Assuming the examination confirms what I think, I would suggest we send a referral to the endocrinologists, who are hormone specialists. Thankfully, this is a treatable problem.
Options ☐	We should also do a few more blood tests, when you come in, to recheck the calcium level as we haven't done this for 3 weeks. I usually also keep an eye on the kidneys to make sure you are not dehydrated. I would also suggest a bone scan, because some calcium will have come out of the bones, which can weaken them.
Empower ☐	You don't need to reduce the calcium in your diet, but it is important to avoid dehydration.
Future ☐	I expect the endocrinologists will see you within the next month. At the hospital they will probably do further tests and may offer an operation to cure the problem by removing the gland. Sometimes no treatment is required, particularly if the calcium level stays below 3.
Safety net ☐	If you ever start to feel thirsty, start passing more urine, have any pains or tummy upset, please come to see me as these may be symptoms of raised calcium. That is a lot of information; may I check I have been clear – what symptoms will lead you to contact the GP straight away? Thank you. See you soon – and please bring any further questions with you.

Patient's Story Hyperparathyroidism

Doctor's notes	Avani Virdee, 57 years. PMH: none. Medications: none.
	Bloods taken for routine health check. Raised calcium and PTH.
	Other bloods normal.
How to act	Keen to know your results and what it means.
PC	*'I was told to have a second blood test and then I've received another letter saying you wanted to speak to me about my tests… What's wrong?'*
History	You have been a little tired but are otherwise very well.
	You had a suspected kidney stone 4 months ago, but the pain settled spontaneously so you didn't go for your USS. You have had no pain since.
Social	You are married with 2 children.
	You are a medical secretary. You are Sikh.
	You are a new grandmother so are often on the road travelling to see the family.
ICE	You thought you were tired because you are busy with work and the family.
	You haven't slept well this week with fear over what the doctor may say.
	You do not know what to expect.
	You have never heard of hyperparathyroidism. You want to know all about it.
Ask the doctor	*'I thought calcium was good for you.'*
	'What has caused it?'
	'Should I stop eating yoghurt and milk?'
Examination	Examination of the neck is normal with no lymphadenopathy.

Learning Points

PTH is released in response to low calcium.

Primary hyperparathyroidism
Causes include an adenoma on the parathyroid gland or familial endocrine disorders (e.g. multiple endocrine neoplasia).

Blood tests show a raised albumin-adjusted calcium + raised PTH + reduced phosphate.

Symptoms[1]		
	Asymptomatic	(often if calcium is below 3).
	'Bones'	Fractures from reduced BMD, fatigue and myopathy.
	'Stones'	Kidney stones.
	'Groans'	Nausea, vomiting, constipation, gastritis and pancreatitis.
	'Moans'	Malaise, confusion, depression or reduced GCS.
	Dehydration	Polydipsia, polyuria and dehydration.

Hypercalcaemia

Differential diagnosis	Investigations required/findings	
Myeloma	Normal PTH	Anaemia + renal impairment + monoclonal gammopathy
Bone metastases	Normal PTH	CT CAP if previous malignancy
Sarcoidosis	Normal PTH	CXR
Paget's	Normal PTH	Raised ALP
Addison's	Normal PTH	Low Na + raised K
Vitamin D toxicity	Normal PTH	Raised vitamin D
Thyrotoxicosis	Normal PTH	Raised T4

Differential diagnosis of raised PTH

Iatrogenic (e.g. lithium)	Normal calcium
Vitamin D deficiency	
Secondary ↑PTH	Low/normal calcium drives the rise in PTH
Tertiary hyperparathyroidism	Similar picture to primary ↑PTH and occurs in CKD[1]

Management of primary hyperparathyroidism[2]
Refer for surgery if symptoms of hypercalcaemia, renal stones, fractures, osteoporosis.

Calcimimetics (cinacalet – check licensing) if surgery unsuccessful or declined or Ca >2.85 mmol/L + symptoms or >3.0 mmol/L.

Consider bisphosphonates (see NICE guideline).

Annual bloods: albumin-adjusted Ca, eGFR.

Imaging: biannual DEXA. USS renal tract if possible renal stones.

Doctor's Notes

Patient	Jayne Fitzpatrick 31 years F
PMH	Wrist fracture
	Recurrent urinary tract infections – three in the past 6 months.
	Tonsillitis
	Chlamydia
	Termination of pregnancy
	Stress at work
Medications	No current medications
Allergies	No information
Consultations	Bloods taken for routine health check
Investigations	No recent results
Household	No household members registered

Example Consultation

Tired All the Time

Open ☐	Tell me more about how you feel. Any other changes? How are you sleeping?
Impact ☐	How is feeling so tired affecting you day to day? In any other ways?
Sense ☐	You seem puzzled as to what may be causing it.
History ☐	What medical problems have you had? How are you now? How is your mood now? Do you take any medicines from the pharmacy or supplements? Any stress in your life or worries? Is anyone at home with you? Do you have family? Are you in a relationship? Do you take any contraception? How did you break your wrist?
ICE ☐	What do you think may be causing this? Is there anything you are particularly worried about or that has crossed your mind? Is there anything you were hoping we would decide today?
Flags ☐	Do you know if you snore or have any pauses in your breathing? Would you have a sleep if you were sitting down quietly in the afternoon, a passenger in a car or in a meeting? Is there any chance you could be pregnant? When was your last period? Was it a normal period? Are they regular? Or heavy? I see you had a urine infection in the past; do you have any symptoms of going more often or burning? Any weight loss or drenching night sweats? Have you felt flushed at times? Any headaches? Have your arms or legs felt different or floppy? Any visual changes? Any recent colds, ear or throat problems? Any problems with your breathing or in the chest? Stomach pain or change in bowels? Have you noticed any unusual dizziness or palpitations? Tell me more about the dizziness: room spinning or feeling lightheaded? What is your eating regime like? Do you avoid any food groups?
Risk ☐	Are there any medical problems that run in the family? Have you travelled in the past couple of years? Or had any recent illnesses or rashes or bites?
Impression ☐	I wonder if this may be a problem originating from the over- or under-production of a hormone, although there are many reasons why one may be tired.
Explanation ☐	The thyroid function, blood sugar level or red cell blood level can all cause tiredness.
SummarICE ☐	To summarise, you have been feeling exhausted for 4 months. It is unlike you to need time off work. You have also noticed a few symptoms: passing urine frequently, weight gain, light-headedness and absent periods. Your skin and hair are different. You believe you may be low and feel your thinking processes are perhaps slower. In the past 6 months you have broken your wrist and had urine infections.
Empathy ☐	It must be a real struggle when you feel so tired.
Examination ☐	I would like to see you at the surgery to measure your height, weight and blood pressure, look at your skin and hands, listen to your heart and lungs, feel your stomach, your neck and legs, look in your eyes and check your vision please. Would you be able to bring a urine sample?
Options ☐	I would also like to arrange a blood test to check for anaemia, check your liver and kidneys, your hormones such as thyroid, the hormones that control your periods, and a blood test which shows the level of your steroid hormone. It would also be helpful if you could collect your urine for 24 hours, again to check for the amount of steroid in your body. I'll give you a container when you come in.
Empower ☐	I would avoid alcohol whilst you are feeling like this and try to go for walks even if you are feeling exhausted.
InCludE ☐	You can of course take a multivitamin if you wish but this is unlikely to make a difference, especially as you are already eating a good diet.
Future ☐	Can we talk again on the phone 3 days after you have handed in your urine and had your blood tests?
Specifics ☐	Once we have the results, I will have a better idea where the problem may lie. Depending on what the first blood test shows, you may need further blood tests or imaging and I may also ask a hormone specialist doctor to see you at the hospital.
Safety net ☐	If you do feel suddenly unwell with new symptoms, for example a headache or vomiting, please see a doctor straight away.

348

Metabolic Problems and Endocrinology–3

Patient's Story

Doctor's notes   Jayne Fitzpatrick, 31 years. PMH: wrist fracture, recurrent UTIs – three in the last 6 months, chlamydia, tonsillitis, termination of pregnancy and stress at work. No current medications.

How to act   Pleasant.

PC   *'I just thought I'd see if there's a reason why I feel tired all the time.'*

History   For the past 4 months you have felt increasingly tired. You sleep well and do not snore or have any pauses in your breathing. You have not fallen asleep during the daytime and even if you do try to rest you would not fall asleep. You already have 8 hours' sleep each night. Your periods are usually regular; however, you haven't had a period for 5 months. Your periods were not heavy. You did a pregnancy test 2 days ago, which was negative. You use condoms but you have not wanted to have sex recently. Being a veterinary nurse, you know about some problems like diabetes and you have noticed a slight thirst and possible increased frequency. You have no symptoms of an infection. You have put on weight but don't know why. You have no night sweats or fevers. You have had no foreign travel other than Europe. You have had no recent rashes. You have had some spots on your face recently. Your bowels are normal. You do not have headaches and have no neurological or visual symptoms but your legs don't feel as strong, e.g. when walking up the stairs. At work you have started to take the lift. You have noticed swelling around your ankles. If asked how this is affecting you – you had to take a day off work last week which you felt guilty about. You have been discussing with the vet how drained you feel. *'I've not needed a day off work since I fractured my wrist 6 months ago – even with urine infections I carry on.'*

You just tripped on the kerb when you fractured the wrist.

Your boss is worried about you; you are usually quite jovial. You feel your thinking is a little slower. You would like your hair to feel nice again. You did feel slightly lightheaded last week. Your ankles swell at the end of the day.

'The vet commented that I've lost my usual spirit.' He encouraged you to take another morning off work to phone the doctor today. If asked about the conversations you have had with the vet: he suggested you need some blood tests and you are hoping the doctor will suggest this today. Straight after the conversation with the vet, you scribbled down a list of what the vet thought the doctor may do. You have this list for the doctor if he/she seems interested in your ideas. *'Anaemia, kidney, thyroid, diabetes, liver, hormones.'* You feel saddened by what the vet said. You don't know why you have lost your spirit. Life should be good. You have not been crying and you don't think you are depressed but perhaps you are a little low.

Social   You are a veterinary nurse. You are in a relationship of 2 years and you plan to move in together soon. Life is not stressful. You drink alcohol occasionally. You do not smoke. You do not currently exercise.

ICE   You are just not sure what has caused it. You wondered if you should take a supplement.

Examination   BMI 27. BP 150/92. Skin – some bruising, acne, abdominal striae.

No palpable thyroid or lymphadenopathy. No hepatosplenomegaly.

HS normal. HR 70 bpm regular. Apyrexial. Hands – no clubbing or nail changes.

Lungs clear. Urine dip negative. Fundi normal.

Metabolic Problems and Endocrinology – 3

Complete CSA's motto 'Common things are common… but what mustn't I miss?'

Have a look at the BMJ Easily Missed series and have a think about how each of these conditions may present.

Cushing's syndrome[1]

Symptoms of Cushing's syndrome arise due to excess levels of glucocorticosteroids (e.g. cortisol). 'The most common cause is the use of exogenous glucocorticoids.'[1]

There are two types of endogenous Cushing's syndrome based on the aetiology:

1. ACTH-dependent, e.g. excessive ACTH production by the pituitary (Cushing's disease), ectopic ACTH production, e.g. malignancy – usually small-cell lung cancer.

2. ACTH-independent, e.g. adrenal adenoma or carcinoma, excess glucocorticoid medication.

Symptoms and signs include: weight gain, buffalo hump, truncal obesity, moon facies, proximal muscle weakness, type 2 diabetes, hypertension, gonadal dysfunction, loss of libido, skin changes (e.g. striae), hypertension, oedema, headaches and visual disturbance if due to a pituitary adenoma.

Investigations:

- 24-hour urinary free cortisol.
- Dexamethasone suppression test. 1 mg oral dexamethasone at 11 p.m. and measure 9 a.m. cortisol.
- Late-night salivary cortisol.

'Tired All the Time'

This is a common presentation in general practice. In the majority of cases no medical cause can be found. Screen for obstructive sleep apnoea, mental health problems, perform a full systemic enquiry and take a detailed social history. If no cause is found, request routine blood tests and advise simple measures such as healthy eating, keeping hydrated, good sleep hygiene, avoiding caffeine and graded exercise can help.

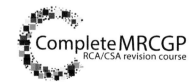

CompleteMRCGP
RCA/CSA revision course

Doctor's Notes

Patient	Fatima Sayed 47 years F
PMH	Graves' disease – 1 year ago
Medications	Carbimazole 20 mg
	Propranolol 40 mg TDS PRN (not issued for 6 months).
Allergies	No known drug allergies
Consultations	12 months ago – goitre palpable, confirmed on USS, no thyroid nodules. Diagnosis Graves' disease. Start carbimazole 30 mg.
	10 months ago – T4 in the normal range. TSH remains low (expected). Decrease carbimazole to 20 mg. Repeat TSH/T4/T3 in 6 weeks. If TSH remains low or T4 increased again increase carbimazole.
	8 months ago – TSH in the normal range. Asymptomatic. Decrease carbimazole to 10 mg.

Investigations

	1 month ago	1 year ago	
TSH	2.2 mIU/L	<0.1 mIU/L	(0.2–4.0 mIU/L)
T4	8.0 pmol/L	32 pmol/L	(10–20 pmol/L)
T3	2.0 nmol/L	3.4 nmol/L	(0.9–2.5 nmol/L)

TSH receptor antibodies positive

Household	Aaqil Sayed 49 years M

Example Consultation

Open ☐ Thank you for phoning. How are you? How are you getting on with the treatment?

Experience ☐ Would you mind taking me back to the start? I'm interested to know what it was like for you before you commenced treatment. What is your understanding of your condition? What is your understanding of the blood results?

ICE ☐ Have you had previous conversations with a GP about when to stop treatment? Have you had anything on your mind that has been worrying you? You mentioned you would like to stop the treatment; is there anything else you were hoping for today?

History ☐ Tell me more about yourself. Have you noticed any new or troublesome symptoms? What dose are you taking of the carbimazole? How often are you taking the tablet? Have you any other medical history? Any medical problems that are in the family? Do you take other medicines or supplements? Any stressors at work or home? Do you drink? Or smoke?

Flags ☐ Is your weight stable? Did you ever have any problem with your eyes or vision?

Impact ☐ And what impact has the Graves' disease had on your life?

Sense ☐ I see you have not seen the GP for 8 months and I'm sensing there may be a reason why you have come to talk to me about the treatment at this time.

Curious ☐ Tell me more about your thoughts about the treatment. I'm wondering why at this stage you feel it would be beneficial to see a specialist.

Examination ☐ Are you able to tell me your pulse and BP? And could you send me a photograph of your face and neck so that I can see your eyes and any swellings in your neck? Thank you.

SummarICE ☐ To summarise, you feel well, all your symptoms of Graves' disease have gone. You started reading about when to discontinue the carbimazole and this led you to forums which discussed the risk of the drug, which has alarmed you and led you to reassess the situation. You are wondering if the benefit of carbimazole no longer outweighs the risk and you would like to discuss stopping treatment with a specialist. Is that correct?

Impression ☐ It does sound like you have had simple Graves' disease, meaning high thyroid levels without signs of eye disease.

Explanation ☐ You are correct; there is a risk of agranulocytosis, 1 in 1000. With any treatment we need to weigh up the benefit of the treatment versus the risk.

Empathy ☐ I can appreciate that when you hear about the frightening risks associated with a tablet and, particularly now that you are well again, it is natural to revisit the decision as to whether the benefits of the tablet continue to outweigh the risks.

InCludE ☐ Looking at your blood tests and feeling your thyroid, a scan would not be helpful now. It was important at the beginning, in order to help make the diagnosis.

Options ☐ We usually treat Graves' disease for about 18 months. I see your recent thyroid levels were in the normal range, and therefore I would usually suggest 5 mg carbimazole for the next 6 months and then, if the blood tests remain normal, aim to stop it when you have completed 18 months of treatment.

Recommend ☐ If you would like to stop it early that is your decision, but there is a risk of your symptoms returning and the disease not being completely treated. I suggest decreasing the carbimazole to 5 mg for 6 weeks, then we can reassess in 6 weeks with a blood test after you have had a chance to think about it. Shall we do that?

Future ☐ If at any stage the TSH drops below the normal range, we need to increase the carbimazole. Once we have stopped the carbimazole I would like to continue to check your TSH level initially after 6 weeks then every 3 months for a year.

Empower ☐ If there were 100 people like you, at the end of the 18 months, 50 of them might need to continue carbimazole.[1] Smoking is a risk factor for this and if you are interested in stopping smoking I would like to help you.

Safety net ☐ If you ever notice a sore throat, rash or infection then arrange a blood test straight away and withhold the medication until you know the blood test is normal.

Patient's Story

Doctor's notes Fatima Sayed, 47 years. PMH: hyperthyroidism – 1 year ago.

Medication: carbimazole 20 mg. Consultations: 1 year ago – goitre palpable, confirmed on USS, no thyroid nodules. Start carbimazole 30 mg.

	1 month ago		1 year ago	
TSH	2.2 mIU/L		<0.1 mIU/L	(0.2–4.0 mIU/L)
T4	8.0 pmol/L		32 pmol/L	(10–20 pmol/L)
T3	2.0 nmol/L		3.4 nmol/L	(0.9–2.5 nmol/L)

TSH receptor antibodies positive.

How to act Pleasant.

PC *'Good morning Doctor. I was hoping to discuss when I could stop my carbimazole please?'*

History Over a year ago you began to lose weight and feel just not yourself. You remember your bowels were loose and you felt quite jittery. Your doctor started carbimazole for high thyroid levels.

Since the treatment you have felt much better. You have always been healthy, take no other medicines and have no FH.

You have read about Graves' disease and have a good understanding of the terms TSH, T3 and T4. You called a month ago and the receptionist said the blood tests were normal.

Social Barrister, married with three children who have now all left home.

You drink no alcohol but smoke five cigarettes a day.

You are active and attend art classes.

ICE *'I should come off it as soon as I can.'* A pragmatic suggestion you believe; however, if the doctor explores your thoughts behind this… You were reading about when to stop carbimazole and came across website forums which reminded you of the risk of the tablet. This led you down the path of reading frightening stories about agranulocytosis and you realised that now you feel well you should stop this tablet. You do not want this problem to happen to you. You wondered whether you should see the specialist again before you finished treatment so she could do a scan again to see if the treatment has to continue. You presume she would rescan and you would like this. You follow the doctor's advice if he or she seems to know what they are doing. Otherwise, you push to see a specialist.

Examination HR 70 bpm regular. BP 120/70. No palpable thyroid.
No sign of eye disease.

Photograph, if sent, shows no enlarged thyroid and no signs of eye disease.

Learning Points

Hyperthyroidism

History: Rapid onset malaise, fever and pain in thyroid (suspect acute thyroiditis)
SOB, hoarseness, dysphagia, neck pressure
Exercise intolerance, fatigue, muscle weakness
↑sweating, heat intolerance. ↑appetite ↓weight
Women: subfertility, oligo-/amenorrhoea. Men: reduced libido, gynaecomastia
See NICE guidelines for full list

Examination: General: agitation, weight loss
Cardiovascular: sinus tachycardia, AF, heart failure, peripheral oedema
Thyroid: enlargement
Hands: fine tremor, palmar erythema
Skin: warm and moist, pruritus, urticaria, vitiligo, diffuse alopecia
MSK: muscle wasting, brisk reflexes
Eyes: exophthalmos, lid retraction, lid lag, chemosis, conjunctivitis, corneal ulceration, strabismus
See NICE guidelines for full list

Next tests: Repeat TSH, T4, T3. FBC (anaemia)
Calcium and LFTs may be raised
Thyroid receptor antibodies (85% positive in Graves')
If positive no need to do a thyroid scintigraphy scan
ESR (raised in Graves' or thyroiditis)
Thyroid scintigraphy scan if unsure on palpation of the thyroid
(GPs may be able to request if antibody negative)

Examine the thyroid

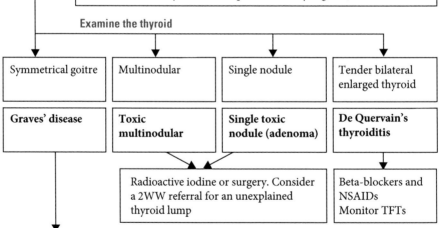

Symmetrical goitre	Multinodular	Single nodule	Tender bilateral enlarged thyroid
Graves' disease	**Toxic multinodular**	**Single toxic nodule (adenoma)**	**De Quervain's thyroiditis**

Radioactive iodine or surgery. Consider a 2WW referral for an unexplained thyroid lump

Beta-blockers and NSAIDs
Monitor TFTs

Emergency admission if thyrotoxic crisis
Refer urgently to endocrinology if pituitary or hypothalamic disorder suspected
For all others with new onset hyperthyroidism: refer to, or discuss with, endocrinology for specialist Ix and management (urgency depends on clinical judgement). Whilst waiting:
• Consider prescribing beta-blocker (titrate dose to clinical response – palpitations/tremor/anxiety/tachycardia). Taper and stop once euthyroid
• If uncertainty about prescribing beta-blocker – seek specialist advice
• Seek specialist advice about starting carbimazole in primary care:
    • If symptoms troublesome despite beta-blocker
    • At risk of complication of hyperthyroidism
    • Taking amiodarone or lithium (liaison with specialist prescribing this drug may be needed)
• Give information leaflet[2]

354

Metabolic Problems and Endocrinology – 4

Doctor's Notes

Patient	Jayne Smith 37 years F
PMH	Type 2 diabetes
	Obesity – last BMI 35
Medications	Metformin 1 g BD
	Gliclazide 40 mg daily
	Rigevidon
Allergies	No information
Consultations	No recent consultations
Investigations	2 months ago HbA1c 51 mmol/mol
Household	No household members registered

Example Consultation

Open ☐	It's great that you are considering this in advance.
Experience ☐	Are you aware of any risks of diabetes in pregnancy?
Sense ☐	I can hear you are keen to control your diabetes. We will look at your diabetes very carefully.
ICE ☐	Is there anything that particularly worries you? What have you been advised so far? Is there anything else you were wondering?
Curious ☐	You seem to have a good understanding. Where has this information come from?
Explanation ☐	Babies can be larger and therefore it's important to control your blood sugar as much as possible. Often babies need delivering a few weeks earlier. They do sometimes initially need help with their blood sugar after birth and some babies need help in the baby unit for a while. In later life, the children can have a higher risk of obesity or developing diabetes themselves. Being overweight can also put you at risk of pregnancy complications so you may need to take other medications such as aspirin when you do become pregnant.
Risk ☐	Do you know what your last HbA1c was?
History ☐	Are you otherwise well? When do you take your medicines? I'm interested to know more about you and your routine.
Impact ☐	How does your diabetes impact on your life? Is there any time you struggle with your diabetes?
SummarICE ☐	To summarise, you have had good control of your diabetes since diagnosis but your HbA1c has crept up and you are hoping for better control as you are planning a pregnancy. You are worried about risks to the baby and are frightened about labour.
Empathy ☐	I appreciate the risks can potentially be scary.
Impression ☐	Being diligent about your health is likely to give a much better outcome for you and the baby. You should be aiming for an HbA1c of <48 mmol/mol. This can be a challenge and we need to avoid hypos – a nickname for hypoglycaemic episodes – which means the blood sugar is too low, putting you at risk.
Explanation ☐	When you do fall pregnant, blood sugars can be more erratic, especially if vomiting.
Experience ☐	Are you aware of the symptoms of a hypo?
Options ☐	Do you have a blood glucose and ketone testing kit? You should start taking 5 mg folic acid, a higher dose than for non-diabetic women, and I will prescribe it for you. You also need extra vitamin D. Let's also arrange your diabetic eye check now. I will ask the secretary to arrange this. You will need more frequent eye checks in pregnancy. We should change your gliclazide to insulin. How do you feel about this? We then need to discuss the benefits of metformin. There is a special clinic which manages women with diabetes in pregnancy and I will refer you to this.
Empower ☐	Continuing exercise will help control your blood sugar. You could see the dietician in case there are any other dietary changes you could make. Any extra weight loss you can achieve will both help you conceive and reduce risk in pregnancy.
InCludE ☐	It is normal to feel anxious and concerned about labour. Is there anything specific that has been going through your mind? The team will be monitoring you and the baby closely and discuss with you when they believe is the safest time to deliver the baby. If you do feel that the worry and anxiety about labour is affecting you, come and see me and we can talk through your options. What are your thoughts?
Future ☐	Shall we look at your blood readings again in a month, then consider insulin together? We should monitor your kidney function and check your chickenpox and rubella status when we take your bloods. Let's do this a couple of days before we meet next time so we can discuss your latest HbA1c then. Please bring a urine sample at the same time to check for protein.
Safety net ☐	Until the HbA1c comes down, are you happy to continue contraception? That is a lot of information, do you have any questions?

Metabolic Problems and Endocrinology–5

Patient's Story

Diabetes in Pregnancy

Doctor's notes	Jayne Smith, 37 years. PMH: type 2 diabetes, obesity. Last HbA1c – 51 mmol/mol. Medications: metformin 1 g BD, gliclazide 40 mg daily, Rigevidon.
How to act	Very interested in your health.
PC	*'My husband and I would like to start a family. I just wanted some advice regarding my diabetes.'*
History	You have had diabetes for 2 years.
	There is a strong history of type 2 diabetes in your family, but you are aware your weight contributed to developing diabetes. The diagnosis provided motivation to make lifestyle changes needed to lose weight and get healthier. You are aware there is some way to go but are proud you have managed to get your BMI down from 46 to 35. You have changed your diet and taken up distance running.
	You take great care but have recently been on holiday.
	You expect your blood sugar may be worse than usual.
	You eat well but often struggle to find time to exercise.
	You have been reading a lot about diabetes and pregnancy.
	You have a BM testing kit which you bought. You know the symptoms of a 'hypo'.
Social	Dental nurse. Married 2 years ago. No alcohol and never smoked.
ICE	You are unsure whether you should stay on your metformin.
	You expect the GP will say start insulin and you are happy with this.
	You are mostly worried about the risks to the baby after birth and in the future.
	You are scared about the labour as you know babies with diabetic mums tend to be big.
	You would like advice about preparing for pregnancy with DM.

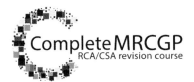

CompleteMRCGP
RCA/CSA revision course

Metabolic Problems and Endocrinology – 5

'Diagnose gestational diabetes if the woman has either: a fasting plasma glucose level of 5.6 mmol/L or above or a 2-hour plasma glucose level of 7.8 mmol/L or above.'[1]

Counselling pre-conception[1]

Book an eye check (unless had one in the last 6 months) and urine ACR.[1]

Folic acid 5 mg/day until 12 weeks.

Offer (up to) monthly HbA1c measurements pre-pregnancy and a BM and ketone kit to all women with type 1 diabetes who are planning a pregnancy.

Advise women with diabetes who are planning to become pregnant to aim for the same capillary plasma glucose target ranges as recommended for all people with type 1 diabetes:

- a fasting plasma glucose level of 5–7 mmol/L on waking **and**
- a plasma glucose level of 4–7 mmol/L before meals at other times of the day.

'Advise women with diabetes who are planning to become pregnant to aim to keep their HbA1c level below 48 mmol/mol (6.5%), if this is achievable without causing problematic hypoglycaemia' 'Reassure women that any reduction in HbA1c level towards the target of 48 mmol/mol (6.5%) is likely to reduce the risk of congenital malformations in the baby.'[1]

Offer a structured education programme as soon as possible if not already attended one.

'Women with diabetes may be advised to use metformin as an adjunct or alternative to insulin in the pre-conception period and during pregnancy, when the likely benefits from improved blood glucose control outweigh the potential for harm. Stop all other oral blood glucose-lowering agents before pregnancy, and use insulin instead.'[1]

Risks[1]

Increased risk of macrosomia and therefore birth complications.

The possibility of temporary health problems in the newborn and possible admission to the neonatal unit.

The risk of obesity and diabetes in the child in later life.

Nausea and vomiting during pregnancy may affect blood sugar control.

Hypoglycaemia unawareness during pregnancy.

Metformin

Discuss the benefits of glycaemic control vs the potential for harm. Refer to http://www.uktis.org/ (UK teratology information service).

Diagnosed gestational diabetes

Refer to:

- 'joint diabetes and antenatal clinic within 1 week'[1]
- a dietitian.

Offer immediate treatment with insulin, with or without metformin, as well as changes in diet and exercise, to women with gestational diabetes who have a fasting plasma glucose level of 7.0 mmol/L or above at diagnosis.[1]

Encourage foods with a low glycaemic index and regular daily exercise.

Targets Do not use HbA1c routinely in the 2nd/3rd trimester.[1]

   Without risking hypoglycaemia, if possible, aim for 'fasting: 5.3 mmol/L and 1 hour after meals: 7.8 mmol/L or 2 hours after meals: 6.4 mmol/L (new 2015).'[1]

Metabolic Problems and Endocrinology – 5

Medication	Metformin	Sulfonylurea	DPP-4 inhibitors
E.g.	Metformin	Glibenclamide, gliclazide, glipizide, glimepiride, tolbutamide	Alogliptin, Linagliptin, Saxagliptin, Sitagliptin, Vildagliptin
Advice – see BNF for full list	Lactic acidosis risk Warn the patient if D&V to stop metformin, ACEI, diuretics and inform the GP Monitor B12	Review at 2 weeks Titrate dose on pre-breakfast BMs	Stop if HbA1c not decreasing, e.g. by >0.5% or 5–6 mmol/mol at 6 months[1]
How given	Oral	Oral	Oral
How it works	↓ glycogenesis ↓ intestinal absorption ↑ insulin sensitivity	↑ insulin secretion	DPP-4 blocks incretin production Incretin ↑insulin
Cautions and contraindications – see BNF for full list	Lactic acidosis risk Recent cardiac, respiratory, liver, renal disease Avoid if eGFR <30 (standard release) or <45 (modified release)[2] Stop if creatinine >150 or eGFR <30[1]	Hypoglycaemic risk Severe liver disease Severe renal impairment Ketoacidosis Acute porphyria Caution in elderly, obese, mild–moderate renal/hepatic impairment[2]	Ketoacidosis Hepatic or renal impairment Heart failure Elderly Pancreatic cancer PMH pancreatitis
Hypoglycaemia risk	Low	Yes	Low unless combined with another Rx with hypo risk[1]
Risks and adverse events – see BNF for full list	<1/10,000 – lactic acidosis D&V, ↓ appetite and abdominal pain[1] Metallic/altered taste[1] B12 deficiency Skin reactions (erythema, urticaria, pruritus)[2]	Hypoglycaemia GI disturbance,[2] photosensitivity, liver function changes and rarely haematological disorders	1–10/1000 – pancreatitis[1] Headache, oedema, infections, GI disturbance[1] Hypersensitivity reactions and rashes[2]

Always use the most up-to-date version of the BNF yourself before prescribing. Ensure you have checked all the cautions, contraindications, interactions and dose regimes.

Medication	SGLT-2 inhibitors	Insulin	GLP-1 agonist	Glitazones
Example options	Dapagliflozin Canagliflozin Empagliflozin		Dulaglutide Exenatide Liraglutide Lixisenatide Semaglutide	Pioglitazone
Advice – see BNF	Seek specialist advice Monitor renal function[1]		Useful if BMI >35 Check U&E and eGFR before and 2 weeks later	Seek specialist advice May improve lipid profile Monitor LFT[1] Stop if HbA1c not decreasing, e.g. by >0.5% or 5–6 mmol/mol at 6 months[3]
How given	Oral	s/c	s/c	Oral
How it works	'Pee out (urinate) sugar'	Replaces insulin	↑ insulin secretion	↑ insulin sensitivity
Cautions and contraindications – see BNF for full list	DKA – stop Rx immediately Avoid if eGFR <60 and stop if eGFR <45 Severe hepatic disturbance Hypotension Elderly >85 Active foot disease		Elderly AKI Caution if eGFR 30–50 and stop if eGFR <30 Caution with DPP4 Pancreatic cancer Gastroparesis Thyroid cancer MEN type 2 Consider stopping after 6/12 if HbA1c hasn't dropped >1% or 10–11 mmol/mol or weight dropped by >3%[3]	Risk of bladder cancer so avoid in smokers and those on chemotherapy or exposed to occupational drugs, or radiotherapy to pelvis[2] (see MHRA alert)[4] Avoid if: Heart failure Liver impairment Bladder cancer Uninvestigated haematuria[1] Caution in: Elderly, insulin users risk factors for bladder cancer, heart failure, bone fracture[2]
Hypoglycaemia risk	Low	High	Low/medium	Low
Weight	Loss	Gain	Loss	Gain
Risks and adverse events – see BNF for full list	UTIs Fournier's gangrene (necrotising fasciitis of genitalia – mainly men) Renal impairment Lower limb amputation (see MHRA alert)[5] Risk of DKA (see MHRA alert)[6] Thirst Constipation Dyslipidaemia[2]	Hypo	Pancreatitis Nausea and vomiting Headache, dizziness Renal impairment AV block/sinus tachycardia Skin reactions – rash, angioedema, urticaria, pruritus	Numbness, visual impairment, weight increase, insomnia[2] Exacerbation of heart failure Bone #s Liver impairment Increased risk of infections Increase in relative risk of bladder cancer (range 1.12–1.33). Increase in absolute risk likely to be small[4]

Always use the most up-to-date version of the BNF yourself before prescribing. Ensure you have checked all the cautions, contraindications, interactions and dose regimes.

Metabolic Problems and Endocrinology

CHAPTER 15 OVERVIEW

Musculoskeletal Health

	Cases in this chapter	Within the RCGP 2020 curriculum: Musculoskeletal Health	Learning points in this chapter include:
1	Low Back Pain	'Spinal disorders including mechanical back pain' 'Examination of back and spine' 'Communicate effectively taking in to account the psychosocial impact of MSK problems on the patient, their family, friends, dependents and employers'	Causes Flags Guidelines Imaging – MRI
2	Knee Pain	'Intervene urgently when patients present with emergencies or red flag symptoms...' 'Sprains, strains and other significant soft-tissue trauma' 'Coordinate care with other health professionals leading to effective and appropriate acute and chronic management'	Osteoarthritis ACL injuries Investigating knee pain NICE CKS on assessing and managing knee pain
3	Osteoporosis	'Osteoporosis – primary and secondary' 'Screening tools and prevention programmes for conditions such as ... osteoporosis' 'Health issues associated with the menopause.... osteoporosis' 'Risk factors for osteoporosis'	NICE Guideline CG146. Osteoporosis: assessing the risk of fragility fracture. February 2017
4	Plantar Fasciitis	'Foot disorders such as plantar fasciitis'	Gout Differential diagnosis of foot pain
5	Shoulder Pain	'Joint pain, stiffness...including individual joints...shoulder' 'Advise appropriately to support the self-care and prevention of problem'	Anatomy Rotator cuff tendonitis Adhesive capsulitis Osteoarthritis Referred pain to the shoulder

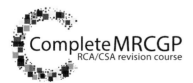

CompleteMRCGP
RCA/CSA revision course

CHAPTER 15 REFERENCES

Low Back Pain

1. Samanta J., Kendall J., Samanta A. Chronic low back pain. *BMJ* 2003; 326: 525. http://dx.doi.org/10.1136/bmj.326.7388.535. Mar 2003.
2. http://patient.info/doctor/low-back-pain-and-sciatica. Oct 2020.
3. https://startback.hfac.keele.ac.uk/. July 2021.
4. https://www.oxfordshireccg.nhs.uk/professional-resources/documents/clinical-guidelines/MSK-and-physio/cervical/MRI-referral-guidelines-for-cervical-thoracic-and-lumbar-spine-for-adults.pdf. Collison K., Russ R. Oxfordshire CCG. Jun 2014.

Useful Resource

https://patient.info/news-and-features/the-best-exercises-for-back-pain

Knee Pain

1. NICE CKS. https://cks.nice.org.uk/topics/osteoarthritis/management/management/. Jun 2018.
2. Kobayashi H., Kanamura T., Koshida S. et al. Mechanisms of the anterior cruciate ligament injury in sports activities: a twenty-year clinical research of 1,700 athletes. *J Sports Sci Med* 2010; 9: 669–75.

Osteoporosis

1. NICE Guideline CG146. Osteoporosis: assessing the risk of fragility fracture. Feb 2017.
2. http://www.shef.ac.uk/FRAX/tool.aspx?country=1
3. http://www.qfracture.org/
4. http://www.shef.ac.uk/NOGG/
5. Michaëlsson K., Melhus H., Warensjö Lemming E. et al. Long term calcium intake and rates of all cause and cardiovascular mortality: community based prospective longitudinal cohort study. *BMJ* 2013; 346: f228.
6. NICE CKS. http://cks.nice.org.uk/osteoporosis-prevention-of-fragility-fractures#!scenario:1. May 2020.
7. http://www.cgem.ed.ac.uk/research/rheumatological/calcium-calculator
8. NICE CKS. https://cks.nice.org.uk/topics/osteoporosis-prevention-of-fragility-fractures/prescribing-information/bisphosphonates/. May 2020.
9. NICE Technology appraisal guidance TA464. Bisphosphonates for treating osteoporosis. Jul 2019.
10. http://patient.info/medicine/alendronic-acid-for-osteoporosis-fosamax. Jul 2020.

Plantar Fasciitis/Differential Diagnosis – Foot Pain

1. Cooper A., Blythe J., Wise E. BMJ Masterclass for GPs. Musculoskeletal Medicine. Course Materials. Apr 2013.
2. http://www.mdcalc.com/ottawa-ankle-rule/
3. NICE CKS. http://cks.nice.org.uk/gout#!scenario. Feb 2018.

Useful Resource

https://patient.info/foot-care/heel-and-foot-pain-plantar-fasciitis

Shoulder Pain

1. http://www.physio-pedia.com/Supraspinatus_tendonitis
2. https://patient.info/doctor/shoulder-pain-pro. Jun 2015.
3. https://patient.info/bones-joints-muscles/frozen-shoulder-leaflet. Dec 2018.

Information taken from NICE guidelines with kind permission. Please note the guidelines change frequently and you should ALWAYS check for the latest updated guidance. Remember that NICE guidance is only applicable to patients in the UK.

Musculoskeletal Health

Doctor's Notes

Patient	Rachel West	43 years	F
PMH	Irritable bowel syndrome		
Medications	No current medications		
Allergies	No information		
Consultations	No recent consultations		
Investigations	No recent investigations		
Household	Arthur West	45 years	M
	Jennifer West	6 years	F
	Timothy West	4 years	M

Open ☐	Rachel, it is a pleasure to meet you and I'm sorry you are in this much pain. What has happened? Tell me more about the pain. Are you having any other symptoms?
Impact ☐	Tell me which important areas of your life are affected by the back pain.
ICE ☐	What do you think has caused this? What did you feel we should do today? Is there anything that you are especially worried about? What pain relief have you tried?
History ☐	Back pain can sometimes be due to kidney problems: any problems passing urine? Is your tummy okay? When was your last period? Tell me more about you. Do you have family? Are you otherwise well? Is everything okay at home?
Flags ☐	I just need to ask a few questions to check that both the spine and you are healthy. Any weight loss? Any fever? Does the pain wake you at night? Have you ever injured your back? Any weakness or numbness in your legs? Any problems controlling your bladder or bowels? Any numbness around your bottom?
Curious ☐	What do you think is keeping you awake all night – the pain or something else?
Sense ☐	I see how much pain you are in. You said this is the 'last straw'. What do you mean?
Risk ☐	Work sounds tough. Have you been feeling low even before this happened?
Empathy ☐	It must be hard with back pain working and looking after children. We can do a work note but your back needs to keep moving or you will stiffen up.
O/E ☐	May I examine your back with you standing and then check your legs on the couch?
SummarICE ☐	So, you developed severe back pain yesterday after bending forward. You have been finding work life difficult, and feel this is the last straw; you need time away from work. You fear the pain will impact caring for your children. You believe this is a slipped disc and you need a scan. Have I understood you correctly?
Impression ☐	It sounds like you have sciatica.
Experience ☐	Have you known anyone with this problem? What do you know about it?
Explanation ☐	In sciatica, the sciatic nerve becomes irritated or squashed which causes pain all the way down your leg. This is probably due to a 'prolapsed disc'. In this situation, the whole disc doesn't usually move, it's just the soft jelly centre.
InCludE ☐	As there are no worrying features – you have not lost weight or had an injury – I do not believe there is anything nasty happening in your spine so I don't think a scan would help.
Future ☐	Back exercises can really help and are important but improvement can take weeks. Do you think you can manage exercises at home or would you like a referral to a physio?
Options ☐	Pain relief options are naproxen, which is an anti-inflammatory or codeine which is a weak form of morphine. Naproxen can cause tummy irritation, whereas codeine can cause nausea, constipation or drowsiness. Which would be better for you? Okay, naproxen is taken 500 mg twice a day. If this isn't helping and your back continues to feel in spasm, there is a tablet called diazepam. I could give you a 3-day supply of this which you can take up to three times a day? This could also make you feel drowsy though and you should not drive. It is not a drug we can continue to use due to its risks. I would expect that over the next few days the intensity of the pain should decrease. If you are not getting back to normal after 4–6 weeks of exercises, please see a doctor, or sooner if you have worsening symptoms.
Empower ☐	This PIL has some exercises, e.g. lying on the floor, knees up and swing them side to side. Avoid lifting the children in the meantime.
Specifics ☐	You can self-certify for a week whilst the pain is severe but let's speak in a week to see how you are. Please book an appointment. If the pain is not coming under control after 3 days of exercises and painkillers, please ask for a telephone consultation with me.
Safety net ☐	If your legs feel different, you need to inform the doctor. Also – I don't expect this to happen – but I tell everyone that, if you lose control of going to the toilet or develop weakness in your legs, you must let a doctor know immediately.

Musculoskeletal Health – 1

Patient's Story

Doctor's notes	Rachel West, 43 years. PMH: IBS. Medications: none.
How to act	You are in a lot of pain.
PC	*'It's my back. I'm in agony.'*
History	You have often had lower back pain in your life.
	It has increased over the past few months.
	Then last night *'I was picking up toys and I felt my back go.'*
	'This is the last straw!' If asked, you mean regarding your work – you need time off.
	The pain goes down your left leg. It doesn't wake you but *'I am awake all night'.*
	You have not had any numbness or weakness. Full control of bladder and bowels.
	There are no abdominal, urinary or gynaecological symptoms. LMP 1 week ago.
	You have IBS but are otherwise well. No weight loss or fever. No injury.
	You have no other symptoms systemically. Paracetamol hasn't helped the pain.
	You have been feeling low but no features of depression.
	You haven't known anyone with this back pain. You don't know what sciatica means.
Social	You work in IT. Your work has been very difficult. Your marriage is good.
	You have two children. Your husband is a director of a building supplies company and busy.
	There are problems with your manager and you do not get on.
	You hope you can find alternative work.
	Work has been very stressful. You think about it through the night.
ICE	You feel you need a scan. You think you have *'slipped a disc'*.
	You expect the doctor will tell you to rest and take time off work.
	You fear it may take months to heal. You would like some strong pain relief. Accept naproxen as you think codeine may make your IBS worse.
	You worry about playing with the children with this pain.
	Your mother is coming to help.
Examination	No spinal tenderness, tender L paraspinal muscles. Slightly reduced ROM.
	Reduced straight leg raise left leg – 50 degrees.
	Normal neurological examination.

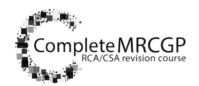

CompleteMRCGP
RCA/CSA revision course

Musculoskeletal Health – 1

Learning Points

Low Back Pain

Causes   Mechanical low back pain, malignancy – primary or secondary, infection (e.g. spinal TB), ankylosing spondylitis, pyelonephritis or kidney stone, or referred pain, e.g. AAA.

Flags[1,2] see also Keele STarT Back stratifying tool[3]

Red flags (*refers to criteria within Oxford guidance – see below)

- Unexplained weight loss*
- Previous or suspected malignancy*
- Drug abuse, HIV, immunosuppression or corticosteroid use
- Abnormal bloods (ESR >50[4])* or fever
- Thoracic or night pain
- Trauma*
- <20 or >55 years (worsening/new onset)
- Disturbed gait or progressive neurological deficit
- Comorbidity or unwell patient
- Abnormal function/control of bladder or bowel or saddle anaesthesia
- Known osteoporosis and suspected crush fracture[3]*
- Severe morning stiffness
- Consider cauda equina syndrome if on examination there is gait disturbance, urinary retention, abnormal perianal sensation or anal tone with lower limb weakness

Yellow flags (psychosocial factors)

- 'A negative attitude that back pain is harmful or potentially severely disabling'[1]
- 'Fear, avoidance behaviour and reduced activity levels'[1]
- 'An expectation that passive, rather than active, treatment will be beneficial'[1]
- History of depression, low mood and social withdrawal[1]
- 'Social or financial problems'[1]

<20 years   consider HLAB27 testing for AS if morning stiffness and pain awakens the patient.

>55 years   Consider an ESR, electrophoresis (myeloma screen), urine dipstick, palpating for AAA, PSA in men and CA125 in women.

So should all >55 years with new onset back pain have an urgent MRI if they have no other red flags and bloods are normal? This is where 'clinical judgement' comes in and follow your local guidance.

Oxford CCG guidance[4]

Cauda equina Widespread neurological deficit or infection	Refer as an emergency to the spinal team.
Red flag symptoms* (no mention of age)	Direct referral for urgent limited MRI.
Suspected osteoporotic crush fracture only	Lateral X-ray then routine MRI.
No red flags and persistent pain >6 weeks	Review diagnosis, conservative Rx and refer to the MSK assessment team.
Progressive deformity (kyphosis) Intractable pain Deteriorating neurology	Review diagnosis and refer to spinal team if patient will consider surgery and is a surgical candidate

Occasionally an MRI will report that it cannot exclude malignancy in which case consider a bone scan.

For simple back pain offer analgesia and exercises. Give a realistic prognosis.

Musculoskeletal Health – 1

Doctor's Notes

Patient	Robert Hayes	27 years	M
PMH	No known medical history		
Medications	No current medications		
Allergies	No information		
Consultations	No recent consultations		
Investigations	No recent investigations		
Household	No household members registered		

Open ☐	What happened? Talk me through the injury in slow motion if you can please. Then what did you notice?
Flags ☐	Did the knee swell straight away? Could you walk on it? Does the knee lock into a certain position stopping you from straightening or bending it? Has it given way?
Risk ☐	Have you injured your knee before? Any other injury?
Impact ☐	And the past couple of days, has it stopped you from doing anything? Do you work? How would a knee injury impact on your work, hobbies or home life?
ICE ☐	What do you think may have happened inside the knee? Has anything else gone through your mind? Anything else you fear about this injury? Is there anything you thought I might say we should arrange? Is there anything else you were hoping we could do? Are there any other thoughts you had about what may be helpful?
Curious ☐	Is there a reason why you would prefer to avoid the orthopaedic doctors?
O/E ☐	I would like to see you at the surgery to examine your knee. That would involve taking off your trousers, having a look at the knee, then doing some movements to work out what may have caused the swelling. If you feel any pain during the examination, I would ask you to tell me where exactly. Is that okay? I have an appointment at 2 p.m. this afternoon. Would that be convenient?
SummarICE ☐	To summarise, you believe you may have torn a ligament and fear needing an operation after your experience with your right ankle. You are hoping that I will organise an MRI scan to guide physiotherapy but would like to get better quickly because you don't want to be sat out for the rest of the season. Is that correct?
Impression ☐	I can't be sure until I examine you but I think you may be right. It sounds as if it could be a torn ligament, and I'm wondering specifically if it is the anterior cruciate ligament. This can be very painful, as you have described.
Sense ☐	You sound disappointed and upset.
Experience ☐	Have you heard of this injury?
Explanation ☐	This ligament in the knee prevents your knee from overstretching, but unfortunately if you have had an injury which causes the leg to overstretch, it can tear.
Empathy ☐	It sounds as if you have been lonely since the end of your relationship so I appreciate that not being able to play football with friends is a huge disappointment.
Options ☐	To get an answer and to get you on the mend as soon as possible, after I have seen you, we should consider referring you to the trauma clinic today.
InCludE ☐	You mentioned you were keen for physio; I think that sounds a good idea but wonder if we should get the orthopaedic opinion first.
Recommend ☐	I suggest that I see you first and then potentially give the trauma registrar a call, if that's okay with you.
Future ☐	If surgery is needed, keyhole surgery may be an option. I can also prescribe some codeine for you for additional pain relief if you need it. Does this sound okay? Perhaps once the injury has settled a little you could still go to matches to support your team and see your friends?
Empower ☐	In the meantime, please keep it elevated with some ice on it to reduce the swelling. Whilst waiting to see the trauma team, I'd recommend paracetamol and an anti-inflammatory like ibuprofen but can prescribe something a little stronger if you need it.

Patient's Story

Knee Pain

Doctor's notes	Robert Hayes, 27 years. PMH: none. Medications: none.
How to act	Pleasant but concerned.
PC	*'I've injured my knee playing football.'*
History	Two days ago you were playing football. You felt something pop as you were changing direction – your studs seemed to stick in the mud. There was no contact with another player at the time. It was extremely painful and you could not continue the game. You applied ice to your swollen knee and the swelling is still present. The knee doesn't lock but has given way. You have had no previous knee injury. You have not been able to drive since the injury despite taking paracetamol and ibuprofen. You also find it painful walking and weight bearing.
Social	You work as a project manager and enjoy running, badminton and football. You live with a flatmate. If the doctor asks you about what impact this may have, you have recently broken up with your long-term girlfriend and it wasn't until the football season started that you began to spend more time with your friends.
ICE	You believe you may have torn a ligament.
	You are worried that you will be *'out for the season'*.
	You also fear you may need an operation. You fractured your ankle falling out of a tree as a child and remember a lot of pain after the operation. You would rather see a physio than be referred to orthopaedics for this reason; however, you will follow the doctor's advice. You would like an MRI of your knee – if asked why, you think this would help a physiotherapist. If the doctor asks you about your understanding of the diagnosis, you remember that Michael Owen couldn't play in the 2006 World Cup due to a cruciate ligament injury. The doctor is giving you terrible news as you fear you will now be isolated from your friends this season.
Examination	The left knee is swollen with an effusion. The knee is not hot or red. There is tenderness along the medial side. The anterior drawer test is positive. The rest of the examination is normal.

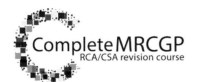

CompleteMRCGP
RCA/CSA revision course

Musculoskeletal Health – 2

Osteoarthritis – new diagnosis

Suspect arthritis if:[1]

- Age >45 years.
- Clinical features are suggestive.
- Alternative conditions have been excluded.

Differential diagnosis includes gout/pseudogout, septic arthritis, inflammatory arthritis, malignancy[1] and injury from trauma.

NICE CKS advise a holistic assessment of a person with OA: social situation and impact, health beliefs, mood, quality of sleep, support network, other MSK pain, attitudes to exercise, influence of comorbidity and a full pain assessment.

GP management options include: NSAIDs, muscle-strengthening exercises, advice about aerobic fitness and footwear, physiotherapy, steroids injection. Consider the additional need for TENS or aids.

Possible referral routes[1]

- Physiotherapy/MSK – strengthening exercises, manipulation, joint supports, joint injections.
- Occupational therapy – advice on helpful devices for DLAs to reduce strain on different joints.
- Podiatrist – biomechanical assessment, orthotics device.
- Orthopaedic surgeon (irrespective of patient's age, BMI or comorbidities and BEFORE severe functional limitations and/or pain if:
  - symptoms (stiffness, joint pain, functional Impairment) are not improving with primary care management.
  - QOL significantly affected.
  - diagnosis is unclear or symptoms are atypical.
  - symptoms suddenly get worse.
- Pain clinic if:
  - pain uncontrolled despite optimised medical and/or surgical management.
  - suspect chronic pain syndrome.
- Psychological services if comorbid depression or anxiety despite primary care management.

ACL injury

Mechanism   Most commonly associated with a non-contact mechanism – 'knee in and toe out'.[2]

The risk is greater in females. [2]

Injury triad   Anterior cruciate ligament + medial collateral ligament + medial meniscus.

Acute injuries

Refer acute injuries to orthopaedics for assessment, imaging and management options.

NB: Immediate effusions following trauma/injury are often due to haemarthrosis which is associated with more significant joint injuries. Have a low threshold for referral of such cases (possibly same day or urgently to trauma/fracture clinic). If presenting as a chronic injury, you may be able to refer for direct access MRI to guide diagnosis and management – check local protocols.

Doctor's Notes

Patient	Shirley Warner	72 years	F
PMH	Wrist fracture		
Medications	Codeine phosphate 30 mg		
Allergies	No information		
Consultations	2 months ago: telephone consultation – codeine prescribed following wrist fracture.		
Investigations	DEXA Score –2.7		
	Corrected calcium 2.36 mmol/L		
	Vitamin D 40 ng/mL		
Household	Tina Wright	76 years	F

Example Consultation

Open ☐	Thank you for phoning. What led to you having this test?
Impact ☐	How is the arm? How has the broken arm affected you day to day?
Flags ☐	How did you fall? I see: when a break occurs after a low-impact injury, we should check the bone strength.
History ☐	Before I explain, may I learn more about you to help me interpret the result and what we may need to do? Are you well? Any medical problems? Any medicines? How do you spend your time? Who is at home? Any family history of medical problems?
ICE ☐	Have you had thoughts yourself about what the scan may show? Do you have any fears about what I may say today? And what did you think I might suggest?
Risk ☐	What age was your menopause? Have you ever taken any steroid treatment? Do you smoke? How much alcohol do you drink? Have you had any other broken bones?
Curious ☐	When you fell, had you been drinking any alcohol?
Sense ☐	You've mentioned your mum a few times. Her experience is important to you; what happened?
Empathy ☐	I understand your fear of another fracture especially after your mother's experience.
O/E ☐	Can you tell me your weight and height?
SummarICE ☐	To summarise, a low-impact fall caused a fracture which led to the scan. You suspect this is due to low calcium which will need replacing and fear another fall, having watched your mother suffer. Is this right?
Impression ☐	The scan has confirmed that you have osteoporosis.
Experience ☐	Do you know anything about osteoporosis?
Explanation ☐	Osteoporosis means the bones are not as strong as they should be. Sometimes calcium tablets are taken but actually your calcium levels are already good. Osteoporosis is a lack of bone strength but not necessarily a lack of the nutrients such as calcium. Many things lead to osteoporosis. In your case, I suspect it is a mixture of things such as being a post-menopausal woman, an ex-smoker, drinking more than 14 units of alcohol a week and having a family history of osteoporosis.
Options ☐	Thankfully there is treatment available which should reduce your risk of more broken bones in the future. Alendronate is a tablet that prevents bone breakdown. It is taken once weekly. Like all tablets there are potential side effects – for this tablet that includes heartburn, diarrhoea or headaches. There are also risks: it can damage the jaw bone. Although this is rare, we recommend seeing your dentist prior to starting treatment. To prevent acid reflux, we advise taking the tablet 30 minutes before your breakfast and any medication, with a full glass of water and remain upright (either sitting or standing) for 30 minutes.
Recommend ☐	I suggest that I prescribe alendronate for you and will give you an information sheet which explains again how to take the tablet. Are you happy to start this medication?
Empower ☐	We also need to consider your calcium and vitamin D. Your calcium blood test was normal but your vitamin D was a bit low. To decide if you need extra calcium, we need to assess your dietary intake of calcium. If it is low, we will give you a tablet with both calcium and vitamin D. If it is adequate, you will only need vitamin D. This is because recent research suggests that too much calcium can be harmful. Could I send you a questionnaire to fill out about your diet? There are other things you can do to protect your bones such as reducing your alcohol intake and doing weight-bearing exercises. I will email you a sheet of these exercises.
Future ☐	Can we talk again in a couple of weeks to go through your questionnaire?
Specifics ☐	We advise taking alendronate for 5 years initially and then we should review whether or not you need to continue. You may be able to stop then, but we would arrange a scan 18 months to 3 years later to reassess.
Safety net ☐	With alendronate if you notice black stools, reflux or heart burn, jaw pain or a loose tooth, inform a GP.

Musculoskeletal Health – 3

Patient's Story

Osteoporosis

Doctor's notes	Shirley Warner, 72 years. DEXA Score –2.7. Corrected calcium 2.36 mmol/L. Vitamin D 40 ng/mL (low). PMH: wrist fracture 2 months ago. Medications: codeine phosphate 30 mg.
How to act	Friendly.
PC	*'Doctor, I'd like my scan result.'*
History	You were referred for a DEXA scan by the hospital doctor.
	2 months ago, you fractured your wrist when you tripped on a kerb.
	Your mother broke her hip when she was in her 80s.
	'Mum was low in calcium and took calcium tablets.'
	You have no other medical history. You have taken no other medicines.
	The arm is improving.
	Your menopause was aged 52 years.
Social	You are a retired seamstress. You live with your partner, Tina.
	You drink 16 units of alcohol a week.
	You *'tripped after the golf party'* (3 glasses of wine).
	You are an ex-smoker.
	You enjoy yoghurt, full fat milk and eat very well.
	You are happy to keep a food diary to calculate your calcium intake.
ICE	You understand that you have weak bones lacking in calcium.
	You are worried you will get a hip fracture like your mother.
	Your mum was in hospital a long time and then had to start warfarin for a DVT.
	You expect the doctor will start calcium tablets.
Examination	Your BMI is 24.

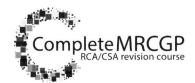

Musculoskeletal Health – 3

Learning Points
Osteoporosis

+ Risk factors[1]   ♀, BMI <18.5, smoking, alcohol (units >14/week ♀ or ♂).

                        Previous fracture or history of falls, immobility, FH osteoporosis or hip #.

                        Medical comorbidity.

++ Risk factors   Corticosteroids, premature menopause, previous osteoporotic fracture.

+++ Risk factors   >7.5 mg prednisolone daily for >3 months (current or recent).

                        Previous major osteoporotic fracture.

                        Multiple fragility fractures.

Who do we screen   ♀ >65 years or <65 years with any risk factor.

                        ♂ >75 years or <75 years with any risk factor.

                        Anyone <50 years with a ++ or +++ risk factor OR <40 years with a +++ risk factor.

How do we screen?

1. History – is the patient at risk?
2. Calculate the FRAX score[2] if aged 40–90 years or Q fracture[3] if aged 30–84 years.
3. Once the data is inserted into the tool, use the link to NOGG[4] to guide management:
   - lifestyle advice (low risk)
   - DEXA scan (intermediate risk) → recalculate risk with BMD
   - start treatment (high risk).

>80 years 'predicted 10-year fracture risk may underestimate their short-term fracture risk.'[1]

Assessment tools underestimate risk in: multiple #s or vertebral #, alcohol abuse, steroid Rx or comorbidities[1]

T score   T score between –1 and –2.5 = osteopenia.

                 T score <–2.5 = osteoporosis.

For reversible causes consider testing: TSH, PTH, Ca^{2+}, vitamin D, testosterone, LH and FSH to investigate for hyperthyroidism, hyperparathyroidism, osteomalacia and hypogonadism respectively.

Who should have calcium and vitamin D replacement?

Due to new studies[5] demonstrating the risks of calcium treatment, consider vitamin D replacement alone if dietary calcium intake is >700 mg/day.[6,7] 'If calcium intake is inadequate:

- Prescribe 10 μg (400 μg) of vitamin D with at least 1000 mg of calcium daily. Prescribe 20 μg (800 μg) of vitamin D with at least 1000 mg of calcium daily for people not exposed to much sunlight.'[6]

Who should have bisphosphonates?

NOGG guidance has indicated treatment is required or following a confirmed osteoporosis diagnosis. For women, all bisphosphonates are licensed but, for men, only alendronate (OD tablets) and risedronate (once-weekly tablets).[6]

The following is recommended reading: counselling prior to bisphosphonate use – see reference.[8]

Also, for information regarding treatment in post-menopausal women – see reference.[9]

Patient.info has a useful patient leaflet on how to take alendronic acid.[10]

Management of osteopenia

Lifestyle: smoking, exercise and weight-bearing exercises.

Test bone profile, albumin, U&E, LFT, FBC, ESR and TSH. Rescan 2–3 years.

Musculoskeletal Health – 3

Doctor's Notes

Patient	Selina Richards	31 years	F
PMH	No known medical history		
Medications	No current medications		
Allergies	No information		
Consultations	No recent consultations		
Investigations	No recent investigations		
Household	Alexander Richards	8 years	M
	Maria Richards	6 years	F
	Amelia Richards	5 years	F

Open ☐ Please tell me the story of the pain from when you first noticed it. Anything else you have noticed? When does the pain come and go?

Impact ☐ And since this problem started, what has the pain stopped you from doing?

Flags ☐ Have you noticed any swelling or redness? Can you move the ankle and foot normally?

Risk ☐ Have you ever had any injury in the past?

ICE ☐ Have you had any thoughts as to what may be causing it? What worries have gone through your mind? Is there anything else you hoped we would arrange today?

History ☐ Any medical problems? Have you tried any pain relief yet? I'm interested to know more about you.

Sense ☐ So this has come at a very difficult time for you?

Curious ☐ What did your friend suggest?

O/E ☐ I would like to see you at the surgery to examine your foot and ankle; I would ask you to remove your socks and shoes and feel the area under the foot. Would that be okay? Are you free at 4 p.m.?

SummarICE ☐ To summarise, you have told me that the pain in the right foot has been building over a month but, especially in this past week, it has stopped you from walking the dog, something that you enjoy, but have also had to do more since you have separated from your husband. You wondered if it was gout.

Impression ☐ I think, from what I have heard so far, that it may be a condition called plantar fasciitis causing your pain. I'll be able to confirm this when I examine you later. Have you come across this condition before?

Explanation ☐ The plantar fascia is a sheet of tissue which supports the bones of your foot. Sometimes it can become painful and inflamed. It may be triggered by an increase in physical activity. Another possibility would be gout but from what you tell me, your foot is not red, hot or swollen. The site of the pain is typical of plantar fasciitis.

InCludE ☐ X-rays do not show this inflammation so are unlikely to be helpful.

Empathy ☐ This is an additional stress, especially as the dog is whining and you have three children to care for. I also hear that you are very fond of the dog. I appreciate why you feel you need to fix this problem straight away. The problem can unfortunately take many months to settle completely. However, if we confirm that this is what is wrong, I would have some suggestions.

Empower ☐ The ibuprofen could be changed for a tablet which is slightly stronger and lasts 12 hours, called naproxen. You take one tablet twice a day but, like ibuprofen, it can irritate your stomach lining so stop it if this becomes a problem. There is a useful exercise for PF too. The exercise aims to stretch the tissue to help the repairing process. It uses a frozen litre drinks bottle. Put the bottle under the arch of your foot and roll the bottle forwards and backwards. The movement helps stretch the tissue and the ice helps reduce pain and swelling. The more you do, the sooner it will improve but, like any exercise, time is needed. Padded footwear can also help.

Options ☐ When I see you, if the examination confirms plantar fasciitis, I can give you a PIL which explains all this. It also mentions steroid injections into the feet, which is an option, but some do not find it effective and there are risks to injecting in the foot, such as infection or injury to the tendons there. We therefore don't recommend the injections as first line. What are your thoughts about what I have said?

Future ☐ How do you feel about coming down at 4 p.m. and we can have a look at your foot and take it from there?

Specifics ☐ Just to let you know about other options if your foot does not start to improve soon – we could think about either physiotherapy, which we can arrange in-house, or the injections, which one of my colleagues can do. See you soon!

Doctor's notes	Selina Richards, 31 years. PMH: none. Medications: none.
How to act	Slightly pushy for the doctor to fix this problem.
PC	*'It's a pain in my foot – it's a nightmare.'*
History	You walk your dog every morning and recently have pain in the right foot whilst walking.
	You have had no injury or swelling.
	You started to notice this a month ago and over the past week you have had enough of this discomfort. You have always been well. Ibuprofen only helps slightly. You drink minimal alcohol and don't smoke.
Social	You do not work. You have three children and a dog.
	Your children are all in primary school.
	Your husband has just left the marriage and he used to walk the dog in a morning.
	You spend your days meeting your friends, doing housework, dog-sitting and food shopping for your mother. Financially you have always been very lucky and have never worked since you were married. You would like to have a job but don't know how or where. You are going to volunteer at the school with cooking classes.
ICE	Your friend told you that the problem may be gout as she had the same thing and you have not had an injury. Therefore, you expect the doctor will give you colchicine, the tablet your friend was given. You would also like a blood test and an X-ray. You plan to pay for a dog walker, but will miss the time out of the house with the dog.
Impact	The dog has been whining as you couldn't walk him and you need to get this sorted straight away. Apart from walking the dog, the pain has not stopped you from doing anything else. You are coping well without your husband; he was always away on business anyway. The divorce proceedings, however, are stressful. You also want to keep the dog and fear your husband will want him if he is not being walked. You have never come across plantar fasciitis.
Examination	No swelling or abnormality of the foot, ankle or Achilles tendon. Tender at the plantar surface of the calcaneus.

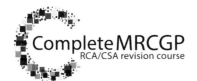

CompleteMRCGP
RCA/CSA revision course

Learning Points

Soft tissue	Chronic heel pad inflammation	'Warm dull throbbing pain over weight-bearing area of the heel… worse when first getting up.'[1]
	Acute synovitis	Throbbing pain made worse by movement.[1]
		Rule out systemic causes.
	Acute inflammation of anterior metatarsal heads	
		Common in women wearing slip-on/heeled shoe.
		Burning and throbbing on walking.[1]
	Plantar metatarsal bursitis	'Throbbing pain under the metatarsal head… persists at rest and exacerbated when the area if first loaded.'[1]
Bone	Fracture	Has there been impact? Use the Ottawa rules.[2]
	Stress fracture (march fracture)	Palpable tender lump.
	Osteoarthritis	Common at 1st MTPJ, tarsus joints and midfoot.[1]
	Rheumatoid arthritis	Swelling and deformity, may describe walking on pebbles due to swelling/subluxation.[1]
	Sever's disease	E.g. boys 8–13 years and exacerbated by jumping.[1]
	Hallux valgus	Great toe moves towards/overlies the 2nd toe.[1]
	Bunion	Inflamed and painful metatarsal head.[1]
Red hot	Gout	
	Septic arthritis	Requires urgent aspiration/culture/Rx.
Nerve	Morton's neuroma	Burning and numbness… often the 3rd/4th toe.[1]
	Peripheral neuropathy	E.g. tarsal tunnel or 2° to ↓B12, alcohol or DM.
Arterial	Ischaemia	Absent pulses, signs of PVD and check ABPIs.

Gout

Risk factors	Thiazides, ACEI, alcohol, obesity.
	Do not start allopurinol during an acute attack.
	But, if already taking allopurinol or febuxostat, do not stop this during an acute attack.[3]
Acute medication[3]	1st line NSAID (diclofenac, indometacin or naproxen) + PPI
	2nd line colchicine
	3rd line if NSAIDs contraindicated – consider systemic corticosteroids

When initiating allopurinol, consider a course of NSAID or colchicine. If in 2/12 you need to ↑ the allopurinol give another overlap of colchicine to prevent an acute attack as the urate levels ↓ again.

| **Uric acid levels** | Measure 4–6 weeks after an acute attack. |

Aim for normal levels of uric acid if the decision has been made to start allopurinol.

| **Self-management**[3] | Rest, avoid trauma, keep the joint cool. Lifestyle: reduce alcohol, weight loss and dietary changes and avoid dehydration. |

Doctor's Notes

Patient	David Meadows	47 years	M
PMH	Cruciate ligament injury		
Medications	No current medications		
Allergies	No information		
Consultations	No recent consultations		
Investigations	No recent investigations		
Household	No household members registered		

Example Consultation

Open ☐	Mr Meadows, how can I help? Shall we start from when you first noticed the problem?
Flags ☐	Have you had an injury? Any pain elsewhere – chest, neck or arm? What are you doing when the pain comes on? Which movements specifically? Does other activity cause pain? Does it wake you?
Impact ☐	Are you having to do anything differently? Is it stopping you do anything else?
Risk ☐	Have you ever damaged the shoulder?
History ☐	I see you have injured your knee. Any other medical problems? Tell me more about you.
ICE ☐	What do you think has caused this? Is there anything else you have been wondering? Is there anything else you are worried about? What did you think I might say we should do today? Is there anything specific you would like to be done today?
Curious ☐	Has someone you know had a shoulder pain that was from their heart?
Sense ☐	You seem very disappointed about having to stop golf.
O/E ☐	Please can you remove your top so that I may feel your shoulder, neck and arm and check their movements?
SummarICE ☐	So, 2 weeks of shoulder pain is now affecting you daily. You wonder whether this may be caused by golf or from arthritis. You wanted to clarify that this is not coming from your heart. You fear it will prevent you from playing in the golf competition. You wondered whether an X-ray would be helpful.
Impression ☐	I believe you have painful arc syndrome. This pain is not coming from your heart. I can reassure you of this because it is painful moving the shoulder joint but not when exercising.
Experience ☐	Other names for it are tendonitis or impingement. Have you come across painful arc?
Explanation ☐	The problem lies within the shoulder at the tendons. Tendons attach the shoulder muscles to the arm. There is a narrow tunnel in the shoulder for these tendons to pass through. Repeated use or an injury can cause swelling of the tendon or wear and tear of the bones that form the tunnel. Both make the narrow tunnel smaller. Lifting the arm makes this space smaller again. This causes friction and is why you get pain with that movement.
Empathy ☐	I appreciate the need to fix the shoulder quickly. I will try but I fear 6 weeks is optimistic.
InCludE ☐	You wondered about an X-ray. As tendons don't show up on X-rays this is unlikely to be helpful at the moment, but further down the line we could consider an ultrasound scan.
Options ☐	Reduce the inflammation with anti-inflammatory tablets. If this doesn't help, a steroid injection may be beneficial. Secondly, I suggest you rest your shoulder from heavy exercise but perform some physio exercises. Holding a weight, like a can of beans, in the right hand directly below the shoulder, leaning to that side and then make circle movements can help. This helps to increase that gap. Should we try a 2-week trial of exercises and anti-inflammatories?
Future ☐	If it is not on the mend, consider the steroid injection guided by an USS and physiotherapy. What are your thoughts? I will send you a PIL with this and other exercises. Any questions?
Empower ☐	With the exercises, the more you do, the sooner you will notice a difference.
Safety net ☐	I will prescribe some naproxen, an anti-inflammatory which is stronger than ibuprofen and lasts longer, so is taken every 12 hours with food. Like any tablet it has its risks, including tummy ulcers, so let me know if it is causing tummy pain. Inform me if you develop shoulder swelling.

Patient's Story

Doctor's notes	David Meadows, 47 years. PMH: cruciate ligament injury. Medications: none.
How to act	Relaxed and pleasant.
PC	*'I've done something to my shoulder doctor.'*
History	Right shoulder pain (no radiation) began slowly 2 weeks ago. No specific injury.
	It is painful inside the shoulder especially when raising the arm: 5/10 severity of pain.
	You have still managed to cycle on your cycling machine to keep fit without discomfort.
	No neurological symptoms in the arm and no problem at the neck or elbow.
	You once injured your knee playing football.
	You have otherwise been well.
	You are very active and never have any chest pains.
	There are no contraindications to starting an NSAID.
Impact	It has stopped you from playing golf. You are right-handed.
	You fear having to pull out of a competition in 6 weeks which you have been looking forward to.
	It is not painful at night.
	You are struggling to wash your hair so you are leaning forward and using your left hand.
Social	Work for local council – the GP practice is near your office.
	Wife and two children at home. Occasional alcohol. Never smoked.
ICE	You wonder if this could be arthritis or maybe you have injured it playing golf.
	At the back of your mind, you hope it isn't your heart.
	You have heard heart pain can be in the shoulder or arm.
	You have heard this from an old boss whilst he was telling you about his heart attack.
	You expect the doctor will send you for an X-ray and give you some pain relief.
Examination	Allow the doctor to examine you.
	No swelling or deformity.
	The shoulder is not hot. Painful arc at 30 degrees.
	Pain on lifting the arm against resisted movement and reaching to the back.
	The neck and elbow are normal.

Learning Points

The three joints of the shoulder Sternoclavicular, acromioclavicular and glenohumeral joint.

The four rotator cuff muscles Supraspinatus (initiation of abduction)

Infraspinatus (external rotation)

Teres minor (also external rotation)

Subscapularis (internal rotation)

These join together to form the rotator cuff tendon which travels through the sub-acromial space.

Rotator cuff tendonitis[1,2] is where inflammation which causes **impingement** (where the tendon becomes trapped) reduces the range of movement, hence a **painful arc**. For example, if there is a supraspinatus tendonitis there is compression of the supraspinatus tendon between the humeral head and acromion.

Causes: tendonitis secondary to an injury or repetitive strain or calcium deposits.

Sub-acromial space narrowing: bony spurs from wear and tear or enlargement of the bursa.

An USS may be helpful to diagnose and guide a steroid injection. It may also diagnose tears in the rotator cuff tendons, some of which require surgical repair. Most tendonitis settles with rest, physio and NSAIDs/steroid injection. Occasionally (e.g. if chronic/bony spurs) arthroscopic decompression is necessary.

Frozen shoulder (adhesive capsulitis)[3] is generalised inflammation within the capsule, which causes pain and limits any ROM of the glenohumeral joint. It usually affects the non-dominant shoulder. Frozen shoulder may occur after rotator cuff injury or spontaneously and the cause is unknown. There are typically three phases:

1.   'Painful freezing' stage – most painful stage with gradual loss of movement, may last up to 9 months.
2.   'Frozen/adhesive stage' – reduced movement but less painful, lasts up to 1 year.
3.   'Thawing/recovery phase' – gradual return to normal function which may take 1–3 years.

Tell patients that symptoms may last between 18 months and 3 years, although the vast majority of patients have recovered by 2 years. The treatment is physiotherapy. A steroid injection may be helpful within the first 8 weeks. Patients with diabetes or thyroid conditions have an increased risk of a bilateral frozen shoulder.

Osteoarthritis: In an older patient it may be helpful to see if there is OA present.

Dislocations usually occur after an impact injury.

Consider **referred pain** from the diaphragm (ruptured ectopic pregnancy) or heart (MI).

If unable to abduct the shoulder the first 10 degrees, consider a complete tear of the supraspinatus and speak to a specialist about arranging a clinic appointment.

If you give a PIL, always describe what is in it.

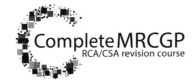

CHAPTER 16 OVERVIEW

Neurodevelopmental Disorders, Intellectual and Social Disability

	Cases in this chapter	Within the RCGP 2020 curriculum: Neurodevelopmental Disorders, Intellectual and Social Disability	Learning points in this chapter include:
1	Need for Procedure	'Be aware of the concept of diagnostic overshadowing...'	Elderly parents Diagnostic overshadowing
2	Down Syndrome	'Genetic causes of intellectual disability... Down syndrome' 'Annual health checks' 'Effects of intellectual disability on the ageing process, particularly in relation to the development and recognition of dementia'	The annual health check Issues specific to the condition/life stage
3	Autism and Transition Process	'Common and important conditions – autism and autism spectrum disorders' 'Support for adolescents transitioning from paediatric to adult care'	Transition Process Model
4	Mental Health and Intellectual Disability	'Atypical presentation of psychiatric problems because of sensory, communication and cognitive difficulties' 'Impact on family dynamics including parenting experiences'	Psychiatric disorders prevalent in the adult with intellectual disability Questions to carers
5	COCP Request	'Safeguarding of vulnerable adults... and the ethics of caring for people with intellectual disability' 'Equal rights of all citizens to healthcare, health information and health promotion' 'Emotional and sexual needs of adults with intellectual and social disabilities and how they may be expressed' 'Risk of sexual... abuse'	Risk factors for safeguarding adults
Extra Notes	Assessing Capacity	'An understanding of legislation and guidance on mental capacity' 'Mental capacity assessment and associated legislation'	Assessing capacity

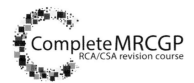

Complete MRCGP
RCA/CSA revision course

CHAPTER 16 REFERENCES

Need for Procedure

1. Hubert J., Hollins S. People with Intellectual Disabilities and Their Elderly Carers. http://www.intellectualdisability.info/life-stages/people-with-intellectual-disabilities-and-their-elderly-carers
2. Dowling S.F. Bereavement in the Lives of People with Intellectual Disabilities. http://www.intellectualdisability.info/life-stages/bereavement-in-the-lives-of-people-with-intellectual-disabilities

Down Syndrome

1. Holland T. Ageing and Its Consequences for People with Down Syndrome. http://www.intellectualdisability.info/life-stages/ageing-and-its-consequences-for-people-with-downs-syndrome
2. Trumble T. People with Down Syndrome at All Ages: Some Tips for Family Physicians. http://www.intellectualdisability.info/life-stages/people-with-downs-syndrome-at-all-age-some-tips-for-family-physicians
3. Dr Matt Hoghton and the RCGP Learning Disabilities Group. A Step-by-Step Guide for GP Practices. Annual Health Checks for People with Disabilities. http://www.rcgp.org.uk/learningdisabilities/~/media/Files/CIRC/CIRC-76-80/CIRCA%20StepbyStepGuideforPracticesOctober%2010.ashx

Autism and Transition Process

1. Barron D.A., Coyle D., Paliokosta E., Hassiotis A. Transition for Children with Intellectual Disabilities. http://www.intellectualdisability.info/life-stages/transition-for-children-with-intellectual-disabilities

Mental Health and Intellectual Disability

1. Department of Health. Valuing People: A New Strategy for Learning Disability for the 21st Century. 2001.
2. RCGP Curriculum 2019 – Clinical Topic Guides: Neurodevelopmental disorders, intellectual and social disability.

COCP Request

1. RCGP Curriculum 2019 – Clinical Topic Guides: Neurodevelopmental disorders, intellectual and social disability.

Useful Resource

https://centralsexualhealth.org/contraception/easy-read-leaflets/

Assessing Capacity

1. https://www.bma.org.uk/advice-and-support/ethics/adults-who-lack-capacity/mental-capacity-act-toolkit

There are many potential social inequalities for a patient with an intellectual disability, including access to healthcare, financial issues and educational opportunities. The potential barriers to healthcare include accessing services, communication, using online services, appointment times, patient's fear or a lack of staff training. The responsibilities of the GP include being proactive with setting up a system which provides patients with equal access to healthcare. This may include a patient register, recall system, a team leader, staff education, regular communication with speciality teams and flexible appointment times. The system should ensure clinicians have the time required to gain an understanding of the patient and their carer's challenges, concerns and needs. The GP should be vigilant for atypical presentations of physical conditions, emotional (fear, frustration and loneliness) or psychological concerns and the potential problems which occur within a time of transition in the patient's life. The systemic enquiry should be appropriate to the patient's life stage.

An understanding of the patient's social circumstances is essential to effectively screen for isolation, neglect and abuse. Health promotion and when and how to seek help should be discussed. Be aware of local services and provide information which is easy to read. The carer's health and well-being should also be explored. In-practice time and follow-ups are needed for a full assessment. Cutting corners cannot be an option.

Remember that the GP may be the only person asking the questions and acting as an advocate for the patient.

Information taken from NICE guidelines with kind permission. Please note the guidelines change frequently and you should ALWAYS check for the latest updated guidance. Remember that NICE guidance is only applicable to patients in the UK.

Neurodevelopmental Disorders, Intellectual and Social Disability

Doctor's Notes

Patient	Henry Sutton	60 years	M
PMH	Hypoxic ischaemic encephalopathy		
	Seizures (seizure-free 30 years)		
	Hearing difficulty. Hearing aids		
	Myopia		
	Learning difficulties (IQ 45)		
	Attention deficit hyperactivity disorder		
	Gastro-oesophageal reflux disease		
Medications	Omeprazole 40 mg		
Allergies	No known drug allergies		
Consultations	Last consultations: 1 month ago when omeprazole was prescribed.		
Investigations	Blood test *Helicobacter pylori* negative.		
	Hb 105 g/L, otherwise FBC normal.		
	U&E, LFT, amylase, CRP, HbA1c, FBG – all normal.		
	Weight 65 kg 1 year ago		
Household	Rosemary Sutton	88 years	F
	Henry attends with mother Rosemary.		

Example Consultation

Need for Procedure

Open ☐	Hello. Thank you for coming to see me. Today we will have a chat about how you are, I will ask you some questions and you can ask me questions at any time. If you don't mind, I may need to examine you, then we will have a chat about what happens next. Is that okay? Who have you brought with you today? Henry, can you tell me what has been hurting you? Can you tell me why you had the tests? When does it hurt?
History ☐	Can you point to where you feel the pain? Does it make you sick? Does it make you burp? When you have the pain, what do you do? Does that help? Do you take any other medicines? Who do you live with, Henry? What do you do during the daytime? Who do you tell if you do not feel well?
Risk ☐	Do you smoke? Do you drink alcohol? Do you like coffee or tea? Is there anyone in the family who has a problem in the tummy?
Flags ☐	Have you lost weight, Henry? Do you ever spit your food out because it hasn't gone down into the tummy? Are you coughing lots? Have you felt shivery or hot and cold? Henry, what colour is your poo? Is it ever red like blood or black? Is your poo hard, soft or like water? When you have a wee is that okay or does it hurt? Do you go to the toilet lots to have a wee, or is it the same as always do you think?
Impact ☐	Have you stopped eating as much since this pain started?
ICE ☐	Henry, why do you think you have tummy pain? Are you worried about it? Why are you worried? What did you and your mum think we may decide today? Rosemary, what do you think may be causing this? What are you mostly worried about? What did you hope I might suggest?
Curious ☐	Henry, do you know what your mum means by the 'big C'? Have you talked about what you think?
SummarICE ☐	To summarise, Henry, you have told me that for a few months you have had pain in the tummy; this has been making you burp but also lose weight. You want some more medicine to make it better. Your mum is worried it could be something serious and thinks you need more tests.
O/E ☐	Can I ask you to step on the scales, Henry? Now, may I feel your tummy and can you tell me if it hurts when I press? Can I feel your pulse and take your temperature?
Impression ☐	It sounds like this could be a tummy ulcer. Have you had an ulcer in your mouth? This is similar but in the tummy. To give us an answer we need to have a look at different parts of the tummy to see where the problem is. Sometimes an ulcer or pain can be there because of a cancer.
Sense ☐	I can see you are upset.
Experience ☐	Have you seen anyone with cancer? What do you know about it?
Explanation ☐	That can happen but we can also fix it and make it better if we know what it is. The bacteria blood test came back normal but you are anaemic which means your blood count is low.
Empathy ☐	Mentioning the big C can be scary, especially when your gran had it. I have to make sure we've done all the right tests to make sure we know what needs to be done to make you better.
Options ☐	I agree that a jelly scan of your tummy will give us more clues. I also think we should look into the tummy.
Recommend ☐	Henry, I suggest we do this by making you sleepy then putting a thin tube with a light into the tummy. Would that be okay? If we see what is causing the pain, we can hopefully make it better.
Future ☐	Whatever it is, we can talk about it again soon.
Empower ☐	If ever you feel hot and shivery please will you tell someone?
Specifics ☐	You should receive the appointment for the jelly scan and tube test within 2 weeks then I will see you the week after. If you don't receive these tests in that time, please let me know. Rosemary – please would you book the appointment to see me? Is that all okay?
Safety net ☐	If you have a high temperature or if you see red or black in the toilet, or you are sick or have really bad pain, you need to tell the warden and they need to call a doctor. Rosemary could you pass that on?

Neurodevelopmental Disorders, Intellectual and Social Disability – 1

Patient's Story

Doctor's notes		Henry Sutton, 60 years. (Attends with mother Rosemary.)
		PMH: hypoxic ischaemic encephalopathy, seizures (seizure-free 30 years), hearing difficulty, hearing aids, myopia, learning difficulties (IQ 45), attention deficit hyperactivity disorder, GORD. Medications: omeprazole 40 mg.
		Blood tests: *H. pylori* negative, Hb 105 g/dL. The rest of the FBC, U&E, LFT, amylase, CRP, HbA1c, FBG – all normal. Weight: 65 kg 1 year ago.
How to act		You are able to answer some questions, but you frequently turn to your mother who either answers for you or repeats the question if the doctor is not being clear.
PC	**Mum:**	*'Henry has come for the results of his blood test.'*
History	**Henry:**	*'I keep getting tummy pain … above the belly button.'* You can't describe a pattern. No vomiting. If the doctor asks, say: *'My poo is normal.'* No melaena or dysphagia.
	Mum:	*'I noticed he was losing weight.'*
		'He keeps telling me he has pain in his stomach.' This has been the case for months.
		Henry came off all his medicines for ADHD in his late teens, followed by his seizure medications. He has been well since. There is no significant family history. He is often belching and he finds this funny. The omeprazole alone doesn't seem to have helped. Henry doesn't drink caffeine or alcohol. He takes no medicines and specifically, no ibuprofen. Henry is happy. When the pain is there, you give Henry Gaviscon. It helps a bit, he says.
Social	**Henry:**	You moved to sheltered accommodation 15 years ago where you made friends.
		Your mother visits twice a week. You do not smoke or drink alcohol. No tea/coffee.
		You do not work but help out in the laundry shop for the residents. There is always a warden on call. You know you can just press the button on the receiver if you need help. You are able to prepare very simple meals such as cereal and sandwiches but have help from staff with hot food.
	Mum:	He eats a very good diet and enjoys going for walks every day with the staff.
ICE	**Henry:**	You don't know why you have the pain. You just want it to stop.
		You think the doctor will give you some more medicine.
	Mum:	*'I am worried it's something serious.'* If asked to explain *'the big C'*.
		You have not told your thoughts to Henry. You would like the doctor to arrange an ultrasound. The other doctor said it might be bacteria, in which case Henry will be given antibiotics. If the doctor starts to talk about the possibility of cancer, Henry becomes distressed. If asked more about this, Henry says, *'People die.'* His granny died in her 80s of lung cancer. If the doctor uses jargon, Henry doesn't want the test. If the doctor empathises and explains why endoscopy is important, Henry agrees.
O/E		Weight 55 kg. Slightly tender epigastrium. Otherwise normal.

Learning Points

When beginning a consultation with a person with intellectual disabilities, it is a good idea to set out what is likely to happen in the consultation. The patient may not be familiar with the consultation process and it can reduce anxiety to explain at the beginning. As with children, address your questions to the patient rather than their carer. Be guided by the language the patient and their carer use, to help you use language and terminology that the patient understands. You may need to slow the consultation pace to allow the patient time to absorb what you have said and think of their answer. Be patient; if you aren't understood at first, think of different ways to explain what you mean rather than giving up. Be aware that some patients with intellectual disabilities take what you say very literally so sometimes using similes/metaphors can add to the confusion! Remember, you can get packs of picture cards which help patients explain their symptoms, e.g. happy/sad faces, body parts, toilets, etc.

Points to be aware of

'Elderly parents are often unaware of community support now available to adults with intellectual disabilities. A mutually dependent relationship may have developed according to their needs and capabilities. Parents may not ask for help for fear their son or daughter will be taken into care. Elderly parents are often socially isolated. They may be less observant of health changes in their son or daughter.

Comorbid medical conditions are common, but easily overlooked unless actively screened for.

Planning for the future should include recognising inevitable separation by death, and the need to anticipate emotional as well as practical needs.

When people with intellectual disabilities have moved to a home of their own, sustained effort by the new carers is needed to support continuing contact with elderly parents.'[1]

'When a person with intellectual disabilities loses a parent through death, it is not only a loss of someone who is loved, but is also the loss of the person most familiar with their needs, their likes and dislikes, and with whom they shared a trusting relationship.'[2]

Diagnostic overshadowing

'Be aware of the concept of diagnostic overshadowing when a person's presenting symptoms are put down to the disability, rather than the doctor seeking another, potentially treatable cause.'[3]

What are the reasons for this?	Time: 10–12-minute consultations, doctor uncertainty, communication barriers, atypical presentations, lack of continuity – the doctor and patient do not know each other.
How can this be prevented?	GP and healthcare education: early screening for physical and mental health problems. Annual reviews. Carer and family education: vigilance for a change in the person and involving the carers in safety netting advice. Time (a recurrent theme) and longer appointments.

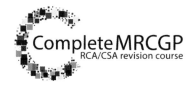

CompleteMRCGP
RCA/CSA revision course

Neurodevelopmental Disorders, Intellectual and Social Disability – 1

Doctor's Notes

Patient	Matthew Dalton	24 years	M
PMH	Down syndrome		
	Closure ASD		
	Sensorineural deafness. Hearing aids.		
Medications	No current medications		
Allergies	No known drug allergies		
Consultations	No recent consultations		
Investigations	No recent investigations		
Household	No household members registered		
	Patient attending for annual review.		

Example Consultation

Open ☐   How are you, Matthew? What is going well for you? What has been difficult this year?

Empathy ☐   I'm sorry to hear that. Do you miss her? Do you cry when you think of her?

Sense ☐   You mentioned your mum told you to see me… is your mum worried about anything?

Curious ☐   Why don't you like going to the doctor? What can you remember? That must have been horrible. Today I would just like to talk and examine you. That's it for today. If either of us is worried about anything we can talk about it and decide together. We won't do anything without your permission. Is that okay?

Sense ☐   Is your ear okay? Why do you keep touching it? Can you hear okay with your hearing aid?

History ☐   Can you remember what health problems you have had in the past? Are you feeling well or is something not right? Can we go through the body to see if you have had any problems? Let's start at the top – do you have any headaches? Can you see everything okay? When did you last have your eyes checked? Can you hear okay? How often do you feel out of breath? Do you have any other strange feelings in your chest? Does your back hurt? Do your arms and legs feel okay? How often do you go for a wee? Does it ever hurt? How often do you have a poo? Is the poo hard like stones, soft or runny? Does anywhere hurt? Have you seen the dentist this year? Who do you live with? What do you do during the day? You have a job: that's great! Do you enjoy it? Do you have friends who live nearby? Do you have a girlfriend or boyfriend? Is it going well? What do you enjoy doing on your own? It sounds like you are very independent.

Flags ☐   Are you happy or sad most of the time? Do you worry about anything?

ICE ☐   What did you think we might talk about today? Why do you think your ear is hurting? Is there anything you would like me to help with?

SummarICE ☐   So it sounds as if you have had an upsetting time with losing your gran but Laura has made you feel happy. Your hearing aid is rubbing and you would like a new one.

O/E ☐   Every year we offer an examination so we can check your health. I would like to check your weight and height, look in your ears, listen to your heart and lungs, take your blood pressure, feel your neck, feel your tummy and check your testicles. Do you know where the testicles are? These are the two round parts that are under the penis. This would involve removing your underpants but it is important so I can check there are no lumps or bumps. Would that be okay? I need a chaperone so I will ask Suzie, our nurse, to come in whilst I examine you. Is that okay?

Impression ☐   Your ear is infected. There is also a little lump on the testicle.

Explanation ☐   We commonly find lumps, most are nothing to worry about, but we need to check it with a scan. The scan is in the hospital. It won't hurt and all you will feel is cold jelly. It is important to make sure that the lump is not a cancer. Usually it isn't.

Options ☐   Can I arrange this for you? For the ear, please use the spray called Otomize three times a day for a week and let me know if it is still hurting in a week. I will write to the hearing aid team to request they see you to talk about a new one.

Empower ☐   Matthew, your weight is a little high. Do you do any exercise? What exercise would you most like to do? Who cooks your meals? Do you know which foods can be bad for you? Would you like to lose weight? Do you think you could cut out some crisps, biscuits and cakes? I will ask our nurse to see you to discuss diet in more detail.

Future ☐   It would also be helpful to do your annual blood test. Oh dear, do you not like blood tests? It is important to monitor your blood to make sure you're healthy. If I ask the nurse to use a small needle would that help? I can give you some cream to make your skin numb so you won't feel it, if you like? It is a good idea to do exercise together with Laura. Would you like me to write down what we have decided to do next?

Specifics ☐   Shall we see you in 3 months to see how you are getting on? I will send you a text message to remind you about the date. If the scan or blood tests show anything more urgent, we will let you know.

Safety net ☐   If you don't receive the appointment for your scan in the next 2 weeks, please speak to me. If you're worried about anything or feel unwell, please let me know.

Patient's Story

Doctor's notes	Matthew Dalton, 24 years. PMH: Down syndrome, closure ASD, sensorineural deafness. Hearing aids. Medication: none.
How to act	Pleasant but quiet. Keep touching your ear.
PC	*'My mum said I have to have my yearly check-up.'*
History	*'I don't like coming to the doctors.'*
	If asked why say: *'Because I always had to go to the doctors.'*
	If asked why, say: *'Operations hurt.'*
	Only if asked about your ear, *'It hurts.'* No other ear symptoms.
	No other symptoms on systemic enquiry.
	You saw the dentist and optician a month ago.
Social	You live with your mum. You do not know your dad.
	You do not smoke or drink alcohol. You work in the hardware store.
	You have been saving money and hope to buy a house one day.
	Your girlfriend's name is Laura. Laura has Down syndrome.
	You met at a party 3 months ago and you look pleased when you tell the doctor this.
	Your gran died earlier in the year. You cried a lot but not since you met Laura.
	Your mum makes your meals. You eat an unhealthy diet. You do not exercise.
	If encouraged to think about how you could be healthier, suggest going swimming with Laura and say you will tell your mum what the doctor said.
	You would be interested in losing weight.
ICE	If the doctor mentions any new medical conditions, say you don't know.
	Have no understanding of any medical problems.
	However, if the doctor says you need tests say: *'I don't want a blood test.'*
	If the doctor explains in simple language why you need tests, agree.
	You are worried that your hearing aid is rubbing. You would like a new one.
	You don't know what the doctor will want to talk to you about.
	Your mum said the doctor will do a blood test. (Wrinkle your nose at this.)
Examination	The ear canal is eczematous and discharging. The tympanic membrane is normal. No surrounding swelling or lymphadenopathy. Apyrexial. HR 82 bpm. BP 116/62. BMI is 31.
	The skin is normal. HS normal. Chest clear.
	There is a <1 cm lump on the lower pole of the left testicle.

Neurodevelopmental Disorders, Intellectual and Social Disability – 2

Practices are encouraged to have a 'Learning Disability register'. This helps ensure that all patients with intellectual disabilities have an annual review. It is a good idea to send out a questionnaire before the appointment for the patient to complete with their carer. If your practice adopts this approach, make sure you ask to see the questionnaire at the appointment!

The annual health check should include:

- Health screening: observations, weight, height, urine dip, discussion about smoking, alcohol, drugs, diet and exercise, breast or testicular awareness, cervical screening, CVD screening (BMI, BP and blood tests).
- Social assessment: dependence and independence. Discussion regarding social skills.
- Vulnerability assessment: risk of abuse (neglect, physical, sexual, emotional).
- Advice regarding check-ups: vision (e.g. for cataracts), hearing (e.g. for SNHL) and dental.
- Systemic enquiry looking for undiagnosed problems (see below).
- Full physical examination: top to toe approach including ears, neck, chest, abdomen, genitalia, skin, nails, etc.
- Mental health assessment.

Discussion of potential issues specific to the condition and life stage, e.g. with Down syndrome:[1,2]

Congenital	Heart disease, hypothyroidism, dislocation of the hip and cataracts.
Childhood	Signs of developmental delay, duodenal atresia, pyloric stenosis, Hirschsprung's disease.
	Constipation and tracheo-oesophageal fistulae.
	Hearing and visual impairment.
	Symptoms of hypothyroidism (may be congenital or acquired). Ongoing cardiac conditions.
	Atlantoaxial instability: have they had X-rays?
	Once diagnosed – neurological assessments.
	Ask about schooling.
Adolescence	Growth and obesity. Dental care.
	Menstruation may be slightly delayed. Annual TFTs. Skin and hair.
Late adult	Glaucoma and dementia screening.
Ongoing	Recurrent URTIs – urine dip and MSU if signs of infection.

Create a **Health Action Plan** at the end of the annual review. This may be fairly simple such as changes to diet/exercise, coming for blood tests or booking a dental review. It is a good idea to write this down for the patient and some may even have a Health Action Plan booklet which you can write this in. The RCGP provides an example of the questionnaires and action plans that can be used, in its document *A Step-by-Step Guide for GP Practices: Annual Health Checks for People with a Learning Disability* by Dr Matt Hoghton and the RCGP Learning Disabilities Group.[3]

'Ageing and the problems of old age are particularly relevant to people with Down syndrome as some of these age-related problems develop earlier in life than would normally be the case.'[1]

'The astute GP will remember that the child with Down syndrome is susceptible to the same range of childhood problems as any other and that not all symptoms will be due to the syndrome.'[2]

Doctor's Notes

Patient	Justin Walton	17 years	M
PMH	Autistic spectrum disorder		
	Behavioural concerns 3 years ago		
	Lower respiratory tract infection		
Medications	None		
Allergies	No known drug allergies		
Consultations	Letter – discharged from CAMHS 2 months ago.		
Investigations	Nil		
Household	No household members registered		

Example Consultation   Autism and Transition Process

Open ☐   Thank you for phoning to speak to me today. Why did you see CAMHS? What did they say was causing you to feel like that? Did they give you a name for the diagnosis?

Impact ☐   Everyone with autism can struggle with different things… what do you struggle with? What is better now? Are you well at the moment? Is anything causing you worry? What does your mum think?

Sense ☐   Do you worry about all the changes that are happening?

ICE ☐   What have you been thinking about recently? Are there any other thoughts that upset you? Or make you feel angry? What do you do when you feel angry? What did you think we may decide today? Is there anything else you were hoping for?

History ☐   Have you had any health problems? Any in your family? Do you take tablets? Drugs? Alcohol? How do you spend your day? Do you do GCSEs? Very good. Were you pleased? What would you like to do next? Who is at home? Are you in a relationship?

Empower ☐   Would you like to earn money? What are you good at? What do you enjoy? Can you think of a job you could try? Would you like to live on your own? What do you do by yourself? When might you be at risk? Does anyone say or do hurtful things to you? Who could you tell if this happened? Yes, your family or your GP.

Flags ☐   When you feel angry do you have thoughts of hurting yourself or anyone else?

Curious ☐   Do you get on with your family? Do you feel life is harder for you than for your sister?

SummarICE ☐   It sounds as if you have had a difficult few years but there are things you are good at: you have gained GCSEs and have, in your words, calmed down. But recent changes have been stressful. Finishing school, being discharged from CAMHS and thinking about what your mum said about finding work and moving out has made you anxious. You have been spending more time alone. You would like to find a girlfriend and feel this would make you happy.

Impression ☐   You are going through a difficult time of change. You mentioned you have autism.

Experience ☐   What do you know about autism? What do you mean by not good at school?

Explanation ☐   Recent changes in your life have put all of the challenges of having autism together: having to speak to new people, having to think about finding work when you don't find it easy learning new skills and having to make changes in your life, like finding work with the aim of becoming independent.

Empathy ☐   Often people feel angry when they are hurt and upset. Your mum has encouraged you to make changes and this is particularly difficult and worrying for you. I recognise you feel upset and stressed. Have you spoken to your mum about this? I suspect she wants you to have a fulfilling life, and finding work and your own place in the world can help with this.

Options ☐   There is an organisation called Restore for people like you who find adapting to work hard. They help build your confidence with areas you are good at. You could tell them you prefer not to work in groups and you are good with your hands. Would you be interested in this?

InCludE ☐   You mentioned a note for the job centre. I wonder: how about I give you a note for the next month, in the short term, and meanwhile we work together to help to achieve your goals of meeting someone and using your current skills in an environment where you are comfortable? I can print this off now and you could come and collect it from our receptionist. You could speak to the Job Centre about your skills and hopes for the future to see what they can suggest too.

Future ☐   Does this sound okay? You could also contact MIND who may point you in the direction of small social events – you may be able to meet a girlfriend.

Specifics ☐   Shall we talk again in a month? In the meantime, could you call Restore to see how they may be able to help you?

Safety net ☐   Please phone a doctor if your anger increases or you are very upset.

Patient's Story

Autism and Transition Process

Doctor's notes   Justin Walton, 17 years. PMH: autistic spectrum disorder, behavioural concerns 3 years ago and lower respiratory tract infection. Medication: none. Documents: discharged from CAMHS 2 months ago.

How to act   Nervous. Your mother told you to talk to the doctor alone. She is in the kitchen.

PC   *'The CAMHS team said I needed to start seeing you now.'*

History   Your mother made the appointment following instructions from CAMHS.

You are physically well and have no current illnesses. No significant family history.

'I have autism. I have learning problems.'

You originally saw the CAMHS team 3 years ago because you were shouting a lot and you were not getting on with your mum. You remember at the time feeling very frustrated that you were struggling at school with friends and the work.

Your mood is okay. You have no thoughts of wanting to hurt yourself or others.

Social   You now get on okay with your mum as you have 'calmed down', but you don't get on well with your father or younger sister. *'She is good at everything.'* There is no violence or abuse in the home or in your past. You left school 2 months ago after gaining three GCSEs in Technology, IT and Geography. You did not make friends easily and became happy being alone. If the doctor mentions a relationship, say you would like a girlfriend to make you happy. You think you would prefer to live with a girlfriend. This is your main aim. You are not sure where to find a girlfriend. You would like money but you don't like being around new people. However, you do feel you have skills – you are good at mending things. There is an old scrapyard near your home and you enjoy restoring broken things. Your dad lets you keep these in the garage. You think you could do a paper-round on your bike.

ICE   You would like a note for the job centre. Your mum has said you can live there for 2 more years but thinks you should start earning your own money and then find a place to live. This has made you feel angry and is always on your mind. Since she said this, you stay in your room. The thought of going to work is making you feel very 'angry' (stressed) and you think your family will force you out the house, but you struggle to verbalise how you are feeling. You expect the doctor will give you a note. If the doctor makes other suggestions, follow his or her advice if explained well and if the doctor is supportive. However, you push for a note if he or she has not explored your skills or do not understand your situation. You know that *'Autism is where you are not good at school.'* If asked to expand, you mean *'not got lots of friends, not clever, don't notice how people feel which can make them angry'*.

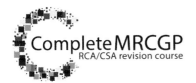

CompleteMRCGP
RCA/CSA revision course

Neurodevelopmental Disorders, Intellectual and Social Disability – 3

'Transitions occur throughout life… from childhood through puberty and adolescence to adulthood; from immaturity to maturity and from dependence to independence… extra transitions as a result of other life events for example, bereavement, separation of parents and being placed in care.'[1]

Complete CSA's Transition Processes Model – grouped into the elements below. First, a few tips…

1. You are not expected to include the whole model in 10–12 minutes! If, however, you spend time practising, you are more likely to be able to ask the appropriate questions in the exam that demonstrate your ability to practise holistically.

2. Keep the questions in a logical order. Even better… signpost! *'I'm interested to hear about changes at school… now questions about what you can do for yourself '*… An excellent way to feel and appear organised.

3. You can also signpost the elements you would like to discuss in a further consultation.

General health	What is their perception of their current health? How could they improve their health?
Health checks	Dental checks, breast awareness, smears or testicular checks.
Physical health	Any current issues? Any ongoing management required? Health awareness?
Mental health	Do they suffer with anxiety, depression or any mental illness?
Life changes	Have they had a change in environment: school, job or home? How did they cope?
Emotional adaptations	How do they feel about the change: excited? scared? isolated?
Challenges	What has been difficult or upsetting? Changes, stress or bereavements?
Strengths	Have they developed skills and strengths? Are they proud of their achievements?
Achievements	Finishing school, leaving home, finding a job, getting married and parenting.
School changes	Are they managing the workload? Future plans? How is the interaction with friends?
Independence	What do they do alone? What do they rely on others for?
Levels of responsibility	What are they currently responsible for? How do they manage this? Current stress?
Logistical challenges	How do they manage money and legal obligations?
Relationships	How are relationships with parents, siblings, friends, sexual partners?
Sexual health	Experiences, contraception and infection prevention? Are they considering a family?
Personal care	Hygiene, managing periods, toileting and cooking?
Ethnic background	Is their religion/background important to them at their current life stage?
'Perception of risk'[1]	Risk of abuse: what is their experience of risk? When are they most at risk? How do they reduce risk? Risk of neglect? Is there vulnerability to exploitation? Social setting: alcohol and drug use? Avoiding dangerous situations.
Needs	What is causing them worry? What are their hopes? What do they need?
Transition services	GPs have a role in providing additional support and bridging the transition between child to adult social services (through a Connexions worker) and health services.

Demonstrate you are being proactive by:

1. Understanding who is currently involved in the patient's care.

2. Offering to liaise with the current/new teams.

3. Providing follow-up and an ongoing point of contact.

Doctor's Notes

Patient	Janine Paton 33 years F
PMH	Cerebral palsy
	Severe learning disability
	Constipation
	Urinary tract infections
	Epilepsy – no seizure for 2 years
Medications	Laxido, sodium valproate and carbamazepine
Allergies	No known drug allergies
Consultations	No recent consultations
Investigations	No recent investigations
Household	No household members registered

Open ☐	Hello Janine, I'm Dr Blount. It is a pleasure to meet you. Who have you brought with you today? (looking to the carer). Can you tell me why you have come to see me today? Let's ask Ruth. Oh dear, what have you noticed? Anything else that has changed? Or changes in behaviour? Or communication? I'm wondering what Janine is like when she is feeling herself?
Curious ☐	Do you use any special ways of communicating?
History ☐	Janine, are you in pain? Does it hurt when you wee? Or in your tummy? Have you been for a poo today? Ruth, have her bowels been normal? How often is Janine opening her bowels? Have either of you noticed a change in going to the toilet? A smell or going more frequently?
Flags ☐	I'm wondering whether you have lost weight Janine? Ruth – how much, do you think? Over how long? Has Janine had a temperature? May I see Janine alone for a moment? Janine – do you like Ruth? Is anyone who lives or works at the home making you feel sad or upset? Thank you. Let's bring Ruth back into the room.
ICE ☐	Ruth, what do you think may be causing Janine to not feel herself? You have mentioned pain; have you had any other thoughts? Is there anything you are worried may be going on? What did you expect we may arrange or decide today?
Sense ☐	Janine, I am wondering if you are normally a quiet person like today or if you are normally smiling and chatty. Ruth, what would you say? Janine, are you feeling happy or sad? Okay, if I draw a picture of a smiling face and a sad face, can you tell me if you are this one… or this one? I'm sorry you are feeling sad.
SummarICE ☐	To summarise what we have said so far: Janine, your carers have been worried about you. You have not had the same energy, you have stayed in your room and not been interested in what you usually enjoy. You tell me you are not in pain but it is not clear what may be wrong. You are feeling sad.
O/E ☐	Janine, may I listen to your chest, feel your tummy, take your blood pressure and temperature and have a look at your throat, ears and neck please? I will also test your wee. I would like to weigh you please. Can we look at all your joints – arms and legs?
Impression ☐	I am not sure what is going on. It seems you are feeling sad at the moment. It could be that there is a physical problem causing you to change or it could be a mental health problem like depression. We will talk about how to help you feel happier, but I need to make sure this is not because you are feeling unwell.
InCludE ☐	I agree we should do so some tests to find out what's wrong.
Empathy ☐	It must be very hard, Janine, when you don't feel yourself but we will try to find out why.
Options ☐	I would like to arrange a blood test. Janine, I will arrange for the teams specialising in seeing patients who, like you, need more time, to perform eye and dental checks. This is to check that it isn't pain from your teeth, or problems with seeing clearly, that are making you feel like this.
Empower ☐	Janine, you can help us in the meantime. Each day, can you tell Ruth or another carer if you are this face or this face? Also, if Ruth points to different parts of your body can you clap your hands if that part doesn't feel okay? For example, if you had a headache and I pointed to your head what would you do?
Future ☐	So we will arrange a few blood tests to look at your blood count, liver, kidney and thyroid, and ask specialists to check your mouth and eyes. I will send your wee sample to the lab to check for any infection.
Specifics ☐	Shall we catch up again in 3–4 weeks to review the blood tests and see how you are? I will also ask a nurse from the learning disability team to see you at home. Ruth, please let me know if you do not receive an appointment in the next 4 weeks to see the specialists.
Safety net ☐	If any new symptoms develop or Janine seems worse, please let me know.

Neurodevelopmental Disorders, Intellectual and Social Disability – 4

Patient's Story   Mental Health and Intellectual Disability

Doctor's notes   Janine Paton, 33 years. PMH: cerebral palsy, Severe LD, constipation, UTIs and epilepsy – no seizure for 2 years. Medications: Laxido, sodium valproate and carbamazepine.

How to act   Attends with carer, Ruth, who does all the talking. Janine looks at the floor unless spoken to and only says yes/no to some questions and not all.

PC   *'We are worried something is wrong. We don't know if she is in pain.'*

History   She usually enjoys sitting in the lounge and watching television shows. Janine also likes it when the music is on. However, over the past 2 months, she has not looked interested and stays in her room. She seems 'weaker' because she has not got the same energy. She does not cry but sometimes makes a wailing sound. You are not sure if this is because she is in pain.

Her urine does not smell abnormal. She is not vomiting. She has required more encouragement to eat her food and she often leaves a lot of it. She has lost some weight over the month. Janine is opening her bowels once daily with Laxido. No rectal bleeding.

Janine has regular periods, the last one being 2 weeks ago. They are not heavy.

Janine does not repeatedly touch her head or ears. She has not had a cough, cold or fever.

Janine does not walk and transfers with the help of two carers between the bed and wheelchair.

The carers have no information on Janine's family.

Social   Janine lives in a home with several other residents cared for by the staff.

ICE   Ruth is worried it may be another water infection.

Ruth also wants to check that there is no abnormality in the stomach causing pain and loss of appetite. Ruth expects she will be given more antibiotics but would like her to have a scan.

Janine only says 'no' when asked about pain. Janine cannot answer about her mood. However, if the doctor asks how best to communicate with Janine, she likes pictures and can respond to pictures with yes or no. Pictures usually used include food, the weather and faces. Janine also likes to clap as another way of saying yes.

O/E   Janine has lost 4 kg in weight since she was last weighed 6 months ago.

HS normal, chest clear, abdomen soft, non-tender, no masses and there is no swelling in any joint. Janine is moving all joints without pain. No lymphadenopathy. ENT normal.

Ruth has brought a sample of urine. Urine dipstick is negative.

Observations are normal.

Learning Points   Mental Health and Intellectual Disability

'In Valuing People (2001) they describe a "learning disability (LD)" as a: 'significantly reduced ability to understand new or complex information, to learn new skills, reduced ability to cope independently, which starts before adulthood with lasting effects on development.'[1]

'Understand the psychiatric disorders prevalent in the adult with intellectual disability and how their diagnosis, detection and management differ...'[2]

The patient may struggle to express or verbalise their emotions. Helpful questions to consider:

Has there been a change in behaviour?

Do they feel angry?

Are there any changes to their routine – sleep or eating?

Is there concern among family members?

Can a collateral history be obtained?

'GPs should be able to recognise the following: atypical presentation of psychiatric or physical illness because of sensory, communication and cognitive difficulties.'[2] Use language without jargon, seek a collateral history; however, also screen for risk of neglect and this includes seeing the patient alone.

Use open screening questions for physical and mental health problems and social challenges. Have vigilance and a high level of suspicion for atypical presentations of conditions.

Have a low threshold for suspicion of mental health problems and be proactive to enquire about subtle changes and atypical presentations.

Other suggestions/tips to demonstrate the RCGP curriculum...

'... community resources, e.g. residential facilities, daytime activities, support groups, advocacy, available to this patient in my practice area, including those provided by the voluntary sector.'[2] Demonstrate your awareness of this by guiding where the patient can go to seek more information.

'Tailored physical and mental state assessments in patients with intellectual disability and those unable to verbalise symptoms.'[2] Tailor the examination to the condition and life stage. A complete assessment should also be performed in the annual health check.

Signpost that following your initial thorough examination, following investigation results you may consider the help of the Learning Disability Team.

'Additional important content... impact on family dynamics, including parenting experiences, bereavement reactions (see also RCGP Topic Guide on *People at the End of Life*; physical, psychological and social morbidity in carers.'[2] Always ask about those who support or care for the patient. How are the relationships? Ask about the carer's health and concerns.

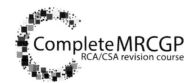

Neurodevelopmental Disorders, Intellectual and Social Disability – 4

Doctor's Notes

Patient	Lilly Young	24 years	F
PMH	Moderate learning disability		
	Constipation		
	Recurrent urinary tract infections		
Medications	No current medications		
Allergies	No known drug allergies		
Consultations	No recent consultations		
Investigations	No recent investigations		
Household	No household members registered		

Example Consultation

Open ☐   Okay. Why would you like to go on the pill? Do you have a boyfriend? How do you know Karl?

Sense ☐   It sounds like you are quite excited about this relationship. Would you like to have sex?

Experience ☐   What do you know about how to have sex? Do you know anything about infections you can catch through sex? What do you know about the pill?

Curious ☐   Do you want to take the pill? What do you think about having a baby?

ICE ☐   Do you know any other ways to stop you from getting pregnant? Do you know how you can avoid getting infections? Is there anything you are worried about? What would you like to take away with you today? Would you remember to take a tablet every day?

History ☐   I see you used to have problems going to the toilet; can you tell me more about that? Are you well now, or not? When was your last period? What are your periods like? Do you have bad headaches? Do you take medicines? Has your mum or your grandparents ever had a health problem? Do you have a dad? Who do you live with? Do you have a job? Do you have a hobby? Who does Karl live with?

Flags ☐   Is Karl making you have sex? Does he ever hurt or upset you? Have you had sex?

Curious ☐   Have you talked to anyone about having sex? What does Julie say? Did she say anything else? Would you like to ask me any questions? Do you get on well with your mum? Can you talk to her about having sex? What does she say? Did she say anything else? Might you have sex before your birthday?

O/E ☐   Lilly – can you tell me how much you weigh? Thank you. I will need to check your blood pressure. Would that be okay? I would need to wrap something around your arm and it will swell up like a balloon and feel tight for a minute – would that be okay? Could you come to see me at 1 p.m. today? Please bring your mum or someone else with you if you would like. Thank you.

Impression ☐   Lilly, you would like to have sex and you have decided not to have a baby yet.

SummarICE ☐   You don't think you will remember a tablet. You don't like having periods. You have decided to talk to your mum again before you decide. You feel excited but Julie has said sex hurts and this worries you.

Explanation ☐   You should only have sex if you want to. You can always say no. Sex should not hurt.

Safety net ☐   If it did hurt, you should tell Karl and tell a doctor too. Do you think you could do this?

Options ☐   The pill is a tablet to stop you having a baby. If you don't think you can remember it every day, there are other options too – an injection every 3 months or a little stick under the arm which is just one injection and lasts three years. What do you think? Okay, there is also a special plaster that you can put on your arm. You leave it there for a week and change it after every week. What do you think to that idea? Do you think your mum would help you with it? The plaster has a medicine inside which goes into your skin. This medicine can make some people very unwell; the risk is small but you would have to remember that if ever your leg hurt or got bigger one day, or if you had a bad headache, you must let a doctor know straight away. This can be a sign that something is wrong. Could you remember this? Would you like to try this plaster? The real name for the plaster is the patch. Do you have any questions?

Empower ☐   After having sex, go to the toilet to have a wee. This stops those wee infections returning. Have you heard of condoms, Lilly? Condoms are important to stop any bugs or infections from Karl going to you. They also help prevent pregnancy too.

Empathy ☐   It is a lot to remember, so are you happy to talk it through with your mum first? When you come this afternoon, I will give you leaflets about the pill, the patch and the implant so you can talk about the choices with your mum.

Future ☐   Next time we can also talk about women's check-ups.

Safety net ☐   Can you remember where in the body you may have pain if the patch is causing you harm?

Neurodevelopmental Disorders, Intellectual and Social Disability – 5

Doctor's notes	Lilly Young, 24 years. PMH: moderate learning disability. Recurrent urinary tract infections. Medications: none.
How to act	You respond well if the doctor uses language which is easy to follow.
PC	*'I would like the pill.'*
History	*'My mum told me I had to, otherwise I can't go camping.'*
	You have known Karl, who is the same age as you, for many years.
	You were in the same class at Rose Hill Special School. *'Karl is like me.'*
	Karl asked you to the cinema a month ago. Now you see each other every evening.
	Karl lives with his parents and younger sister. They are all family friends.
	He wants to take you camping for your 25th birthday.
	You've not had sex but would like to when you go camping (not before).
	Karl says you will only have sex if you want to.
	You are well. No contraindications to the pill. You have light periods 3/28.
	No IMB.
	'I don't like periods.'
	'Going for a poo and wee is okay now.' You take no medicines.
	Your mum has told you the doctor will want to know if there are any problems in the family and there are none. If the doctor wants to know what your mum thinks, say your mum said you will talk about what the doctor says at home. You forget this if the doctor does not ask.
Social	You live with your mum. You do not know your dad. You have a friend, Julie.
	You like going to the cinema and going out to eat pizza. You do not drink or smoke.
	You work in the local garden centre cafe serving the tea and coffee.
ICE	*'We talked about sex in class.'*
	You don't know anything about the pill or any other contraception.
	You are vaguely aware that you can become ill from having sex, i.e. STIs.
	Your mum is happy for you to have sex; you have talked about it but promised her you would take the pill. You hate having periods.
	You don't think you will remember a tablet every day.
	You feel *'scared but excited'*. Julie has had sex and tells you sex hurts.
	You don't want any procedure or needles. You would like a baby. But your mum told you not yet. Your mum said she would have to help you look after a baby and she can't do this until she retires.
Examination	BP 110/60. Weight 60 kg. BMI 23.2

Risk factors for safeguarding concerns:

Dependence on others: learning or physical disability.

Lack of family support/confidantes.

Social isolation.

At risk of neglect.

Partner dominance/unequal relationships.

The impact of multiple negative events.

How do we pick up on risk?

Sensing: behavioural changes, low mood, annual reviews, MDT, awareness of DNAs or the opposite – multiple attendances. Building the relationship.

How to demonstrate the RCGP curriculum, which includes:

'Additional important content… emotional and sexual needs of adults with intellectual disability and how they may be expressed.'[1]

You can demonstrate this by respecting the patient's request and providing education, an opportunity to ask questions and choices. Do not make assumptions but check their understanding. Support them by offering safe options and helping the patient to consider different scenarios which may guide them to a decision they feel comfortable with.

The common pitfall with this consultation may be forgetting the routine medical checks, e.g. common contraindications, missed pill rules and safety netting advice. Do not avoid this conversation but instead adjust the language to ensure how you deliver it is effective and allows the patient to reach an informed decision.

From the RCGP curriculum you need to think about service issues: 'Health promotion including sexual health, contraception, cardiovascular disease risks, cancer screening and smoking cessation.'[1]

Always remember to 'Empower' the patient and take every opportunity to provide health promotion advice – in this case the UTI prevention, STI prevention and signposting the discussion about cervical screening. Find out if your area has an Intellectual/Learning Disability team or specialist nurse you can ask for advice. These teams/nurses should have awareness of local services available and may be able to help with capacity assessments and challenging behaviour. They can often support patients and provide advice to practices about improving access for those with ID. Sometimes they can also provide tips on encouraging patients to attend for blood tests, etc.

BMA's Mental Capacity Toolkit
See the **Link Hub at CompleteMRCGP.co.uk** for a useful link to the BMA's Mental Capacity Toolkit with series of very useful cards.

Information from the BMAs Mental Capacity Toolkit

Card 4 covers 'assessing capacity'. In brief:

- As part of your assessment of whether or not an individual can consent to treatment or care, you may need to assess whether or not they have capacity to make the decision or not.
- There are four aspects to consider and, if an individual fails any one of these, they are deemed not to have capacity to make a decision:
  - Understand information relevant to the decision.
  - Retain the information relevant to the decision.
  - Be able to weigh up or use the information.
  - Be able to communicate their view – in any way/by any means.[1]

You need to listen, where appropriate, to relatives or friends who may be able to provide useful additional information but must not be influenced by the views of the third party regarding the decision.

If you decide that someone lacks capacity, this should be based on your 'reasonable belief' and backed up by objective reasons.

The assessment of capacity relates to a specific decision at a specific time. If there is a change in the situation, capacity should be reassessed.

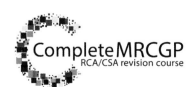

Neurology

	Cases in this chapter	Within the RCGP 2020 curriculum: Neurology	Learning points in this chapter include:
1	Peripheral Neuropathy	'Sensory and/or motor disturbances (peripheral nerve problems) including mono- and poly-neuropathies such as nerve compression and palsies'	Causes, blood tests, red flags
2	Normal Pressure Hydrocephalus	'Common and important conditions – dementia... normal pressure hydrocephalus' 'Tests of cognition and interpretation in relation to memory loss, dementia, delirium and associated disease'	Symptom triad Cause Differential diagnosis
3	Migraine	'Headaches including migraine' 'The effect of... migraine on vision' 'Treatments for migraine'	Red flags, differential diagnosis, management options
4	TIA	'Stroke including transient ischaemic attacks'	FAST Initial management of stroke and TIA Secondary prevention
5	Multiple Sclerosis	'Demyelination such as multiple sclerosis'	Epidemiology Symptoms Diagnosis Differential diagnosis Blood tests

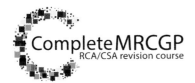

CHAPTER 17 REFERENCES

Peripheral Neuropathy

1. https://patient.info/brain-nerves/peripheral-neuropathy-leaflet#nav-2. Jul 2017.

Normal Pressure Hydrocephalus

1. https://patient.info/doctor/normal-pressure-hydrocephalus. Jan 2016.

Migraine

1. NICE CKS. https://cks.nice.org.uk/topics/migraine/. May 2021.
2. http://patient.info/doctor/giant-cell-arteritis-pro. Nov 2016.
3. https://clinox.info/clinical-support/local-pathways-and-guidelines/Clinical%20Guidelines/Ox%20Migraine%20Acute%20Therapy%20Guidelines%20Adult.pdf?UNLID=2551633772020617112816
4. https://clinox.info/clinical-support/local-pathways-and-guidelines/Clinical%20Guidelines/Migraine%20Adult%20Prophylactic%20Therapy%20Guidelines.pdf?UNLID=2551633772020617113019

Useful Resource

https://patient.info/mental-health/cognitive-behavioural-therapy-cbt-leaflet. Nov 2019.

TIA

1. NICE Guideline NG128. Stroke and transient ischaemic attack in over 16s: diagnosis and initial management. May 2019.
2. https://www.stroke.org.uk/what-is-stroke/what-are-the-symptoms-of-stroke
3. NICE CKS. https://cks.nice.org.uk/stroke-and-tia. Aug 2020.
4. Royal College of Physicians. *National Clinical Guideline for Stroke*. 5th edition. 2016.
5. Gent M., Beaumont D., Blanchard J. et al. A randomised, blinded, trial of clopidogrel versus aspirin in patients at risk of ischaemic events (CAPRIE). CAPRIE Steering Committee. *Lancet* 1996; 348(9038):1329–39.
6. Rothwell P.M., Algra A., Chen Z. et al. Effects of aspirin on risk and severity of early recurrent stroke after transient ischaemic attack and ischaemic stroke: time-course analysis of randomised trials. *Lancet* 2016; 388: 365–75.
7. https://www.sign.ac.uk/assets/pat108.pdf. Leaflet for patients following stroke.

Multiple Sclerosis

1. http://patient.info/doctor/multiple-sclerosis-pro. Mar 2020.
2. NICE CKS. https://cks.nice.org.uk/topics/multiple-sclerosis/. Aug 2020.

Information taken from NICE guidelines with kind permission. Please note the guidelines change frequently and you should ALWAYS check for the latest updated guidance. Remember that NICE guidance is only applicable to patients in the UK.

Doctor's Notes

Patient	Maggie Freestone	72 years	F

PMH	Bereavement. Death of husband 2 years ago.
	$2 \times$ NVD
	Gastritis
	Miscarriage
Medications	No current medications
Allergies	No information
Consultations	No recent consultations
Investigations	No recent investigations
Household	No household members registered

Open ☐	Tell me about this problem from the beginning. Then what did you notice? Anything else that isn't right?
Curious ☐	When you say you don't trust your feet, what do you mean? Have you fallen?
Sense ☐	I can see you are a positive person but I'm worried how this is affecting you.
Impact ☐	Has this changed how you live or your behaviour? Or your mood?
ICE ☐	What do you think has caused this? What has been on your mind? Is there anything you are worried about? What did you think or hope we may do today?
History ☐	Any other symptoms? Are you otherwise well? Any other medical conditions yourself or which run in the family? I'm sorry that I am not aware, but what caused your husband's death? How are you getting on without him? Who else is in your life? Do you take any medicines? Did anyone in your family have a similar problem?
Risk ☐	Do you drink alcohol? Have you been unwell recently or had a cold or sore throat?
Flags ☐	Is it painful? What does it feel like? How are you on the stairs or rising from a chair? Any weight loss? Any change in your bowels or change in control of going to the toilet? Any episodes of sweating? Or weakness? Have you felt lightheaded on standing? Do you still feel hot and cold where the numbness is? Any dry mouth or problems with the skin or joints?
O/E ☐	May I examine you; check the sensation and strength in your arms and legs, check your reflexes and watch you walk then check the spine for tenderness and movement please? I'd just like to look at the muscles in the legs now. Can I check your weight, pulse and blood pressure? Now I'd like to feel the pulses in your feet. May I feel your abdomen and the lymph glands in your neck, under the arms and groin? Lastly can I ask you to go to the toilet for a urine sample please?
SummarICE ☐	To summarise what you have told me, your feet have been gradually becoming more numb over the last year. This has stopped you cycling and you have fallen. You have been concerned about what may have caused this and so has your son. You sometimes have pain in your feet too. You weren't sure what I'd say today. Have I understood?
Empathy ☐	I imagine it knocks your confidence when you can't trust your feet, especially after a fall.
Impression ☐	I think you have peripheral neuropathy.
Experience ☐	Have you known anyone who has had a similar problem?
Explanation ☐	Peripheral means the parts of us furthest from the heart, and neuropathy means a problem with the nerve. Unfortunately, though, this is only a description of the problem rather than telling us the cause. There are several things that might cause it but no clues so far from what you have told me.
InCludE ☐	You told me you've been lying awake worrying about this and it's important we help you to sleep better by finding out what's wrong.
Recommend ☐	I'd like to start by doing a blood test for your routine health including for anaemia, your kidneys and liver, blood tests for inflammation, also check your cholesterol, your sugar level and vitamins called B12 and folate which, when low, can cause this. I would also like to check your urine for protein and sugar. Could I ask our falls team to see you, to help rebuild your confidence?
Options ☐	We can try different pain relief – would you like to hear about the options?
Empower ☐	Have you any thoughts about what may give you more confidence on your feet? Perhaps something to give you some support when walking?
Specifics ☐	After we've finished today, please tell reception that you need two appointments – one for a blood test as soon as convenient and then another to see me a week later.
Future ☐	When we meet up again after the blood tests, I should have more information and it is likely that I will, at that point, ask the neurologists – the nerve specialists – to see you. I expect they may talk to you about nerve conduction studies – a test which looks at the electricity flow in your nerves.
Safety net ☐	If ever you notice any weakness or new symptoms, or if you fall, please contact a doctor straight away as you would need to be examined again. I don't expect this to happen but if you ever notice a change in the control of your bladder or bowel or a new back pain or difficulty breathing, please let a doctor know straight away so we can make sure it is nothing serious.

Patient's Story

Doctor's notes   Maggie Freestone, 72 years. PMH: bereavement. Death of husband 2 years ago. 2 × NVD. Miscarriage. Gastritis. Medication: none.

How to act   Chirpy and chatty.

PC   *'Hello Doctor. Well, it's my feet. Often, I can't feel them. Very strange. What do you think it is then?'*

History   You have always been very healthy. About a year ago you started to notice your left foot felt a bit odd at times and then the right started about 6 months ago. Now both feet don't really feel normal most of the time. You therefore watch your feet as you walk. You have no symptoms of diabetes. You drink no alcohol. You have never smoked. You take no medicines. Your memory is good. You have had no head injury. You have no back pain or bladder/bowel dysfunction. Your strength is good apart from when you can't feel what you are doing. You have no problems in the proximal muscles. You wouldn't describe it as pins and needles but *'peculiar … like my feet have become sponge'*. You can still feel warm water. You have no other symptoms. No FH.

Social   You miss Des but you get on with life and love seeing people. Des died of prostate cancer which had spread to his bones and caused his kidneys to fail. You remain very active for the church, often raising money. You are very proud of how good you are for your age. You enjoyed riding your bike until last year when it became a problem.

'Now, I don't trust my feet.' Say this with laugh.

You live on your own.

ICE   You try to laugh this off; however, you have been lying awake wondering what this is. But you like to stay positive and you shrug it off when your children mention it. Your son is worried since you fell and banged your shoulder. The shoulder recovered but it did knock your confidence. Only if the doctor specifically asks you, you mention the burning pain the problem causes but you do not want any medicine for this. Your son bought you a mobile phone just in case you ever fall.

Examination   There is decreased sensation in both feet to just above the ankle. Arms are normal. The power in the legs is normal until L5/S1 which is 4/5 strength. Reflexes absent. Plantars downgoing. No muscle wasting. There is no spinal tenderness. BMI 25. BP 130/60. HR 62 bpm regular. Normal ROM spine and straight leg raise. Sensory ataxic ('stomping') gait. Abdomen normal, no masses and no lymphadenopathy. Normal urine dipstick. Normal peripheral pulses.

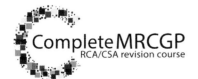

Learning Points

As well as sensory and motor symptoms, ask about features of autonomic dysfunction, which may include a change to the bowels, sweating, sphincter disturbance and postural hypotension.

Prevalence   About 1 in 50 people have some form of peripheral neuropathy.[1]

Causes   Diabetes or diabetic amyotrophy (most common cause in Europe)

Alcohol

B12/folate deficiency

Chronic kidney disease

HIV

Shingles

Rheumatoid arthritis

Lyme disease

Sjögren's syndrome

Amyloidosis

Uraemia

Guillain–Barré syndrome/chronic inflammatory demyelinating polyneuropathy (CIDP)

Porphyria

Charcot–Marie–Tooth disease

Malignancy or paraneoplastic syndrome

Vasculitic neuropathy

Side effects of chemotherapy including drugs used to treat HIV and more.

Remember Complete CSA's motto: **Common things are common… but what mustn't I miss?**

Ensure you are aware of how the rare conditions above may present.

Blood tests   FBC, U&E, LFT, GGT, TFTs, CRP, ESR, ANA, B12, folate, serum and urine electrophoresis.

Urine dipstick for protein and glucose.

CXR – sarcoidosis, malignancy.

Consider – Lyme or HIV serology, urinary porphyrins and an autoimmune screen.

Red flags   Always look out for cauda equina syndrome.

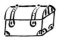
Gait
See the Link Hub at CompleteMRCGP.co.uk for a link to a helpful guide on the assessment of different gaits.

Doctor's Notes

Patient	Lionel Moore	84 years	M
PMH	TIA 3 years ago		
	Atrial fibrillation		
	Hypertension		
Medications	Warfarin		
	Atorvastatin 40 mg ON		
	Indapamide 2.5 mg OM		
	Ramipril 5 mg OM		
	Bisoprolol 5 mg OM		
Allergies	No information		
Consultations	No recent consultations		
Investigations	BP 130/70 1 month ago		
Household	Sandra Moore	79 years	F

Example Consultation **Normal Pressure Hydrocephalus**

Open ☐ Tell me, when did either of you first notice something wasn't right? What symptoms followed? Has anything else changed with your health?

History ☐ I am interested to hear your story, Lionel. Sandra, feel free to add anything. Lionel, how do you feel? In what way 'not right'? Have you felt like this before? What happened when you had the TIA? Your tablets, please talk me through when you take each one. Let's now go through the different parts of the body. Any headaches? How did it start? Any nausea or vomiting? Any changes in the arms or legs? Any problems with your speech or swallowing? Eyesight problems? Any breathing difficulties or chest problems? Pain in the tummy? Have you had a temperature? Any back pain? Any changes passing urine? Can you tell me about the accidents?

Curious ☐ What do you mean by wobbly exactly?

Risk ☐ Has your INR been in the normal range? Have you fallen or banged your head?

Flags ☐ Have you lost weight over recent months? Have you had any change in behaviour?

Sense ☐ Lionel, you keep looking at Sandra, is that because you are struggling to tell me?

Impact ☐ How has your memory affected you day to day, Lionel? Sandra, in what way have Lionel's memory troubles been difficult for you?

ICE ☐ Lionel, what did you think may be causing your symptoms? Is there anything you are particularly worried about? What did you think I may suggest today? How about you, Sandra – what have you been wondering? Did you hope I would do anything particular today?

SummarICE ☐ To summarise, the unsteadiness came first 9 months ago and for 6 months your memory has been patchy. Sandra, you have been worried about what this may mean for the future; however, with recent urinary incontinence you both wondered if you have a water infection and thought we needed to prescribe antibiotics for this.

O/E ☐ I would like to take a good look at you: listen to your heart, take your BP, pulse, temperature, check the nerves to your face, arms and legs, and look at the back of your eyes. Now please stand up and walk across the room, turn around and return. Can you move your neck up and down? Now, lying down, please lift your head and now raise your legs. May I check on the edge of the back passage to see if the nerve supply is normal? Could you provide a urine sample?

InCludE ☐ I see why you worried about a urine infection and dementia but, with the additional symptom of feeling wobbly, I think it may be something else.

Impression ☐ I believe it is possible that the diagnosis may be normal pressure hydrocephalus. If I'm right, prompt treatment should quickly improve your symptoms, especially your walking.

Experience ☐ Have you come across the term hydrocephalus?

Explanation ☐ 'Hydro' means water and 'cephalus' refers to the brain. Fluid surrounding the brain is continuously made then reabsorbed. If the reabsorption stops, this leads to less fluid being produced but overall, the pressure increases. Usually three things happen: a change in mobility, followed by memory trouble then urine incontinence. The treatment involves redirecting the fluid so that it moves away from the brain to reduce the pressure. Sometimes there is no cause found, but a previous bleed in the brain is possible. Your age and drinking alcohol put you at risk of a bleed, but your headache symptoms are not typical.

Empathy ☐ I appreciate this must have come as a shock when you were expecting just antibiotics.

Options ☐ I think we need to ask the hospital doctors to see you today. I expect they will arrange a head scan and may insert a needle into your back to check the fluid pressure. I think this problem has been building for many months rather than a sudden change like a stroke. Sandra, do you feel comfortable driving Lionel to the hospital? I will call the specialist.

Specifics ☐ Lionel, when you are back home, please message reception to let me know and also book an appointment to see me.

Future ☐ We can then reassess your memory and walking to see if there are any ongoing concerns and check your general health.

Empower ☐ We could also discuss the link between alcohol and risks to the brain and talk about practical steps you could take to protect your brain health.

Safety net ☐ I don't expect problems en route but if any problems arise, stop and call 999.

Doctor's notes	Lionel Moore, 84 years. PMH: TIA 3 years ago, atrial fibrillation and hypertension. Medications: warfarin, atorvastatin 40 mg ON, indapamide 2.5 mg OM, ramipril 5 mg OM and bisoprolol 5 mg OM. BP 130/70 1 month ago.
	You attend with your wife, Sandra, today.
How to act	You are quiet and often turn to Sandra to answer for you.
PC	Your wife Sandra is with you; she speaks first.
	'Lionel has been incontinent the past few days.'
History	**Sandra** You have found that he is damp and feel guilty that you shouted at him for wetting on the sofa. There has been no faecal incontinence. When the incontinence happened a third time you thought you had better see the doctor.
	'Lionel's memory hasn't been too good.' For example, he can't remember if he has had dinner and repeatedly asks if the dog has been fed. He has not wandered and there have been no safety concerns.
	'Over the last week he is not quite right.'
	Lionel had a TIA. His INR levels have been good and were last checked 1 week ago.
	There have been no further neurological signs unlike last time when, for 8 hours, his left side was weak. He has been *'a bit wobbly'*. You remember this started 9 months ago.
	Lionel You feel *'not myself'*. By this you mean you feel muddled. Your vision is normal.
	No abdominal pain or dysuria. You can't remember any increased urinary frequency.
	No prostate symptoms. You have no back pain. You have lost no weight.
	You have no cardiac or respiratory symptoms. Your bowels are normal.
	You have not fallen or had a head injury. You have a *'bit of a headache'* of gradual onset and no vomiting or nausea.
Social	Lionel enjoys two glasses of whisky every night. He stopped attending the pub quiz 6 months ago, as it started to become embarrassing that Lionel's memory was fading. Lionel used to be a solicitor and has three children, grandchildren and now great-grandchildren.
	Lionel smoked until he was 38 years old.
ICE	Neither of you are worried that this may be another TIA as Lionel has had no weakness.
	You suspect a UTI. You expect antibiotics.
	Sandra Worried if he has the 'big D'. You have been very worried how this will progress.
Examination	BP 128/72. HR 68 bpm irregularly irregular. RR 14. Sats 97%. Temperature 36.6 °C.
	Urine dipstick leucocytes only. HS normal. Abdomen soft, non-tender.
	Normal neurology apart from reflexes which are brisk bilaterally. CN normal examination. Unsteady gait. No other cerebellar signs. Fundi are normal. Brudzinski/Kernig's negative. No neck stiffness.
	Normal anal tone and sensation.

Learning Points

Normal Pressure Hydrocephalus

Significance	A potentially reversible cause of dementia, possibly accounting for up to 6% of all dementias.[1]
Triad	Apraxia, progressive memory disturbance and sphincter disturbance/ incontinence.
Cause	Idiopathic meningitis, subdural haematoma, head injury and radiotherapy.

Differential diagnosis in this case: all are possible and the scan will help differentiate.

Subdural haematoma	Secondary to age and alcohol.
TIA/cerebellar stroke	Secondary to risk factors but history and examination not typical.
Dementia, postural hypotension and UTI	
	All common. The symptoms and dipstick do not support a UTI.
	With the above triad, normal pressure hydrocephalus needs to be excluded.
Metastases	However, there was no reported weight loss or vomiting.
Cauda equina syndrome	However, no back pain or associated red flags.

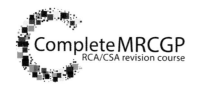

CompleteMRCGP
RCA/CSA revision course

Doctor's Notes

Patient	Yasmin Small 23 years F
PMH	Migraines
Medications	Amitriptyline 25 mg ON
	Desogestrel 75 μg OD
	Sumatriptan 50 mg PRN. Max 2 daily.
Allergies	No information
Consultations	3 months ago. Migraines occurring twice a week. Commenced amitriptyline. No abnormal bleeding with desogestrel.
Investigations:	No recent investigations
Household	No household members registered

Example Consultation

Open ☐ Tell me more about your headaches please. Any other symptoms you've noticed? Can you talk me through a typical headache episode? Thank you.

History ☐ Is there one type of headache? A pattern or relation to periods? How often are they occurring? What time of day do they start? Do they wake you? Where on the head? What does it feel like? Severity from 1 to 10? What makes it worse? Or better? Does lying down help? Any medical problems? Sinus trouble or increased headache learning forward? What medicines are you taking at the moment? Do they help? Any changes in your life that may have triggered them? Are work and home okay? Any stress?

Sense ☐ You sound tense; are you in pain now?

Impact ☐ How does it feel living with all these headaches? Please tell me more about your anxiety.

Curious ☐ What does your mum think? Why did you decide to talk to me on this particular day?

ICE ☐ Have you read about anything that can help?

Flags ☐ Any visual disturbance? Do the arms or legs feel different or weak? Any weight loss? Nausea? Vomiting? Are you ever confused or unusually sleepy? Has anyone said your behaviour has changed? Do you now struggle with anything you could easily do a few months ago? Any fevers? Does the light bother you? Any neck stiffness? Any head injury?

Risk ☐ Any FH? Do you have much alcohol, caffeine, cheese, chocolate or citrus fruits? How is your sleep? Do you have much screen time? Do you drink plenty of water?

SummarICE ☐ Your headaches affect your life and this is frustrating. You suffer with anxiety and worry about a serious cause like a brain tumour and would like specialist advice. Sumatriptan helps but you want to prevent their onset. Your friend suggested topiramate. Anything else I've missed?

O/E ☐ It would be helpful to arrange an examination, where I check your HR, BP and your eyes, arms and legs? Would it be possible to come to see me today at 2 p.m.? Great.

Empathy ☐ I appreciate why you want to check that this frequent headache is nothing serious.

Impression ☐ I agree with you and the previous GP who diagnosed that these headaches are migraines.

Experience ☐ What do you know about migraines? Do you know anything that can trigger them?

Explanation ☐ A one-sided headache which takes you to bed is typical of a migraine. The cause of the migraine is not completely known but theories include chemical and blood vessel changes.

InCludE ☐ It sounds like you thought seeing a specialist may be helpful for two reasons: to ensure there is no tumour and find the cause. I don't expect to find anything concerning when I examine you and I am reassured that you have no symptoms of a brain tumour. The headaches do not occur when the pressure is at its highest in the morning, you don't feel sick and have not vomited. Your nerves appear to be working normally.

Recommend ☐ You mentioned feeling groggy on amitriptyline. Your friend's right, topiramate is an option but we'd need to change your contraception as it can cause serious problems in pregnancy. I think a tablet called propranolol may be useful as it helps with migraine and anxiety. Potential side effects can include tiredness. However, many feel fine on it and we could start at a low dose. What are your thoughts? Okay I'll check your BP and HR at 2 p.m. before starting it. May I check, have you ever had asthma or used inhalers? I would suggest we start with a 40 mg tablet daily to make sure there are no side effects and after a week increase to 40 mg twice daily. Regarding your amitriptyline – let's wean your body off this by prescribing a 10 mg tablet at night for a month. Meanwhile could you keep a headache diary? The features/timing and any triggers for the headache would be very helpful.

Empower ☐ Could you try to avoid caffeine, citrus, chocolate and alcohol? Be prepared for rebound headaches initially. Also, general lifestyle measures – including regular healthy meals, a good sleep pattern and exercise – can all help. Next time we could discuss other ways to help your anxiety and later I'll give you a leaflet about anxiety and a therapy called CBT.

Safety net ☐ If at any time you start vomiting, feel unwell, have any new symptoms or the headaches wake you or change, see a GP as we would have to reassess your migraine diagnosis.

Specifics ☐ Okay have a think about what I've suggested and I'll see you at 2 p.m. to examine you and provide you with prescriptions.

Doctor's notes	Yasmin Small, 23 years. PMH: migraines. Medications: amitriptyline 25 mg ON. Desogestrel 75 µg daily. Sumatriptan 50 mg PRN.
How to act	Currently in discomfort. Keep touching your head if face to face.
PC	*'I keep getting these headaches.'*
History	You have suffered with migraines for years but they started becoming more frequent 4 months ago. You can't think of any triggers. Now they occur at least twice a week. It is always the same headache. Left side or frontal. Onset usually mid-afternoon. It develops over an hour and reaches 8/10 severity. Apart from occasional nausea, only during the headache, you have no associated symptoms.
	You have not been under pressure; you are not stressed or depressed.
	The headaches are not related to your periods.
	You have no medical history and take no medicines. Your mum had migraines.
	You don't take any other pain relief.
	When the headache comes on you lie down in a dark room and sumatriptan helps.
Social	You work in a clothes shop which you enjoy. You live with your boyfriend of 2 years.
	You drink a couple of glasses of wine weekly. You do not smoke.
	At work you take it in turns to buy each other a coffee and chocolate.
	You have had to have time off work. Your healthy anxiety has also been running wild with the headaches happening so frequently. The anxiety stops you from focusing on tasks.
ICE	*'Well, I suppose you always worry you may have a brain tumour, don't you?'*
	You saw a programme 3 nights ago about a girl who had a brain tumour.
	Your friend told you that you should be on topiramate.
	You would like to see a specialist, your reason being that the headaches keep coming back and you want to know what is wrong.
	You don't really know anything about migraines other than they are bad headaches.
Examination	BP 110/60, Fundi normal. Visual acuity 6/6. Normal neurological examination.

Please use your own judgement and refer to the full NICE guidance and BNF for further advice.

Red flags   Neurological or raised intracranial pressure symptoms or seizures.
Changes in behaviour, memory or skills.
Unilateral deafness or pulse synchronous tinnitus.
Drowsiness or loss of consciousness.
Ataxia.
Sudden visual loss.
Migraine with aura using OCP.

Diagnosis   See NICE guidelines for full details. Can diagnose migraine without aura if there are at least five attacks that fulfil criteria (duration, characteristics, associated symptoms, photophobia/phonophobia, no other explanation). Diagnose migraine with aura with at least two attacks that fulfil criteria (typical fully reversible symptoms, characteristic features of aura, no other explanation for headache).

Differential diagnosis

Tension headache.
Trigeminal autonomic cephalgias, e.g. cluster headache.
Primary cough headache and cold-stimulus ('ice-cream') headache.
Secondary headache, e.g. from trauma to head or neck.
Subarachnoid haemorrhage: 'thunder-clap headache' – severe, sudden onset.
Subdural haemorrhage: risk factors include alcohol, being elderly and falls.
Temporal arteritis: >50 years + pain on chewing or combing your hair? Temporal artery: 'absent pulse, beaded, tender or enlarged'.[2]
Exposure to, or withdrawal from, substances: carbon monoxide, cocaine, alcohol. Also medication overuse headache.
Infections, e.g. ear, sinuses, meningitis, encephalitis, cerebral abscess.
Hypoxia/hypertension – including pre-eclampsia and eclampsia.
Head/neck problems such as angle closure glaucoma or temporomandibular joint dysfunction.
There are many more – see guidance for the full list.

Migraine management options to consider[3]

Medication options   Ibuprofen.

Aspirin.

Metoclopramide or prochlorperazine. Migraines cause gastric stasis so patients are likely to benefit from prokinetic treatment (with acute therapy) to assist absorption and decrease nausea. There is a risk of extrapyramidal side effects.

Triptans   Avoid if uncontrolled HTN and vascular disease.

Check licensing: >60 years and children.

Migraine prophylaxis   Propranolol. Amitriptyline or topiramate.[4]

  See the Link Hub at CompleteMRCGP.co.uk for links to a very useful one-page Summary of:
Migraine – Acute Therapy Guideline
Migraine – Prophylactic Therapy Guideline

Doctor's Notes

Patient	Ahmed Hidad	58 years	M
PMH	Hypertension		
	Hypercholesterolaemia		
Medications	Indapamide 2.5 mg		
	Atorvastatin 40 mg		
Allergies	No information		
Consultations	No recent consultations		
Investigations	BP 3 months ago 132/80		
	Blood tests 1 year ago HbA1c 5.8% (40 mmol/mol)		
	Lipids – normal range		
Household	No household members registered		

Open ☐	Tell me the story of what happened. How are you now? How is your health generally? Did you notice any other symptoms? How long did it last? What do the arm and leg feel like today? How do you feel today? Are you still affected in any way?
Flags ☐	Did the left side feel weak? Did you notice any changes in your vision or speech? Did you feel lightheaded, the heart racing or in pain at the time? Headache or vomiting? Has anything like this happened before?
Sense ☐	I see you are worried. It sounds like you were hesitant about calling for help.
Curious ☐	Why did you not call for help? What was going through your mind?
ICE ☐	What do you think the problem was? Is there anything else that you have been concerned about? What did you think I may suggest today?
History ☐	Talk me through when you take your medicines. Who is important to you in your life? Since your wife died, how are you doing on your own? Do you drink any alcohol?
Risk ☐	Has anyone in your family had a heart attack or stroke? Have you ever smoked? Do you have any pain in the chest or legs when walking? Have you had a fall or hit your head? Have you ever had a stomach ulcer?
SummarICE ☐	To summarise, you are usually well. You are worried that you have had a stroke as last night the left side felt weak, you lay in bed for hours uncertain whether to call for help but what stopped you is the fear that the ambulance crew would take you to hospital, which is a frightening thought.
Empathy ☐	You are a man who likes peace and quiet. It sounds as if you would have liked some support, but didn't feel there was a good option – your daughter was 2 hours away, is that correct?
O/E ☐	May I feel your pulse, listen to the heart and neck vessels, take your blood pressure, check the nerves in the face, arms and legs please. Please may I see you walk across the room?
InCludE ☐	You wondered if this was a stroke like your neighbour had and that it might leave you lasting problems. Thankfully I don't think that's the case.
Impression ☐	It sounds as if you had a mini-stroke called a TIA: transient ischaemic attack. Transient means short-lived and ischaemic means a lack of blood supply, in this case to the brain.
Experience ☐	Have you come across any of these terms before?
Explanation ☐	Several factors increase the risk of having a stroke or mini-stroke. In your case it includes the high cholesterol and high blood pressure.
Recommend ☐	I would like to refer you to the hospital where you will be seen as an outpatient within 24 hours. Would that be okay?
Specifics ☐	Please let me know if you are not seen within 24 hours. I would also like to give you some aspirin to take until you have seen the specialist: 300 mg right away and then 75 mg daily. Let's get a heart tracing and some blood tests to help the specialist; could you book in for these at reception?
Empower ☐	There are things you can do whilst waiting to be seen such as ensuring you remember to take all your medication regularly, including the aspirin.
Future ☐	At the hospital they will examine you and then discuss further tests such as a special brain scan or a jelly scan of your neck arteries. When you have been seen by the hospital doctor, please return so we can discuss your general health and update your medicines.
Safety net ☐	There is risk this may happen again. I'm pleased that your symptoms went away which is why we call it a mini-stroke, but a TIA can be a warning of a larger stroke and you could be left paralysed like your neighbour. This would greatly affect your life around the home and in the garden.
Specifics ☐	Therefore, if this happens again, I would like you to call 999 straight away. The benefit of this is that they could give you treatment to help the blood supply to the brain and prevent some damage to the brain. Do you think you will call 999 if it happens again? Because of the risk of another episode like this, you must not drive until you have been told it is safe to do so.

Doctor's notes	Ahmed Hidad, 58 years. PMH: hypertension and hypercholesterolaemia. Medications: indapamide 2.5 mg and atorvastatin 40 mg.
How to act	Pleasant and respectful.
PC	*'Last night I couldn't use my arm and my leg felt weak.'*
History	You have always been well. You attend the doctors yearly for your blood pressure and cholesterol check. Last night you were sweeping the garage and your left arm dropped the brush. It felt as if it had gone limp and your left leg also felt strange and possibly weak. You went to sit down in the kitchen and weren't sure whether to call your daughter but it went away after 10 minutes. You lay awake for many hours unsure what to do but relieved it had gone away. Eventually you fell asleep. No symptoms this morning.
	You have never had anything like this before.
	You often forget to take your cholesterol medicine at night but you remember the blood pressure medicine with breakfast.
	Your vision was normal and you didn't speak to anyone. You didn't feel muddled in any way.
	You have not had a fall or head injury. You didn't call an ambulance as you thought they would send you to hospital and you have always preferred being alone and hate the thought of hospitals.
Social	You lost your wife to leukaemia 10 years ago.
	Your daughter lives 2 hours away so you didn't want to worry her.
	You used to be a gardener and still enjoy looking after your large garden for when the family is around. Your son lives abroad but tries to see you with his family every few months.
	You are independent with your ADL. You have never smoked and do not drink alcohol.
ICE	You are worried that you may have had a stroke.
	You expect the doctor may give you aspirin.
	Your neighbour had a stroke many years ago. He needed to be in a wheelchair afterwards.
	You follow all of the doctor's advice.
Examination	Normal examination of the arms, legs and cranial nerves. BP 132/88. HR 72 bpm regular.
	No carotid bruit. Normal gait.

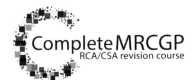

Neurology – 4

Prompt recognition of symptoms of stroke and TIA

Outside hospital, use a validated tool (e.g. FAST) to screen for TIA or stroke in people with neurological symptoms that have come on suddenly:[1]

- Face – Can the person smile? Has their face fallen on one side?
- Arms – Can the person raise both arms and keep them up?
- Speech – Slurred speech? Can the person speak clearly and understand what you are saying?
- Time – If ANY of these three signs, phone 999.[2]

Initial management of suspected TIA[3]

- Aspirin 300 mg immediately (with PPI if appropriate), unless contraindicated (e.g. already taking, or known bleeding problem).
- If the suspected TIA occurred within last 7 days, refer people to be seen for specialist assessment and investigation within 24 hours.[1]
- Admit to hospital if patient is taking anticoagulant or has bleeding disorder.

Initial management of suspected stroke[3]

- 999 ambulance.
- Tell ambulance control and the hospital that you suspect a stroke.
- Do not give aspirin until possibility of haemorrhagic stroke excluded.
- While waiting for an ambulance, monitor ABC and give O_2 if SATS <95% and no contraindication.

Secondary prevention

- Control of blood pressure. Reduce BP gradually aiming for systolic <130, unless severe bilateral carotid stenosis.[3]
- Antiplatelet agents – see below.
- Atorvastatin 20–80 mg.[3,4]
- Diet and lifestyle advice (smoking, alcohol, daily exercise, good diet, etc.).

After the CAPRIE trial[5] which recommends clopidogrel following atherosclerotic vascular disease, the 2016 Royal College of Physicians guidelines suggest that 'patients with a non-disabling stroke should receive treatment for secondary prevention as soon as the diagnosis is confirmed' – including clopidogrel (300 mg loading dose then 75 mg daily).[4]

A study published in *The Lancet* (May 2016), 'Effects of aspirin on risk and severity of early recurrent stroke after transient ischaemic attack and ischaemic stroke: time-course analysis of randomised trials', suggests that the benefit of aspirin given as soon as possible after TIA has been underestimated in terms of preventing further stroke or severity of further stroke.[6]

Primary care management after discharge following stroke or TIA[3]

Consider:

- Optimise management of risk factors such as:
  - Diabetes
  - OSA
  - Contraception – no COC for patients who have had stroke or TIA
  - Annual flu immunisation
- Driving. Patient must notify DVLA. See DVLA 'Assessing standards for fitness to drive'.
- Work – can the person return to work? Will rehabilitation be needed?
  - Job centre can arrange for referral to specialist in employment for people with a disability or to specialist vocational rehab, team.

TIA booklet for patients

Available at https://www.sign.ac.uk/assets/pat108.pdf[7]

Doctor's Notes

Patient	Lydia Cooper	25 years	F
PMH	Tonsillitis – 3 years ago		
Medications	No current medications		
Allergies	No information		
Consultations	No recent consultations		
Investigations	No recent investigations		
Household	No household members registered		

Example Consultation

Open ☐ Tell me what you've noticed from the beginning. Anything else that is unusual? How do you feel?

Impact ☐ Have your symptoms stopped you from doing anything?

History ☐ Are you well usually? Have you had any recent illnesses or viral symptoms? Tell me more about you? Who are you close to? Do you work? What do you like to do – do you have hobbies?

ICE ☐ Have you had any thoughts about what may have caused this? What is going through your mind? Did you have any ideas about what I may say or suggest today?

Sense ☐ I can see you are upset and very worried.

Curious ☐ Tell me about your grandpa's experience.

Risk ☐ Has anyone in your family had similar symptoms in the past? Have you been abroad or noticed any insect bites? Have you ever had an infection through sex?

Flags ☐ Has your vision changed recently? What have you noticed? Has your speech changed? What about any weakness in the body where a leg or arm actually feels floppy? Have you noticed any difference in your control when going to the toilet? Have you lost weight? Any headaches or vomiting? Is your back painful? Have you had an injury?

SummarICE ☐ To summarise, you have noticed unusual sensations now in both legs and your vision has been troubling you. You became very concerned when you realised you were wobbly on your feet. You have been passing urine more urgently. You fear it may be a similar problem to your grandpa's, but you are puzzled and worried by your symptoms. Is that correct?

O/E ☐ I would like to examine you please, take your pulse, blood pressure, breathing rate and temperature, look at the nerves supplying the face, arms and legs and in the back of the eyes. Is that okay? May I check the nerve supply to the bottom? Because you mentioned urgency of urine, testing the sensation in the bottom is important. May I see you walk across the room… and can you do a sample of urine please?

Empathy ☐ I appreciate it is frightening when you have symptoms which you cannot explain, especially when they come quickly together and it has made you wonder if this is similar to your grandpa's condition.

InCludE ☐ I don't believe it is the same, however, as firstly your symptoms are different and secondly the causes of problems in older people are usually very different from those in young people.

Impression ☐ However, I do think we need to ask the nerve doctors to have a look at you. I am questioning whether your nerves have become a little swollen, but the exact cause for why this has happened is not yet clear.

Explanation ☐ This can happen for several reasons: following an infection, low vitamin B or where the nerve supply is irritated by something pushing against the nerve. The body can also attack itself by mistake and affect the nerves so they become weak and lose their protective layer. Instead of this protective layer, scar tissue forms and it blocks the normal signals from the nerves, which is why you may be feeling the strange sensations. I think the last reason may be the most likely but we need to do some tests to get the answer to why this has happened. Do you have any questions? You may find your symptoms go away and then come back again. Before we can give you the exact answer, we need to know what we are dealing with.

Specifics ☐ I would like to ask you to sit in the waiting room where a nurse will call you through for a blood test. Meanwhile I'm going to give the nerve doctors at the hospital a call to ask if they want to see you today or in their rapid-access clinic.

Future ☐ At the hospital I expect they will examine you like I have done today and, if they feel it is necessary, they may arrange an MRI scan. There may still be further tests you need before we have the answer.

Doctor's notes	Lydia Cooper, 25 years. PMH: tonsillitis – 3 years ago. Medications: none.
How to act	Nervous and anxious.
	Start to cry when you explain your symptoms.
PC	*'I've got this strange feeling in my leg – it's the second time I've had it.'*
History	Six weeks ago you noticed your right foot was tingling within the shoe. You thought it must have been your tight trainers but you noticed it again in bed last week but this time on the left foot and lower leg and today it has gone above your knee. You feel wobbly when you walk today. You feel like you are going to fall over. A couple of months ago you realised that you needed glasses. Your right eye has been blurry this week.
	No headache or weight loss.
	You have noticed urgency of urine and nearly missed the toilet yesterday but no other urinary symptoms. Your bowels are normal.
	No other symptoms on systemic enquiry.
Social	You live with your boyfriend of 1 year. You are looking for work.
	You left college aged 16 years. Since then, you've found temporary work in offices.
	You smoked in your teens. You do not drink alcohol.
ICE	You don't know what may be causing it.
	You hope you haven't had a stroke like your grandpa 2 years ago.
	Your grandpa lost all movement on the right side and his speech was different.
	You don't know what the doctor will say today.
Examination	BP 120/60. HR 72 bpm regular. Apyrexial. RR 14.
	No nystagmus, fundoscopy normal.
	Visual acuity reduced right eye.
	CN otherwise normal.
	Reduced sensation from the left toes to L3.
	Weakness L4/5/S1–3/5.
	Knee/ankle jerk increase, clonus and extensor plantar response – left side.
	Abnormal gait.
	Reduced perianal sensation.
	Urine dipstick normal.
	Ask the doctor *'Will it get better?'*

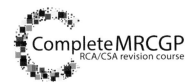

MS may take the course of relapsing-remitting, primary or secondary progressive.[1]

MS is usually a progressive disease.

Relapses may be triggered by infections, stress and post-partum.[1,2]

Epidemiology	Incidence >M; common in young adults.
Risk factors[2]	Genetic.
	EB virus infection.
	Cigarette smoking.
	Obesity/poor diet in adolescence.
	Low levels of vitamin D.
	Latitude – prevalence increases with distance from the equator – north or south – ?due to lower average levels of vitamin D because of lower levels of sunlight.
Symptoms[1]	Visual changes, e.g. acuity, colour vision, visual fields (optic neuritis).
	Reduced vision, loss of vision or double vision.
	Hearing loss.
	Facial weakness.
	Altered sensations.
	Limb weakness, gait problems.
	Bladder and bowel control may be affected.
	Altered temperature regulation, e.g. sweating.
	Altered sexual function/impotence.
	Lhermitte's phenomenon: the feeling of electricity down the spine on neck flexion.
	Cerebellar symptoms: ataxia, nystagmus, dysarthria and vertigo.
	Cognitive dysfunction (late symptoms).
Diagnosis	Relapsing, remitting – ≥2 demyelinating lesions in the brain/spinal cord occurring in different places at different times.[2]
	Primary progressive – progressive deterioration over 12 months.[2]
	Investigations may include MRI, lumbar puncture and visual evoked potentials.
Differential diagnosis[1]	Sarcoidosis
	Spinal cord compression
	Vitamin B12 deficiency
	Neurosyphilis
	SLE
	Cerebrovascular disease
	SOL/tumours
	Lyme disease
Blood tests	FBC, U&E, LFT, calcium, glucose, TFTs, ESR, CRP, vitamin B12, ANA (antinuclear antibody), HIV ± syphilis.

CHAPTER 18 OVERVIEW

Population Health: Promoting Health and Preventing Disease

	Cases in this chapter	Within the RCGP 2020 curriculum: Population Health: Promoting Health and Preventing Disease	Learning points in this chapter include:
1	Immunisation Refusal	'Disease prevention programmes for common important communicable ... conditions' 'Risk–benefit conversations in relation to health protection (e.g. child immunisation)'	MMR refusal, other reasons for immunisation refusal and legal considerations
2	Cervical Screening	Promote health – including cervical screening	Cervical cytology, results and counselling
3	Inappropriate Use of Services	'The health of minorities and marginalised populations'	Educating families with regards to how to use local services
4	High Cholesterol	'Cardiovascular health screening including ... cholesterol checks'	Cardiovascular risk scores Statin discussion
5	Wants to Lose Weight	'Approaches to behaviour change and their relevance to health promotion and self-care'	The importance of understanding the patient to help guide behaviour change See also The Motivational Interview in the Introduction
Extra Notes	UK Immunisation Schedule	'Immunisation programmes including: • childhood immunisation schedules • immunisation in pregnancy, travellers and other important situations, e.g. contact tracing • vaccinations available on the NHS • mandatory vaccinations for travel to certain areas'	Current immunisation schedule Live attenuated vaccines
	Immunisation/ Vaccine Preventable Diseases	'Disease prevention programmes for common important communicable conditions'	Immunisation/vaccine preventable diseases Symptoms, complications and mortality rates
	Cervical Screening Programme	'Promote health – cervical screening'	Who should be screened
	Other NHS Screening Programmes	'NHS screening and immunisation programmes' 'Disease prevention programmes for common and important communicable and non-communicable diseases'	Bowel cancer, breast cancer, diabetic retinopathy, AAA, newborn and antenatal screening
	Diet and Exercise Advice		NICE Guideline CG181. Cardiovascular disease: risk assessment and reduction, including lipid modification. September 2016
	Statins		Primary and secondary prevention

CHAPTER 18 REFERENCES

Immunisation Refusal

1. https://www.nhs.uk/conditions/vaccinations/mmr-vaccine/. Apr 2020.
2. Harmsen I.A., Mollema L., Ruiter R.A.C. et al. Why parents refuse childhood vaccination: a qualitative study using online focus groups. *BMC Public Health* 2013; 13: 1183. http://bmcpublichealth.biomedcentral.com/articles/10.1186/1471-2458-13-1183
3. https://www.nhs.uk/conditions/consent-to-treatment/children. Mar 2019.
4. https://www.gov.uk/government/publications/consent-the-green-book-chapter-2

Cervical Screening

1. https://www.who.int/news-room/fact-sheets/detail/human-papillomavirus-(hpv)-and-cervical-cancer. Nov 2020.
2. NICE CKS. https://cks.nice.org.uk/topics/cervical-screening/management/managing-hpv-cervical-cytology-results/. May 2021.

High Cholesterol

1. NICE Guideline CG181. Cardiovascular disease: risk assessment and reduction, including lipid modification. Sep 2016.
2. https://qrisk.org/three/

Wants to Lose Weight

1. NICE Guideline CG189. Obesity: identification, assessment and management. Nov 2014.

UK Immunisation Schedule

1. https://www.nhs.uk/conditions/vaccinations/. Apr 2020.
2. https://assets.publishing.service.gov.uk/government/uploads/system/uploads/attachment_data/file/899422/PHE_Routine_Childhood_Immunisation_Schedule_Jun2020_03.pdf

Immunisation/Vaccine Preventable Diseases

1. https://patient.info/doctor/measles-pro
2. http://www.who.int
3. http://www.cdc.gov/
4. https://patient.info/childrens-health/acute-diarrhoea-in-children/rotavirus#nav-0. Oct 2017.

Cervical Screening Programme

1. http://patient.info/doctor/cervical-screening-cervical-smear-test-pro. May 2021.
2. Cervical cancer screening. https://www.cancerresearchuk.org/about-cancer/cervical-cancer/getting-diagnosed/screening. Feb 2020.
3. Human papillomavirus (HPV) and cervical cancer. Nov 2020. http://www.who.int/mediacentre/factsheets/fs380/en/ Nov 2020.
4. NICE CKS. https://cks.nice.org.uk/topics/cervical-screening/management/managing-hpv-cervical-cytology-results/. May 2021.
5. https://www.cancerresearchuk.org/about-cancer/screening/trans-and-non-binary-cancer-screening#screening40

Other NHS Screening Programmes

1. http://patient.info/doctor/screening-programmes-in-the-uk. Apr 2014.
2. https://www.gov.uk/guidance/fetal-anomaly-screening-programme-overview. Contains public sector information licensed by the Open Government Licence v3.0. Apr 2021.

Diet and Exercise Advice

1. NICE Guideline CG181. Cardiovascular disease: risk assessment and reduction, including lipid modification. Sep 2016.
2. https://assets.publishing.service.gov.uk/government/uploads/system/uploads/attachment_data/file/559044/CMO_Drinking_Gov_Resp.pdf. Contains public sector information licensed by the Open Government Licence v3.0. Aug 2016.

Statins

1. NICE Guideline CG181. Cardiovascular disease: risk assessment and reduction, including lipid modification. Sep 2016.
2. https://www.nice.org.uk/guidance/ta385. Feb 2016.

Information taken from NICE guidelines with kind permission. Please note the guidelines change frequently and you should ALWAYS check for the latest updated guidance. Remember that NICE guidance is only applicable to patients in the UK.

Population Health

Doctor's Notes

Patient	Bhakti Shukla	12 months	F
PMH	No information		
Medications	No current medications		
Allergies	No information		
Consultations	Last appointment with practice nurse 2 weeks ago.		
	'Attended for 12-month vaccinations. Hib/MenC, PCV, Meningitis B given. Mum refused MMR. Asked to book telephone appointment with doctor for discussion.'		
Investigations	No information		
Household	Talika Shukla	60 years	F
	Laksha Shukla	32 years	F
	Aaditya Shukla	32 years	M

Example Consultation
Immunisation Refusal

Open ☐   Thank you for taking the time to talk on the phone today. I understand you have concerns about the MMR vaccine? Can you tell me more about what has been going through your mind about this vaccination? Let's discuss it today so you have all the information you need to help you decide.

Sense ☐   I can hear you want to ensure you are making the best decision for Bhakti.

History ☐   First, can you please tell me more about your family and their health? I see Bhakti has had her other vaccinations. Did she have any problems with them?

Risk ☐   Does Bhakti have any allergies? Is she otherwise fit and well?

ICE ☐   What do you know about the vaccination? Do you know what the letters MMR stand for? Correct. Would you like me to explain more about those diseases? Okay, we will go through that. How much do you know already? Was there any other information you were hoping to gain today? Was there anything else you were hoping for? Is there anything else that worries you apart from autism?

Experience ☐   What is your experience of autism? So you fear this condition in your children?

Curious ☐   How do you feel about vaccinations in general? What does Bhakti's father think?

SummarICE ☐   So, generally, you are all for vaccination but you remember a lot of bad press about the MMR vaccination in the news, in particular about a link between the MMR vaccine and autism. It is important to you that Bhakti has the best education and, having seen another child with autism, you hope to protect her as best you can. You would like some more information about the MMR vaccination.

Explanation ☐   The MMR vaccine is designed to protect against measles, mumps and rubella. This followed a piece of research which was published in 1998.

InCludE ☐   You're right, there was a scare about the MMR vaccination a few years back but this has been discredited and I hope I can put your mind at rest about this.

Explanation ☐   There has been a lot of research into the possible link between autism and the MMR vaccination, and no link has been found. After reviewing all the available information, the World Health Organization recommends that the MMR vaccine is given. Is there anything I have said that doesn't make sense so far?

Explanation ☐   Measles is a virus which causes cold-like symptoms, high fever and a rash. It is often a mild illness but can have serious complications such as pneumonia, deafness, blindness and inflammation of the brain called encephalitis. Thankfully the death rate is low but there are about 1–2 deaths per 1000 cases. Mumps is a viral infection which affects the salivary glands of the cheeks. It usually gets better on its own but can affect the testicles and ovaries which, rarely, affects fertility. It, too, can cause deafness and can also cause meningitis. Rubella is another virus which causes high fever, a rash and cold-like symptoms. The main worry with rubella is for women who are pregnant catching it, as it can cause problems with the baby's development.

Options ☐   As a parent you have the right to refuse vaccinations, but I hope I have reassured you that the MMR vaccination is safe and that it is there to protect against some serious infections.

Recommend ☐   I recommend the vaccination to protect against these diseases as, after reading the studies myself, I am confident there is no link to autism.

Empathy ☐   I understand it can be scary to make decisions which may put our children at risk.

Empower ☐   Would you like some information that you can read in your own time? I can email it to you so you can discuss it with your husband. What are your thoughts at this time?

Future ☐   Let me know when you've made a decision and we can arrange an appointment if you wish Bhakti to have the vaccination.

Specifics ☐   Our nurse-led vaccination clinic is held every Tuesday afternoon from 1 p.m. to 2 p.m. and you would just need to phone reception, or call in, to book an appointment.

Safety net ☐   If you have any concerns or wish to discuss anything further, please give me a call.

Population Health – 1

Patient's Story

Doctor's notes	Bhakti Shukla. 12 months. No information in medical history. Last appointment with practice nurse 2 weeks ago.
	'Attended for 12-month vaccinations. Hib/MenC, PCV, Meningitis B given. Mum refused MMR. Asked to book in with doctor for discussion.'
How to act	Concerned
PC	*'Hi Doctor, your nurse asked me to call you. I don't want Bhakti to have the MMR vaccination. I've heard it can cause autism.'*
History	Your name is Laksha Shukla. You are 32 years old and live with your husband, mother-in law and your daughter Bhakti. Generally, you are all for vaccinations. You grew up in India and saw the damage polio can do. You moved to the UK when you were 12 years old. You remember reading about the MMR vaccination causing autism so you don't want Bhakti to have this. Bhakti is developing well, and she has recently started walking. She has been well up until now and you have no concerns about her health.
Social	You are a full-time mum. Your husband feels Bhakti should have the vaccination but thought you should get some more information first to put your mind at ease. You have Hindu faith.
ICE	You believe there is a link between the MMR vaccination and autism. You would prefer Bhakti not to have the vaccination. You aren't sure what diseases the MMR vaccine protects against, but you suspect they aren't as bad as autism. You expect the doctor to be able to give you information about the link between the MMR vaccination and autism. You would also like to know more about measles, mumps and rubella. Your neighbour's son has autism and you have heard from his mum that he has real difficulties at school. He struggles to learn and you are very keen that Bhakti has a good education.

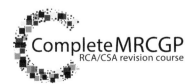

CompleteMRCGP
RCA/CSA revision course

Population Health – 1

The immunisation schedule is included in the Extra Notes section, along with information about the recent changes and some further points.

MMR and autism?[1]

The scare regarding the MMR vaccine and autism came about in 1998 after a study was published in *The Lancet*. The study claimed that the MMR vaccine had been linked to regression (loss of skills), autistic spectrum disorders, inflammation of the small intestine (enterocolitis) and that children with autism had higher levels of measles antibodies in their bloodstream. Since this study was published, the claims have been widely discredited in follow-up studies. There were flaws in the original study which could have led to bias. Based on the subsequent trials, there is no reason to suspect that the MMR vaccine is linked to autism, and therefore the MMR is recommended by the World Health Organization because it is more effective than giving the separate vaccines for measles, mumps and rubella. Interestingly, the rates of autism continued to increase in Japan even after the vaccine had been withdrawn, adding further evidence of no causal link.

Other reasons for vaccination refusal

There is a multitude of reasons for parents refusing vaccination. Consider the following and how you would discuss these with the parents. One study[2] found the following were often cited:

- Perceptions about the child's body and immune system – too young for immune system to cope with immunisation or child already protected by breast feeding.
- Perceived risks of disease. The belief of a low risk of catching the illness, the belief that conditions can be easily treated and the belief the diseases are not serious.
- Vaccine efficacy. The belief that the vaccines don't work.
- Side effects.
- Perceived advantages of experiencing the disease.
- Prior negative experience with vaccination.

Legal considerations[3,4]

Although the consent of one person with parental responsibility for a child is usually sufficient (see Section 2(7) of the Children Act 1989), if one parent agrees to immunisation but the other disagrees, the immunisation should not be carried out unless both parents can agree to immunisation or there is a specific court approval that the immunisation is in the best interests of the child.

Doctor's Notes

Patient	Chloe Atherton 25 years F
PMH	Tonsillitis aged 22 years
	Viral respiratory tract infection aged 14 years
	Urinary tract infection aged 4 years
Medications	Rigevidon
Allergies	No information
Consultations	Last appointment with practice nurse 3 weeks ago. Cervical smear taken.
Investigations	Recent cervical cytology result: high risk HPV detected, mild dyskaryosis. A colposcopy referral has been made.
Household	No household contacts

Example Consultation

Cervical Screening

Open ☐   Firstly let me reassure you that the test result has not found cancer. Before we discuss it in more detail, may I ask you a few background questions to ensure I understand what has happened so far? This will help me interpret your result.

History ☐   What led to you having the test done? Are you otherwise well? Any problems with your periods or bleeding pattern? Do you smoke? Do you work? Regarding your women's health, when was your last period? Have you any abnormal bleeding? Have you ever been pregnant? Do you have a sexual partner? Do you have any abnormal vaginal discharge? Have you ever had a sexually transmitted infection?

Risk ☐   Any bleeding between periods or after sex? Have you had any pain? Have you ever had a smear test before? Is there any family history of cervical cancer or women's problems? I'd like to reassure you this is not connected to the ovary.

ICE ☐   You have mentioned that you are worried about cancer. Is there anything else that has been concerning you? Were you hoping I would do anything in particular today?

SummarICE ☐   So you have no worrying symptoms, but received a letter telling you that your smear was abnormal and that you have been referred to the hospital. You are worried that you have cancer and whether this could be related to your aunt's cancer. You are concerned about the colposcopy test and whether it will be painful.

Experience ☐   What do you know about colposcopy tests already? Have you known anyone who has had it done? Or had problems with the cervix?

Explanation ☐   The cervix is the neck of your womb. I can see from your record that HPV was found. So, the cells from your cervix were looked at under a microscope and the middle of the cells looked a little abnormal. In your case, the changes are only mild. Often, in cases like yours, the cells will go back to normal all on their own. However, we know that cervical cancer is caused by HPV, so we offer a further test called colposcopy to look at the cervix in more detail. Smear tests look for HPV and changes in the cervix, which if left, may develop into cancer. We can then monitor the cervix or treat it to prevent cancer. Is there anything I have said that you are unclear about or that I haven't explained well enough? Would you like to know about colposcopy?

Explanation ☐   Colposcopy is a procedure in which a doctor looks at the cervix under a microscope directly. You will be asked to undress from the waist down and usually sit in a special chair which supports your legs. A speculum is put into the vagina so the cervix can be seen, like when you had the smear test. The doctor will usually put a special stain on the cervix which shows any abnormal cells. If any are found, the doctor will often take a biopsy or offer to treat the cells there and then by removing them after giving a local anaesthetic. If this happens, the doctor will explain this to you.

InCludE ☐   I know you were concerned about this – like a smear test, it can be uncomfortable but you really shouldn't experience pain. I can reassure you this is a very different condition to ovarian cancer.

Options ☐   How do you feel about the colposcopy now? Do you feel you will go?

Empathy ☐   I understand getting abnormal results is scary, especially if there is a possibility of cancer. But hopefully there are just some abnormal cells which can be taken away.

Empower ☐   Would you like me to email some information to read in your own time?

Future ☐   We will get a letter from the hospital after your appointment, but I would be happy to talk to you after the appointment if you'd like to discuss what happened.

Specifics ☐   You should receive a letter for the colposcopy within the next 2 weeks. Please let me know if you haven't heard by then.

Safety net ☐   In the meantime, if you do have any bleeding not during your period or pain please let me know. Please don't hesitate to contact me if you have questions.

Doctor's notes	Chloe Atherton, 25 years. PMH: tonsillitis aged 22 years. Viral respiratory tract infection aged 14 years. Urinary tract infection aged 4 years. Medication: Rigevidon.
How to act	Concerned.
Investigations	Recent cervical cytology result: mild dyskaryosis, high-risk HPV detected. A colposcopy referral has been made.
PC	*'Hi Doctor, I've recently had my smear done but the results have come back abnormal. Do I have cancer?'*
History	You attended for your first cervical cytology test 3 weeks ago following receiving an invitation after your 25th birthday. You were unsure about going for the test but discussed it with a friend who is older than you and she said the test was fine, so you booked in. The nurse doing the test explained that if the results were abnormal you would be referred to the hospital for more tests. You are worried about this. Before the test you had no symptoms; no intermenstrual bleeding, no post-coital bleeding and no dyspareunia. There is no family history of cervical cancer but your aunt died of ovarian cancer and you thought this could be related. You take the oral contraceptive pill so feel pregnancy is unlikely; you always remember to take it. Last menstrual period 1 week ago.
Social	You work as a barmaid and waitress. You have a boyfriend. You have been together 3 years. He knows about the result and how worried you are, so has offered to go to the hospital with you.
	You don't smoke and only drink alcohol at weekends.
ICE	You think you may have cervical cancer. You are concerned about the colposcopy test as you don't know what this will involve. You hope the doctor will be able to reassure you that you don't have cancer and explain the colposcopy test to you. You fear it will be painful.

Details of the cervical screening programme can be found in the Extra Notes section.

Important counselling points

- The screening test is a test for HPV and not cancer cells. The purpose of the test is to find out if you have high-risk HPV so that you can be treated before cancer develops.
- Colposcopy is a procedure to look at the cervix in more detail. It is similar to having a smear in that a speculum is inserted to make the cervix visible, but then the doctor will look at the cervix using a microscope called a colposcope. The colposcope itself doesn't enter the body. The doctor will usually put a special stain on the cervix to show up any abnormal areas.
- If abnormal areas are found, biopsies may be taken or the doctor may decide to treat the cells there and then. If that is the case, the doctor will explain what they would like to do. Any removal of tissue is usually done with local anaesthetic.

Results[1]

- HPV primary screening. Cells are first tested for high-risk HPV – HPV-16 and HPV-18.
- There are 100 different types of human papillomavirus (HPV) but only these two are considered high risk for cervical cancer. These cause 70% of cervical cancers.

Management of cervical cytology results[2]

Result	Management
No HPV found = no high-risk HPV	Recall – 3 or 5 years' time depending on your age
HPV found with no cell changes = high-risk HPV present but no changes to cells	Recall – 1 year to check HPV gone
HPV found with cell changes = high-risk HPV + cervical cell changes	Colposcopy

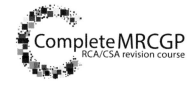

Doctor's Notes

Patient	Sara Azmeh	28 years	F
PMH	No information		
Medications	No current medications		
Allergies	No information		
Consultations	No recent consultations		
Investigations	No information		
Household	Yusuf Azmeh	29 years	M
	Lilah Azmeh	7 years	F
	Najm Azmeh	5 years	M
	Akram Azmeh	4 years	M
	Rasha Azmeh	6 months	F

During a recent 'Unplanned Admissions Review' your practice has noted that this family have been attending A&E and out-of-hours services regularly. You have sent a letter to the parents to ask them to come in to discuss the health of the family and the services available.

7 A&E attendances in 2 months with viral URTI symptoms between four children.

1 A&E attendance with eczema (Akram).

1 A&E attendance with vomiting (Rasha).

1 out-of-hours attendance due to running out of salbutamol inhaler (Lilah).

1 attendance to out-of-hours with hay fever symptoms (Yusuf).

No admissions required, discharged back to GP care after each attendance.

Example Consultation   Inappropriate Use of Services

Open ☐ Thank you for talking on the phone. I wanted to discuss your family's health and offer help and support. As you have recently joined our practice, could you tell me more about your family? Welcome to Nottingham. How are you settling in? What were your experiences in Syria? I'm sorry to hear what your family has been through.

Impact ☐ How have you coped with the stress of the move? We are here to help your family.

History ☐ Are you well physically and mentally? And your husband? Have you made friends? Did you work in Syria? Giving yourselves time to settle in is important, but do you have any plans? Ah, best of luck with your future studies. Are your children in school? Tell me about each member of your family; how they are coping and their health.

Sense ☐ I sense you are particularly worried about breathing problems in the children.

Curious ☐ Have you had any bad experiences with asthma or chest infections?

ICE ☐ How do you feel the children are at present? Do you have any particular worries about yourself, your husband or your children? Have you had any thoughts about what could help? Was there anything you were hoping I would do today?

Experience ☐ Do you know where you can get help from if someone in the family is poorly?

SummarICE ☐ To summarise, your family have moved away from where you felt in great danger and it has been hard for you all. You feel exhausted and miss your loved ones, your husband has the stress of trying to find work and your children have been quiet. You feel this is from the shock of what they have experienced. You worry about Lilah's asthma, Akram's eczema and don't know where to get Rasha weighed. You would like some information about healthcare in England. Let's make a plan together.

Empathy ☐ I cannot imagine what you have been through, but I am glad you now feel safe.

Explanation ☐ In the UK there are lots of different ways to seek help. For problems like hay fever or colds, you can go to a pharmacy where there are medications which you can buy. The pharmacists are experienced in giving advice for these problems, so they are often a good first point of call. You may be able to sign up to 'Pharmacy First' which enables you to get free prescriptions for some things like paracetamol for the children. At the practice we can offer emergency appointments if your family are unwell. Please phone our receptionist who will provide you with an appointment. We also have doctors and nurses at the practice who help to manage long-term conditions like asthma or eczema. When the practice is closed and your problem cannot wait, you can phone 111. This includes evenings, night-time and weekends. They will provide advice or arrange an appointment with another GP. If someone is very poorly or has been in a bad accident, this is when you should go to A&E or call 999 on the telephone. This is a lot to take in. Any questions so far? It must be difficult when things are so different in a new country.

Recommend ☐ I recommend we book Akram in to assess his eczema and also see Lilah for her asthma?

Specifics ☐ I'd also like to refer you to our health visitor service. Health visitors look after families with children under 5 years old and can advise you on minor problems and do health checks like weighing children. You can just turn up with Rasha to the health visitor's clinic once a week to get Rasha weighed. The health visitor can also put you in touch with other services like Sure Start which supports mums and runs mum and baby groups. Does any of that sound helpful? If you continue to worry about your children, we could arrange counselling for them.

Empower ☐ Would you like me to email you an information sheet with the practice information? Helpful website addresses include NHS choices and patient.info.

Future ☐ Shall I book those appointments for you? I look forward to meeting your family.

Safety net ☐ If you are ever worried about a health problem, don't hesitate to give us a call.

Patient's Story

Doctor's notes	Sara Azmeh, 28 years. PMH: no information. During a recent 'Unplanned Admissions Review' your practice has noted that this family have been attending A&E and out-of-hours services regularly. You have sent a letter to the parents to ask them to book a telephone consultation to discuss the health of the family and the services available.
How to act	Confused.
PC	*'Hello Doctor, you have asked me phone to discuss this letter I have received.'*
History	You, your husband and four children moved to the UK 4 months ago. You are Syrian asylum seekers. You are unsure how the healthcare system works in the UK. You love your children dearly and get frightened when they are unwell. You and your husband are both well. Over recent years you have had very little access to healthcare in Syria and worry about Lilah's asthma which isn't well controlled. You have had an inhaler from the practice which helps but she keeps running out. You also have trouble managing Akram's eczema; although you know it isn't life threatening, it often becomes sore and stops him sleeping. You are aware that you have been to A&E quite a lot but are unsure what else you should do when the practice is closed or if you can't get through on the phone. After you had been to hospital a couple of times, they told you to ring 111 next time, so you did when you required the extra inhaler for Lilah and they helped your husband when he had problems with his nose.
Social	Your asylum request is being processed at present but you are very hopeful that it will be granted. Your husband used to work in local government in Syria. Since having children, you have been a full-time mum but do hope to train as a nurse in the future. You have met a nice elderly lady who is your neighbour and has been helping to look after the children if you need to run errands. You hope your children can start school soon and your husband will find work.
	In Syria you were very frightened and your family walked for days to safety. You feel exhausted but you are thankful that you are safe. You cry when you think of home. You left your elderly relatives who were not able to travel. You lost contact with your parents but believe they are safe as they were with you until you crossed the border. The children have become very quiet since you left. You imagine they are shocked but you give them lots of love and tell them they will be okay now.
ICE	You feel that if the children are poorly you should take them to A&E where they can see a doctor and will be safe. You are concerned about Lilah's asthma and Akram's eczema. You also wonder where you should get Rasha weighed. You expect the doctor to tell you off for going to A&E too much but you worry about your children and didn't know what else to do. You hope that the doctor may help your children's chronic problems but you do not feel you should tell the doctor what to do. You knew a few babies in Syria who died of chest infections as they didn't get seen by a doctor quickly enough, so you worry if any of the children start coughing.

Learning Points

Avoiding unplanned admissions and directing appropriate use of services can be quite difficult. It is important that patients are given as much information as possible to allow them to make the right decisions regarding their health.

Make sure you are aware of what is available in your area

- How do you access your health visitor/midwife/community nurses/community mental health services? How can patients access these in an emergency or out-of-hours?
- Does your practice offer extended opening hours or is there an NHS walk-in centre nearby?
- Do your patients know about the 111 helpline?
- Is 'Pharmacy First' available in your area? (Scheme running in certain areas to allow patients to receive prescription medicines for some conditions without the patient seeing a GP.)

Chronic conditions

In patients with chronic health problems such as asthma, COPD and heart failure, it is good practice to develop a care plan or action plan with the patient. For example, an asthma action plan would be based on symptoms and peak expiratory flow rate and include when the patient should go to see a GP or phone an ambulance. Likewise, does the COPD sufferer have clear instructions about when to start antibiotics or steroids? These care plans can be effective in reducing hospital attendances by empowering the patients to manage their condition themselves and giving them good advice about which signs and symptoms need routine, urgent or emergency attention.

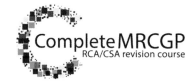

Doctor's Notes

Patient	Vincent Riley	60 years	M
PMH	Hypertension		
	Ex-smoker		
Medications	Amlodipine 10 mg daily		
Allergies	No allergies		
Consultations	Nurse appointment for bloods and blood pressure.		

Consultations (continued)

Letter to patient. 'Dear Mr Riley. Thank you for having your blood tests for your medication review. I would be grateful if you could please make an appointment to speak to the doctor on the phone to discuss your cholesterol. Best wishes. Dr Emily Blount.'

Investigations

BP 124/80

Height 185 cm

Weight 70 kg

BMI 20.4

Cholesterol/HDL ratio 5.8

QRISK3 15%

Household

No household members registered

Open ☐	Thank you for phoning. Is there anything else that you would like to talk about?
History ☐	Your cholesterol is a little high but what we need to do about this depends on your general health. I'm interested to know more about you. How do you feel your health is? You have an active lifestyle… How often a week are you doing exercise? When did you stop smoking? How much alcohol do you drink? Who is in your life?
Flags ☐	Do you ever become breathless or have any chest or leg pains?
Sense ☐	I sense you feel this is a waste of time but, if there is anything we can do to protect you from having angina, a heart attack or stroke, I want to offer help. Are you interested in discussing ways to prevent problems down the line?
Risk ☐	Do you have a family history of angina or heart disease in relatives when they were under 60 years old?
ICE ☐	Since reading the letter we sent you, have you been concerned? Has anything else gone through your mind? Do you have an idea about what I may talk about today?
Curious ☐	I'm interested… Tell me more about how you have come across statins?
Impact ☐	It sounds as if you are healthy but is there anything more you can try, do you think, to improve your diet? Do you avoid saturated fats in your food?
SummarICE ☐	To summarise, you feel well and your blood pressure is well controlled. Your cholesterol is slightly high. Your friends have had bad experiences with statins.
O/E ☐	It would be helpful if you could come into the surgery so I can feel your pulse and listen to your heart for a check-up. Could you book an appointment later this week? Thankyou.
Empower ☐	Assuming that your pulse and heart are normal when I examine you, I would want to ensure you have the information you need to make an informed decision.
Impression ☐	We put all the information into a medical calculator. It is not perfect but it is based on research so we can share with you, if you wish, your predicted risk of having a heart attack or a stroke in the next 10 years. Are you interested in knowing your risk? We take into account if your vessels may have been affected by cigarettes or require blood pressure treatment. Your risk is predicted to be 15%. This means that if there were 100 people just like you, about 15 of them would have a heart attack or stroke in the next 10 years. This is not extremely high but we want to do everything we can to bring that down. Your cholesterol was 5.8, which is higher than it should be. Research advises that if your risk if greater than 10%, you may benefit from a statin treatment. What are your thoughts?
Empathy ☐	I appreciate I am being pessimistic when talking about events like heart attacks and strokes, which is not what you want to hear when you do all you can for your health. I appreciate this is a big decision as it involves taking a tablet every day.
Experience ☐	What do you know about statins? Do you know how they work?
Explanation ☐	Statins lower cholesterol, but seem to have extra benefit above what we would expect from just lowering cholesterol, potentially stabilising or even reversing furring of the arteries. Because you already lead a healthy lifestyle and have stopped smoking, the only other thing we can change to reduce your risk is lower your cholesterol.
Recommend ☐	I recommend we start atorvastatin 20 mg, taken at night. Like all tablets there are potential side effects that can include feeling unwell with stomach and muscle aches. Rarely, statins can cause muscle breakdown. Statins can also affect the liver but we monitor this and if it occurs we stop the statin. Many people feel well on statins and they usually do lower cholesterol. Whether you choose to take the statin or not will depend on your own perception of the risk versus the downsides of taking a tablet every day.
Options ☐	What do you think? You are always welcome to come to discuss this again, perhaps when I see you to listen to your heart and check your pulse and we will of course continue to invite you for an annual health check. Are you interested in reading material? I can email this to you to read at home. Do you have any questions?
Future ☐	I respect your decision. Thank you for taking the time to listen to me today and let's see you soon to check your heart and pulse. If you ever want to talk more about cholesterol, please don't hesitate to make another telephone appointment.

Doctor's notes	Vincent Riley, 60 years. PMH: hypertension and ex-smoker. Medications: amlodipine 10 mg daily.
	Consultations: Nurse appointment for bloods and blood pressure. Letter to patient. 'Dear Mr Riley. Thank you for having your blood tests for your medication review. I would be grateful if you could please make a telephone appointment with the doctor to discuss your cholesterol. Best wishes. Dr Emily Blount.'
	Investigations: BP 124/80. Height: 185 cm. Weight: 70 kg. BMI: 20.4. Cholesterol/HDL ratio: 5.8. QRISK3 15.0%.
How to act	Apprehensive about why the doctor has called you today.
PC	*'I had a letter asking me to talk to you about cholesterol treatment.'*
History	You feel very well. Apart from well controlled high blood pressure you have no other medical history. No-one in your family has had a heart attack, angina or a stroke.
Social	You are a semi-professional golfer but are starting to spend more time helping around the clubhouse. You remain active, usually playing a few rounds a week and you also enjoy running and cycling. You eat a healthy diet. You are divorced and have a new female partner since last year. Things are going well and you are very happy. You used to smoke until the age of 48 years, on average 10 cigarettes a day. You drink 1–2 beers a couple of nights a week. You have three children with your ex-wife and they live in different parts of the world.
ICE	You are not concerned about your health. You feel very fit and active.
	You ask the doctor: *'Is this a box-ticking exercise, Doc?'*
	You have heard about statins. Several of your friends have tried them and felt awful on them.
	You are interested to hear what the doctor has to say but you do not accept any cholesterol treatment.
Examination	HS normal. HR 64 bpm regular. No stigmata of hyperlipidaemia.

Notes from NICE Guideline CG181. Cardiovascular disease: risk assessment and reduction, including lipid modification. September 2016.

Who should we screen using CVD risk score (e.g. QRISK3*)?[1,2]

Use a systematic strategy to identify people who are likely to be at high risk.

People with estimated 10-year risk of CVD of 10% or more should be prioritised for full formal risk assessment. Use the QRISK risk assessment tool to assess CVD risk for the primary prevention of CVD in people up to and including age 84 years.

Exclude type 1 diabetics and those with inherited disorders of lipid metabolism.

Exclude eGFR <60 mL/min/1.73 m^2 and/or albuminuria – see CKD guidance.

Both the above groups are considered to be at increased risk of CVD.

Consider people aged 85 or older to be at increased risk of CVD because of age alone, particularly people who smoke or have raised blood pressure. 'For people 85 years or older consider atorvastatin 20 mg as statins may be of benefit in reducing the risk of non-fatal myocardial infarction. Be aware of factors that may make treatment inappropriate.'[1]

CVD risk scores will underestimate risk in people with...

HIV, serious mental health conditions, taking immunosuppressants, antipsychotics and corticosteroids and with autoimmune and systemic inflammatory disorders... Those taking antihypertensive or lipid modification therapy or who have recently stopped smoking.[1]

Investigations

'Treat comorbidities and secondary causes of dyslipidaemia.'[1]

Address smoking, alcohol, obesity and hypertension.

Investigations: lipid screen (non-fasting), HbA1c, eGFR and renal function, ALT and TSH.

Screening for familial hypercholesterolaemia

Ask about 'the likelihood of a familial lipid disorder rather than the use of strict lipid cut-off values alone and consider if: a total cholesterol concentration more than 7.5 mmol/L and a family history of premature coronary heart disease...

Refer if the total cholesterol concentration >9.0 mmol/L or a non-HDL cholesterol concentration of >7.5 mmol/L even in the absence of a first-degree family history of premature coronary heart disease.'[1]

For information about managing raised cholesterol and triglycerides – see Extra Notes.

*QRISK3 is in use at the time of publication but new versions are released each Spring, so keep a look out for these.

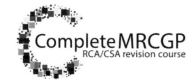

CompleteMRCGP
RCA/CSA revision course

Doctor's Notes

Patient	Kirsten Cameron	40 years	F
PMH	Gastro-oesophageal reflux disease		
	Gallstones		
	Depression		
	BMI 40		
	3 × NVD		
	Tonsillitis		
	Mild OA knees		
	Menorrhagia		
Medications	No current medications		
Allergies	No information		
Consultations	Recent consultations for OA knees and directed to physiotherapy.		
Investigations	X-ray knees – mild OA		
Household	Richard Cameron	46 years	M
	Winnie Cameron	7 years	F
	Grace Cameron	6 years	F
	Thomas Cameron	4 years	M

Example Consultation Wants to Lose Weight

Open ☐   Tell me more about what has led to you phoning me today? What has triggered the call this week in particular? There can be emotional or social stress that can all lead to weight gain. Are either of these factors something you can relate to?

Sense ☐   I'm hearing from you that this has now become a priority, is that correct?

Impact ☐   What impact has this problem had on your life? Anything else?

Curious ☐   You say it gets you down, what do you mean? What triggers feeling this way?

ICE ☐   What is your goal? What do you think will be the challenges to you achieving that? Do you have any ideas or wishes about how you would like to achieve this? What did you think I would suggest today? I can see it is important we tailor our plan to your busy life otherwise we are swimming against the tide.

History ☐   It's helpful to know more about you and the stressors in your life so we can plan around them. Tell me about past problems with your health. And now? What have you tried? With a job and three children, what exercise do you manage to do at the moment? Do you smoke? How much alcohol do you drink? Who else in your life might support you?

Empathy ☐   It sounds like being overweight has affected your confidence, which was perhaps already low following the depression.

Empower ☐   Usually we need to put several things in place to help, as well as medication. What other steps could be squeezed into your schedule if your husband and friend support you? Are there any health professionals you might find helpful?

Impression ☐   It sounds as if you have taken what the doctor said, about losing weight to help your knees, seriously – and you now feel this has become a priority for your mental and physical well-being. This problem has contributed to your pain, feeling down and low confidence with your partner. Can you think of any other problems it has led to?

Experience ☐   What problems might it also cause in your future?

Explanation ☐   You are right; the health of vessels supplying the heart and brain can be at risk.

Risk ☐   I would like to do some tests to make sure there is no medical issue contributing to your weight gain. I would like to test your ovulation hormones and thyroid. Also, can we do a health check of your cholesterol, sugar level, kidney function and BP?

SummarICE ☐   To summarise, your knee pain and your friend's encouragement have led you to think about the impact your weight has had on your life. It is important for you to gain some control back, because your big fears are that your depression may return and further knee pain. You have a good relationship with your husband but you feel sad that you do not have a sexual relationship.

InCludE ☐   You worried that I may say you should eat less and exercise more or join a programme, which is not practical advice for your circumstances, and you enjoy food and cooking. You believe your husband and friend will support you and can offer the flexibility you need, time-wise. Your goal is to run up that hill and meanwhile you plan to enjoy learning some new healthy recipes. Have I got it?

Recommend ☐   I recommend a tablet called orlistat which reduces fat absorption. Your bowels become loose and it may give you a tummy upset as you pass more fat in the stool. Is this something you would like to try?

Specifics ☐   Please take orlistat 3 times daily at meal times. Can you make an appointment with the nurse for the blood tests, BP and an up-to-date weight?

Future ☐   We will check your weight again in 3 months' time and you may continue this tablet if you have lost 5% of your current weight. It can also help to use calorie counting apps on your phone to keep track of what you're eating, and some women find exercise videos, which they can do at their convenience at home, helpful.

Safety net ☐   If your mood does drop, or you are concerned about anything, please phone again.

Patient's Story

Doctor's notes   Kirsten Cameron, 40 years. PMH: gastro-oesophageal reflux disease, gallstones, depression, 3 × NVD, tonsillitis, mild OA knees, menorrhagia. BMI 40. Medications: none. Recent consultations for OA knees and directed to physiotherapy. Investigations: X-ray knees – mild OA.

How to act   Quiet and embarrassed.

PC   *'Doctor, I would like help to lose weight please.'*

History   Your knees are becoming increasingly painful. Originally you were worried about arthritis but, following an X-ray, the doctor explained that treatment for osteoarthritis is either anti-inflammatories, injections or exercises. You were told they are not bad enough for surgery but have been advised to lose weight. You do not have time to do the physio exercises or lose weight. You have three small children at home. You do the school run after work. You have had multiple health problems, but currently only your knees are bothering you. Your depression resolved about a year ago but you don't have any confidence. It is obvious that your husband does not find you attractive as he has no interest in having sex. *'It gets me down.'* You remain good companions. He would be supportive of you losing weight and would help with the children if you asked. It has just become routine that you run the home. Reading women's magazines gets you down. You used to be a size 12 and, over the past decade, you have gradually gained weight; especially when you were depressed and you used to binge eat. You spoke to your friend and she told you to see the GP. Your friend said she would help with the kids or go on a walk with you at night. There's a lovely view from the top of the hill near your house and you have laughed with your friend that in a year you will run up it. You also know you comfort eat. You would like to get into healthy eating and might start searching for new recipes on websites. You enjoy cooking.

Social   Your husband is an undertaker. You are a milliner. You do not smoke. You rarely drink alcohol as money is tight and you save where you can.

ICE   You are aware that you are at risk of heart attacks and increasing knee pain. You know that you have to eat less and exercise more; easier said than done. You are tired at the end of the day. Your big fear is your depression returning. You felt at rock bottom at the time and it impacted on enjoying life with your children. Then you felt guilty that you were missing out on their precious years. (Your mood is generally okay at present.) You would like the doctor to provide a weight loss tablet rather than tell you to go to an exercise class which you have never been able to commit to. You would like practical solutions for your personal circumstances and feel other doctors have just told you to join Weight Watchers or go to classes. If the doctor explores options with you, you will agree to increase your exercise but you cannot commit to an exercise programme as you need to be at work or home.

Notes from NICE guideline CG189. Obesity: identification, assessment and management. Nov 2014.

'Tailor the components of the planned weight management programme to the person's preferences, initial fitness, health status and lifestyle.'[1]

'The main requirement of a dietary approach to weight loss is that total energy intake should be less than energy expenditure.'[1]

Asian family origin	Consider lower threshold for intervention.
Children	'Clinical intervention should be considered for children with a BMI at or above the 91st centile… Encourage parents (or carers) to take main responsibility for lifestyle changes in children…'[1] Multicomponent interventions include behaviour change strategies for activity and eating behaviours.
Multicomponent interventions	The treatment of choice. These include behaviour change strategies for increasing activity, improving eating behaviour and diet quality and reducing energy intake.
Examination	BP, waist circumference.
Investigations	Lipid and HbA1c
Orlistat	'Only prescribe orlistat as part of an overall plan for managing obesity in adults who meet one of the following criteria: a BMI of 28 kg/m^2 or more with associated risk factors or a BMI of 30 kg/m^2 or more.'[1]
	'Continue orlistat therapy beyond 3 months only if the person has lost at least 5% of their initial body weight.'[1]
Exercise	Encourage adults to do at least 45–60 minutes of moderate or greater intensity physical activity on 5 or more days a week. However, higher amounts may be needed to prevent obesity without dietary changes.[1]
Diets	Suggest 'diets that have a 600 kcal/day deficit…
	Consider low-calorie diets (800–1600 kcal/day), but be aware these are less likely to be nutritionally complete.'[1]
	Beware of free sugar content in fruit, juices and drinks.
Bariatric surgery	'Consider if: BMI >40 or BMI >35 + comorbidities or BMI >30 + recent onset DM as long as they are also receiving or will receive assessment in a tier 3 service or equivalent.'[1]
	Consider a lower threshold in the Asian population.
	'All appropriate non-surgical measures have been tried but the person has not achieved or maintained adequate, clinically beneficial weight loss…
	The person has been receiving or will receive intensive management in a tier 3 service …
	The person is generally fit for anaesthesia and surgery…
	The person commits to the need for long-term follow-up.'[1]

Age	Immunisation
8 weeks	DTaP/IPV(polio)/Hib/HepB – diphtheria, tetanus, pertussis, polio, *Haemophilus influenzae* type B, hepatitis B Rotavirus gastroenteritis, oral drops Meningitis B
12 weeks	DTaP/IPV(polio)/Hib/Hep B – 2nd dose Rotavirus gastroenteritis, oral drops PCV (pneumococcal – 13 serotypes)
16 weeks	DTaP/IPV(polio)/Hib/Hep B – 3rd dose Meningitis B – 2nd dose
1 year old (on or after 1st birthday)	Hib/MenC = 4th dose of Hib and 1st dose of MenC MMR – measles, mumps and rubella PCV booster (pneumococcal) Meningitis B – 3rd dose
Eligible paediatric age group	Influenza (each year from September). Given to all at-risk children and other specific age cohorts. See relevant Public Health publications for national childhood flu immunisation programme details
3 years 4 months	DTaP/IPV(polio) MMR – 2nd dose
Boys and girls aged 12–13	HPV – 2 doses, 6–24 months apart
14 years old (school year 9)	Td/IPV (tetanus, diphtheria and polio) Meningitis ACWY Check MMR status
High-risk children	Hep B – at birth, 4 weeks and 12 months, if mother infected with Hep B TB – at birth, if local incidence ≥40/100,000 or parent/grandparent born in high incidence country Influenza – at-risk children, from age 6 months to 17 years
Pregnant women	Influenza – during flu season, at any stage of pregnancy Pertussis – from 16 weeks' gestation
Adults	MenACWY. If not received offer to students up to 25 years Influenza and pneumococcal for those aged over 65 years and those in high-risk groups Td/IPV(polio) – for those not fully immunised as a child or travelling to high risk areas Shingles vaccine for adults either aged 70 or 78 (plus catch up for adults born after 2/9/1942 if aged <80 years and not previously immunised)

Live attenuated vaccines: MMR, chickenpox, rotavirus, yellow fever, oral polio, BCG, typhoid, Japanese encephalitis, rabies and cholera. They should not be given to immunosuppressed or pregnant patients.

Information collated from Patient.info,[1,4] WHO,[2] NIH Centers for Disease Control and Prevention[3]

Measles[1] – cold-like symptoms, high temperature, white/grey spots inside cheeks, red/brown diffuse rash starting on head and neck then spreading to body. Serious complications: pneumonia, encephalitis, blindness, deafness.

Mumps – painful swelling of the parotid glands. May cause testicular pain/swelling and can also affect ovaries. Serious complications: meningitis, fertility problems, deafness.

Rubella – red/pink rash of small spots with fever, viral symptoms and enlarged lymph nodes. Can cause complications in pregnancy (fetal abnormalities).

Diphtheria – high fever, thick grey/white coating back of throat with sore throat and breathing difficulties. Bacterial infection. Serious complications: myocarditis, problems with nervous system. 5–10% mortality rate despite treatment,[2] especially patients aged <5 or >40 – can be 20%.[3]

Tetanus – wounds contaminated with soil or animal manure. High fever, muscle spasms and lockjaw. Bacterial infection (*Clostridium tetani*). Complications: PE, pneumonia. Mortality rate 11%.[3]

Pertussis – whooping cough. *Bordetella pertussis*. Persistent cough with secretions in airways, distinctive 'whoop' at end of cough. Complications: pneumonia, seizures, encephalopathy, apnoea. In infants <12 months, half need treatment in hospital.[3]

Polio – viral infection, often asymptomatic but can cause paralysis, which is life threatening. There is no cure. Although most cases pass without being noted, 1 in 200 with the condition have some degree of paralysis,[3] muscle atrophy, joint contractures and bony deformity such as twisted legs.

Haemophilus influenzae B – potentially serious bacterial infection. Can cause epiglottitis, meningitis, pericarditis, pneumonia, septicaemia, septic arthritis, cellulitis and osteomyelitis. Most serious complication is meningitis.[3]

Pneumococcal – bacterial. PCV protects against 13 types of *Streptococcus pneumoniae*. Typically causes respiratory tract infection (bronchitis, sinusitis) and otitis media but can cause invasive infection such as pneumonia, meningitis and septicaemia.

Rotavirus – virus causing gastroenteritis. Although rarely fatal, 1 in 10 cases in infants cause dehydration that requires hospitalisation – 18,000 infant hospital admissions in England and Wales each year.[4]

Meningitis B, ACWY – protection against meningococcal groups B, A, C, W and Y. Causes meningitis and septicaemia. Complications include hearing damage, epilepsy, brain damage, limb amputation and death. Group W is most aggressive form. Symptoms: fever, headache, vomiting, muscle pains, cold hands and feet, non-blanching rash (petechial or purpuric).

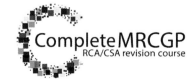

CompleteMRCGP
RCA/CSA revision course

Population Health

Overview of Cervical Screening Programme

All women* between 25 and 64 years

- 25–49 years have 3-yearly recall.
- 50–64 years have 5-yearly recall.
- Over 65 years are entitled to screening if they haven't been screened since they turned 50 years or if they have had recent abnormal results requiring follow-up.

Should screening be offered to younger women?

- In all four countries of the UK, screening starts at 25 years. This is because:
  - Younger women are more likely to have abnormal cytology.
  - The abnormal cells are more likely to return to normal by themselves in younger women, making the development of cancer less likely.
  - Therefore, if the screening age was brought down this would likely result in an increase in unnecessary invasive tests/biopsies, i.e. would lead to more harm than benefit.

Who doesn't need cervical screening?

- Women with symptoms of cervical cancer should be referred directly via the suspected cancer pathway: cervical cytology should not be done (it is a screening test not a diagnostic test).
- Unless under active follow-up for a previous abnormal result, pregnant women should wait until 3 months after delivery before having their routine cervical screening test.
- Women who have never been sexually active are at very low risk of cervical cancer so can choose not to be screened.
- Women who have had a total hysterectomy (i.e. cervix removed) do not require screening. However, in certain situations 'vault smears' are done – if this is required the patient's gynaecologist should arrange it.

*'Women' includes people with a cervix including trans men and non-binary people assigned female at birth.

What	Who	Comment
Bowel cancer	60–74 years old Plan to extend programme to >50s	FIT testing. Positive results referred for colonoscopy Tested every 2 years
	Information from https://www.gov.uk/guidance/bowel-cancer-screening-programme-overview (updated March 2021)	
Breast cancer	Women* 50–71 (Plan to extend to 47–73 years)	3 yearly mammography
	https://www.gov.uk/guidance/breast-screening-programme-overview (updated March 2021)	
Diabetic retinopathy	Annually (>12 years of age with diabetes)	Digital retinal photography
	Information from https://www.gov.uk/guidance/diabetic-eye-screening-programme-overview (updated May 2021)	
Abdominal aortic aneurysm	Men** aged 65 years	
	Information from https://www.gov.uk/guidance/abdominal-aortic-aneurysm-screening-programme-overview (updated March 2021)	
Newborn / infant	All newborns (hearing, bloodspot, physical examination)	Blood spot tests for: sickle cell, cystic fibrosis, hypothyroidism + six metabolic disorders (phenylketonuria, MCADD, maple syrup urine disease, isovaleric acidaemia, glutaric aciduria type 1 and HCU)
	Information from https://www.gov.uk/guidance/newborn-blood-spot-screening-programme-overview (updated November 2018)	
Pregnancy	Pregnant women (fetal anomaly, infectious diseases, sickle cell/ thalassaemia)	**Examination** – height, weight, fundal height, urine dip, BP **Blood tests** – blood-borne viruses, anaemia, blood group, rhesus status, sickle cell, thalassaemia **Scans** – dating 8–14 weeks, anomaly 18–21 weeks **Down screening** – bloods 10–14 weeks. Best test is combined test (β-hCG, PAPP-A and nuchal translucency) Cut off for further investigation is 1 in 150. Also Edwards' syndrome and Patau's syndrome now screened for[2] Non-invasive pre-natal testing for Down syndrome is available – currently private. Based on maternal blood sample, tested for fetal DNA. Said to be 99% accurate in detecting Down, Edwards' and Patau's syndromes
	Information from https://www.gov.uk/guidance/infectious-diseases-in-pregnancy-screening-programme-overview (updated June 2020) https://www.nhsinform.scot/healthy-living/screening/pregnancy/non-invasive-prenatal-testing-nipt	

*'Women' includes trans men and non-binary people assigned female at birth who have not had an operation to remove their breasts and trans women and non-binary people assigned male at birth and who have taken feminising hormones.

- If registered with a GP as female, will automatically be called for screening.
- If registered with a GP as male, will not automatically be called for screening and should organise mammogram through GP or by booking appointment with screening service.

** 'Men' includes trans women and non-binary people assigned male at birth.

Information from NICE guideline CG181. Cardiovascular disease: risk assessment and reduction, including lipid modification. September 2016.

Cardioprotective diet recommendations[1]

Total fat intake <30% daily intake.

Saturated fats <7% daily intake.

Reduce/replace animal or saturated fats with monounsaturated or polyunsaturated fats.

Olive oil and rapeseed oils or spreads based on these oils are healthy substitutes.

Reduce intake of sugar and products containing refined sugars such as fructose.

Choose wholegrain varieties of starchy food.

'Eat at least five portions of fruit or vegetables a day' (however, fruit may be high in sugar).

Fish at least twice a week (one portion of oily fish). Pregnant women should limit oily fish to two portions and avoid marlin, swordfish and shark.

'Eat at least four to five portions of unsalted nuts, seeds and legumes per week.'

Exercise recommendations

'At least 150 minutes of moderate intensity aerobic activity or... 75 minutes of vigorous intensity aerobic activity' a week.

'Muscle-strengthening activities on 2 or more days a week that work all major muscle groups.'

Encourage patients with a comorbidity, medical condition or personal circumstances to 'exercise at their maximum safe capacity.'

Alcohol consumption: Department of Health, January 2016[2]

Recommends maximum limit of **14 units** per week for **both men and women**. Those 14 units should be spread over 3 or more days.

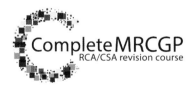
CompleteMRCGP
RCA/CSA revision course

Population Health

Information from NICE guideline CG181. Cardiovascular disease: risk assessment and reduction, including lipid modification. September 2016.

Secondary prevention   80 mg atorvastatin and repeat lipid profile 3 months later. Lower dose if potential drug interactions, high risk of adverse effects or patient preference. Do not delay managing modifiable risk factors, do not delay if acute coronary syndrome.

Primary prevention   Offer lifestyle changes and retesting

Offer 20 mg atorvastatin if: ≥10% 10-year risk of developing CVD.

>85 years (but be aware of factors that might make Rx inappropriate)

CKD

Consider in all T1DMs and offer if either:

>10 years of DM

>40 years

Established nephropathy

Other CVD risk factors

Type 2 diabetes and ≥10% 10-year risk of developing CVD

Advise of risks and adverse effects – an example explanation: *'Side effects include muscle pain or weakness, stomach problems or pain, and statins can affect the function of the liver. Rarely, they can cause muscle breakdown. (See BNF for full list.) If muscle pain or weakness develops seek help. Attend for another blood test to check the liver at 3 and 12 months. Avoid grapefruit juice when taking statins.'* Check no pre-existing generalised muscle pain and check CK level if present before starting. Remember to change simvastatin to atorvastatin if on amlodipine.

Measure liver transaminase enzymes at 'baseline, 3/12 months… 12 months, but not again unless clinically indicated'.[1]

Follow-up for both primary and secondary prevention includes a lipid retest after 3/12. If >40% reduction (non-HDL) is not achieved discuss compliance, timing, diet, lifestyle. Consider increasing dose if started on <80 mg and at higher risk due to risk score, comorbidities or using clinical judgement. Annual medication review to discuss compliance, lifestyle and address CV risk factors. 'Consider annual non-fasting non-HDL cholesterol to inform discussion.'[1]

If eGFR <30 mL/min/1.73 m^2 discuss with a renal specialist first.

If intolerance of statins, treat with maximum tolerated dose. Consider stop/restart, 'reducing the dose… or changing the statin to a lower intensity group.'[1] If there is muscle pain or weakness, check the CK.

Triglycerides

>20 mmol/L   Refer urgently if not secondary to alcohol or poor glycaemic control.[1]

10–20 mmol/L   Repeat day 5–14 (fasting sample) then refer after considering secondary causes if remains ≥10 mmol/L.[1]

4.5–9.9 mmol/L   CVD risk may be underestimated by risk assessment tools. Optimise CV health and seek advice if non-HDL cholesterol >7.5 mmol/L.[1]

Ezetimibe monotherapy may be used in primary hypercholesterolaemia if the patient is intolerant of statins or if drug interactions prevent the use of statins.[2]

Seek specialist advice before considering fenofibrates (e.g. for hypertriglyceridemia).

Lipid management
See the **Link Hub at CompleteMRCGP.co.uk** for a link to helpful information about lipid management.

Population Health

Respiratory Health

	Cases in this chapter	Within the RCGP 2020 curriculum: Respiratory Health	Learning points in this chapter include:
1	Pneumonia	'Lower respiratory tract infections' 'Diseases scoring tools, e.g. CURB for community-acquired pneumonia'	Management of pneumonia CRB-65 score and AMTS
2	Acute Asthma	'Common and important conditions – asthma: acute and chronic' 'Specific procedures such as PEFR'	Acute asthma management
3	COPD	'Common and important conditions – COPD' 'Local and national guidelines to manage… COPD' 'The importance of lifestyle changes, particularly smoking cessation and pulmonary rehabilitation'	Management of COPD
4	Snoring	'Snoring and sleep apnoea' 'CPAP for sleep apnoea'	Risk factors, assessment and management of OSAS/OSAHS
5	Lung Cancer	'Respiratory malignancies' 'Indications for chest X-rays, CT and MRI scans'	Causes of coin lesions Lung cancer 2WW referral criteria
Extra Notes	Spirometry	'Primary care investigations such as … spirometry' 'Interpretation of spirometry results'	Spirometry Reversibility testing Restrictive lung disease

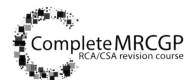

CompleteMRCGP
RCA/CSA revision course

Pneumonia

1. NICE CKS. Chest infections – adult. https://cks.nice.org.uk/chest-infections-adult#!scenario:1. Jun 2021.
2. BMJ Best Practice – Community-acquired pneumonia. https://bestpractice.bmj.com/topics/en-gb/3000108/management-recommendations
3. Lim W.S., van der Eerden M.M., Laing R. et al. Defining community-acquired pneumonia severity on presentation to hospital: an international derivation and validation study. *Thorax* 2003; 58: 377–82.
4. Hodkinson H.M. Evaluation of a mental test score for assessment of mental impairment in the elderly. *Age Ageing* 1972; 1: 233–8.

Acute Asthma and Acute COPD

1. BTS/Scottish Intercollegiate Guidelines Network (SIGN). British guideline on the management of asthma. https://www.brit-thoracic.org.uk/quality-improvement/guidelines/asthma/. Jul 2019.
2. NICE CKS. Asthma (Acute asthma section). https://cks.nice.org.uk/topics/asthma/management/acute-exacerbation-of-asthma/. May 2021.
3. NICE CKS. Chronic obstructive pulmonary disease. https://cks.nice.org.uk/chronic-obstructive-pulmonary-disease#!scenario:1. Jul 2021.

COPD

1. 2020 GOLD Report (2020 Global strategy for prevention, diagnosis and management of COPD). https://goldcopd.org/gold-reports/
2. NICE CKS. Chronic obstructive pulmonary disease. https://cks.nice.org.uk/chronic-obstructive-pulmonary-disease#!scenario. Jul 2021.

Snoring and OSAHS

1. http://patient.info/doctor/obstructive-sleep-apnoea-syndrome-pro. Jul 2020.
2. http://www.britishsnoring.co.uk/sleep_apnoea/epworth_sleepiness_scale.php
3. https://www.gov.uk/government/publications/assessing-fitness-to-drive-a-guide-for-medical-professionals. Contains public sector information licensed under the Open Government Licence v3.0.

Useful Resource

Tiredness can kill. https://www.gov.uk/government/uploads/system/uploads/attachment_data/file/503534/INF159_150216.pdf. Contains public sector information licensed under the Open Government Licence v3.0.

Lung Cancer

1. NICE Guideline NG12. Suspected cancer: recognition and referral. Jan 2021.
2. https://radiopaedia.org/articles/coin-lesion-lung?lang=gb
3. NICE CKS. https://cks.nice.org.uk/lung-and-pleural-cancers-recognition-and-referral#!scenario. Feb 2021.

Spirometry

1. https://www.blf.org.uk/support-for-you/breathing-tests/spirometry-and-reversibility

Information taken from NICE guidelines with kind permission. Please note the guidelines change frequently and you should ALWAYS check for the latest updated guidance. Remember that NICE guidance is only applicable to patients in the UK.

Doctor's Notes

Patient	Lionel Morgan	82 years	M
PMH	Parkinson's disease		
Medications	Sinemet		
	Entacapone		
Allergies	No information		
Consultations	Medication review 3 months ago. No concerns.		
Investigations	No information		
Household	Betty Morgan	80 years	F

Wife Betty also present and talks on the phone.

Open ☐	A chest infection? Anything else you have noticed? How do you feel about your health generally?
Flags ☐	Are you feeling SOB? Have you had a fever? Do you have any pain? What colour are you spitting out? Any blood? Any cold or sore throat at the moment?
Risk ☐	Are you managing to swallow food and tablets without coughing? Do you smoke? Have you suffered with lung trouble in the past? Have you been exposed to asbestos?
History ☐	I see you take Sinemet and entacapone for your Parkinson's; is there any other medical history? Is it just the two of you at home?
ICE ☐	Any other concerns? Is there anything specific you were hoping I would do today?
Impact ☐	I'm interested to know how your Parkinson's is affecting you at the moment. How does it impact on your day? Since this cough, have either of you noticed any other changes?
Sense ☐	Lionel, you have asked Betty to answer for you a few times, are you feeling slightly muddled?
Curious ☐	Are you or your family worried about your memory?
O/E ☐	Can I test your memory by asking a few questions (AMTS). Would you normally be able to answer these questions more easily? Betty, please can you check Lionel's temperature for me? Does he look as if he is breathing quicker than usual?
SummarICE ☐	So, for 4 days you have been struggling with your breathing and coughing up green phlegm, felt feverish and slightly more muddled than usual. You are both concerned this could be an infection.
Impression ☐	I think you could have pneumonia, Lionel.
Experience ☐	Pneumonia is an infection of the air sacs in the lungs which is usually significant enough to show up on a chest X-ray.
Explanation ☐	I think this is the case as you have been coughing up green phlegm, you have a fever and are more breathless and muddled than normal.
InCludE ☐	I appreciate you said you are well cared for at home and prefer not to go to hospital but I think it may be necessary.
Recommend ☐	When someone has a fever and confusion, we usually ask the hospital doctors to see them. The other option is I could see you in the surgery to examine you. By listening to your chest, checking your BP, heart rate and oxygen levels it will be clearer just how much this infection is affecting you. If your numbers seem okay, we could consider giving you antibiotics at home and keep a very close eye on you over the next couple of days. However, I suspect my recommendation will still be to go to hospital for some oxygen and antibiotics into the blood to speed up your recovery.
Empower ☐	What do you both think? Lionel and Betty, it sounds as if the two of you are looking after each other very well; however, should you need any help with carers then please let me know.
Specifics ☐	How quickly can you get to the surgery? Great, I will see you shortly. When you are feeling better, let's have another chat about your memory and Parkinson's in more detail: if you could please book an appointment in about 2 weeks and I will see you then. Betty, it would be helpful to talk to you too about how you feel things are going. Perhaps you could book a separate appointment for yourself.
Safety net ☐	If, en route, you have pain or feel more short of breath or feel more poorly, please stop the car and call 999 for an ambulance.

Doctor's notes	Lionel Morgan, 82 years. PMH: Parkinson's disease. Medications: Sinemet and entacapone.
	Wife Betty also present.
How to act	Betty, your wife is with you. You turn to ask your wife Betty for answers. Betty likes to answer for you.
PC	*'Doctor, I think I've got a chest infection.'*
History	**Betty** Lionel is more muddled than usual.
	Lionel has been coughing green phlegm for 4 days.
	He looks breathless but isn't wheezy. He is not choking on his food.
	No blood seen. No other viral URTI symptoms. His fever was 102 °F.
	Lionel You have no pain. Your spit is green.
Social	**Lionel** You live with your wife, Betty, who does all your ADL and takes care of your medicines.
	You are well looked after at home and your three children live close by.
	You have never smoked. You drink no alcohol. No asbestos exposure.
	Your son is on his way over and would be able to take you to the surgery or hospital.
ICE	**Lionel** You worry you have a chest infection.
	'I would prefer you don't send me into hospital.'
	However, you will do as the doctor suggests – if they insist on calling an ambulance accept this. If they offer to see you in surgery, state you would prefer this to see if there's any chance of avoiding hospital.
	Betty You wonder if this is pneumonia.
	'You will do as you are told, Lionel.'
Examination	Bronchial breathing and crackles in the left base. Temperature 38.2 °C. HR 90 bpm regular. Sats 95%. RR 24. BP 120/68.
	AMTS score 6/10.
	If telephone – AMTS 6/10, sounds breathless. Betty able to tell you his temperature is 102 °F.
	Betty states he would usually answer memory questions more easily.

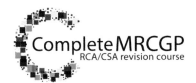

CompleteMRCGP
RCA/CSA revision course

Pneumonia	An infection of the lung parenchyma (alveoli).

. NICE states 'clinical judgement must always be used to diagnose CAP because no combination of symptoms or signs is clearly diagnostic'[1]

Calculate CRB-65 score	This gentleman's CRB-65 was 2.
	1 point each for: confusion (AMTS ≤8/10), RR ≥30/min, systolic BP <90 or diastolic ≤60, age ≥65 years.

Score = 0	'Low risk'[2]	<1% mortality risk[2,3]
Score = 1–2	'Intermediate risk'[2]	1–10% mortality risk[2,3]
Score = 3–4	'High risk'[2]	>10% mortality risk[2,3]

Sputum culture	'Do not routinely recommend microbiological tests for people with low-severity community-acquired pneumonia.'[1]
CRP testing	Consider if clinically a diagnosis of pneumonia is not clear or uncertainty about whether antibiotics are indicated.[1]
<20 mg/L	'Do not routinely offer antibiotic therapy.'[1]
20 mg/L–100 mg/L	'Consider a delayed antibiotic prescription.'[1]
>100 mg/L	'Offer antibiotic therapy.'[1]

NB: A fever is 100 °F (= 37.8 °C). Many older patients still use Fahrenheit.

[4] to save time, ask the hard questions first, once they have got >2 wrong then move on.

Address to remember (42 West Street), age, time, year, where are we, 2 persons, DOB, queen, First World War, 20–1 backwards, ?recall address correct.

Treatment of pneumonia

Score = 0	5 days antibiotics. See your local guidance. E.g. Amoxicillin 500 mg TDS or doxycycline 200 mg day 1 then 100 mg daily or clarithromycin 500 mg BD (erythromycin in pregnancy if penicillin allergy).
Score = 1–2	Consider hospital admission, particularly if score 2. 5 days amoxicillin + 5 days clarithromycin (erythromycin if pregnant). If penicillin allergy, doxycycline or clarithromycin alone.
Score = 3–4	Admit urgently to hospital.[1]

Recovery

Useful to explain to patients that the recovery can take a long time. Fever usually resolves within 1 week, chest pain and sputum should settle by 4 weeks, cough and breathlessness by 6 weeks, fatigue by 3 months, full resolution by 6 months.[1]

Safety net

See your GP if no response within 3 days and sooner if worsening symptoms.

Practising holistically

In this scenario, asking about swallowing demonstrates you have considered the chronic comorbidities in this acute situation and thought about aspiration pneumonia.

When a carer is present, acknowledge them and their role.

If there is no time to discuss the impact of a chronic disease (Parkinson's) in this first consultation then signpost that you will do so later.

Doctor's Notes

Patient	Daisy Fitton	24 years	F
PMH	Asthma		
Medications	Clenil 100 2 puffs BD		
	Salbutamol PRN		
Allergies	No information		
Consultations	Last attended 9 months ago for asthma review with nurse. Peak flow 450 L/min.		
Investigations	No information		
Household	No household members registered		

Open ☐	Oh dear, tell me more. What else have you noticed?
Flags ☐	How often have you been using your blue inhaler? With a spacer? How often do you usually use the blue one? What about the brown one?
Risk ☐	Have you ever been admitted with your asthma? Have you ever been in intensive care? Do you smoke? Has your asthma ever been as bad as this? Do you have a personalised asthma action plan?
History ☐	I understand that you are otherwise well, and taking no medicines, is that correct? Is there anyone at home with you?
ICE ☐	What do you think has caused this? From your experience of your asthma, what do you believe is necessary?
Sense ☐	I can see you are struggling.
O/E ☐	May I examine you, listen to your chest, check your pulse and oxygen levels and your temperature and do the blowing peak flow test? May I ask you to take off your top: is that okay?
SummarICE ☐	To summarise, you have had a cold and sore throat and now you are struggling with your asthma despite regular use of your blue inhaler. You think this may have been caused by the weather and that you may need antibiotics and steroids.
Impression ☐	Your peak flow blowing test and your breathing and heart rate suggest this is a severe asthma attack.
Explanation ☐ InCludE	There is no sign of a pocket of bacteria in the lung. You have not had a fever.
	I think this has been caused by a viral infection. You are not coughing green phlegm and your sore throat and cold are typical of a virus so, although I agree that steroids will help, I don't think that antibiotics will be of any use.
Empathy ☐	Normally, you have been able to manage the asthma at home so it is frightening when your asthma is so much worse than usual.
Recommend ☐	May I give you a nebuliser and then see how you respond? I will also give you 40 mg of prednisolone, a steroid. I will ask the nurse to give you a nebuliser in the treatment room and I will see you again in 10 minutes. Let's see how your chest responds to that and make a decision then about whether you need to go to hospital. What are your thoughts about that? I would want you to be able to manage at least an hour without the inhaler, and then 4-hourly at home. Hopefully, you will respond to treatment and will be able to go home.
Specifics ☐	If that is the case, I will see you again in 2 days' time to check you are getting on okay. I will book you an appointment for 9 a.m. if that is convenient.
Future ☐	When you are feeling better, I'd like to meet up again to optimise your inhalers. In future, if you are using your blue inhaler more than twice a week this suggests we need to increase the preventer, the brown inhaler. We can write all this down for you in your own asthma plan.
Safety net ☐	If you feel your breathing is deteriorating in the treatment room, please tell us and we'll call an ambulance.

Doctor's notes	Daisy Fitton, 24 years. PMH: asthma. Medications: Clenil 100 2 puffs BD, salbutamol PRN.
How to act	A little distracted by your breathing.
PC	*'My asthma isn't very good.'*
History	You've had a cold and sore throat and for the past 2 days you've become wheezy.
	You are not coughing any phlegm and have no pain but feel tight in the chest. No fever.
	Your chest always feels like this at this time of year.
	You were admitted once as a child but no ITU admissions.
	You use the Clenil BD and usually your salbutamol 6 times a week, especially after hockey.
	You have a peak flow meter but don't use it very often.
	You last took four puffs of salbutamol 1 hour ago.
Social	You are a solicitor. You live with your boyfriend. You have never smoked. All is well.
ICE	You believe the weather has caused this exacerbation. You are not too concerned.
	You expect the doctor will give you steroids and antibiotics – if the doctor suggests you don't need antibiotics, question them about why – you usually get given them.
	You will follow the doctor's advice regarding admission, stating: *'You are the doctor.'*
Examination	Peak flow 210 L/min. RR 24 Sats 95%. HR 104 bpm. Temperature 36.9 °C.
	Good air entry, R = L. Vesicular breaths and wheeze throughout, expiration > inspiration.

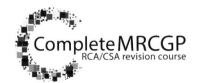

Life-threatening asthma

Peak flow <33% or asthma with the following features: Sats <92%, silent chest, cyanosis, poor respiratory effort, arrhythmia, hypotension, confusion or exhaustion.[1]

Acute severe asthma

Peak flow 33–50%, RR ≥25, HR ≥110 bpm in people >12 years and not able to complete sentences (no features of life-threatening asthma).[1]

Moderate asthma

Peak flow 50–75%, normal speech and no signs of acute severe/life-threatening asthma.[1]

Management of acute asthma – adults

All: oxygen to keep the saturations between 94 and 98%.[1]

Prednisolone 40–50 mg stat then daily to complete minimum of 5 days.[1]

Follow up patients at home within 2 working days.

Life-threatening asthma: admit the patient **immediately**. Call 999. Give salbutamol 5 mg + 0.5 mg ipratropium nebuliser. May repeat salbutamol if required whilst waiting for the ambulance.

Severe asthma: consider admission. Give 5 mg salbutamol via nebuliser or spacer if nebuliser not available. If not response or still has features of acute severe asthma, admit.[1]

Moderate asthma: give up to 10 puffs (1 every 60 s) of salbutamol via spacer, if no response give nebulised salbutamol, consider admission. If good response, continue or increase usual treatment and continue prednisolone for minimum of 5 days. NICE suggest can quadruple inhaled corticosteroid treatments in some patients to reduce oral steroid use.[2]

In a CSA exam situation, if the actor is really struggling to answer your questions, advise a nebuliser +/– phone ambulance early in the consultation. It is kinder to the patient to ask them more questions after their breathing feels better. You can always indicate to the examiner that you know you require more information by stating that you will need to ask some more questions once their breathing has improved.

Safety netting

On discharge. If requiring more than 10 puffs of salbutamol through a spacer within 4 hours, they will then need to see a doctor again or go to hospital. Arrange follow-up within 2 days, e.g. F2F or telephone call.

Acute COPD[3]

Consider admission if severe breathlessness, inability to cope at home/lives alone, poor or deteriorating general condition, rapid onset, acute confusion/impaired consciousness, cyanosis, saturations <90%, worsening peripheral oedema, new arrhythmia, already on LTOT, failure to respond to initial treatment or changes on CXR. Give supplemental oxygen whilst awaiting emergency transfer aiming for saturations of 88–92%.[3] Provide oxygen through a Venturi 24% mask at 2–3 L/min or Venturi 28% mask at 4 L/min or via nasal cannula at 1–2 L/min if Venturi mask unavailable.

Where admission not required treat increased cough and/or breathlessness with 30 mg prednisolone, once daily for 5 days. Discuss adverse effects of long-term treatment and consider osteoporosis prophylaxis if >3 or 4 courses of steroids per year. Treat change in colour or increased volume of sputum with antibiotics (e.g. amoxicillin, doxycycline or clarithromycin).

Doctor's Notes

Patient	Chao Lin	82 years	M
PMH	COPD		
	Current smoker		
Medications	Salbutamol		
	Tiotropium		
Allergies	No known drug allergies		
Consultations	COPD review 1 year ago with the nurse – no changes made. Using salbutamol on hills. Tiotropium daily. Saturations 96%. MRC dyspnoea scale: 2.		
	Weight 72 kg.		
	Spirometry 1 year ago.		
	FEV1 48%, FVC 80%, FEV1/FVC 0.6		
	FEV1 following salbutamol 50%.		

Letter to patient

'Dear Mr Lin. Please make an appointment to speak to me at the surgery. I would like to discuss your breathing and inhalers to see if any adjustments are required and take this opportunity to discuss your general health and if there is anything that you may need. Best wishes. Dr Blount.'

Flu and pneumococcal vaccines up to date.

Investigations	No information
Household	No known household contacts

Example Consultation COPD

Open ☐ Thank you for calling Mr Lin. How are you? This is the first time we have spoken so please tell me about your health. What is most difficult? What has changed?

ICE ☐ Is there anything you wanted to talk to me about? Has anything been on your mind or worrying you? What is your biggest fear? Did you have any thoughts about what we may talk about today?

Sense ☐ I noticed when you first answered the phone your breathing was harder but seems to have eased now. Have you been struggling with your breathing whilst moving around?

Impact ☐ What are you not able to do? How long can you walk for? Do you have stairs in your home? Do you do your meals and shopping? Are you able to keep the home clean?

History ☐ Apart from your breathing, have you had any other medical conditions in the past? Or other parts of your body which don't work as they used to? Tell me more about your breathing. When do you take your inhalers? Every day? Do you use a spacer with your blue inhaler? Any allergies? Who else is important to you in your life? I'm sorry, that must still be very painful. How are you managing on your own? How often do you see your son? What did you do at work?

Risk ☐ Did that involve exposure to asbestos? Are you still smoking? Growing up, were you exposed to much pollution or smoke? Did your family in China have any health problems?

Flags ☐ Do you cough up any phlegm or blood? Do you ever have any chest pain? Do you feel breathless at night? How many pillows do you use? Do your legs swell up? Have you lost or put on any weight? When did you last have a chest infection? You seem concerned about infections.

Curious ☐ Why might that be? How is your mood? Do you feel isolated? Or depressed? Do you ever want to not wake up? Do you have a faith? With your faith is there anything important to you that I should know about now or in the future?

SummarICE ☐ Mr Lin, you have noticed that, for the past 6 months, you struggle to walk as far as before without having a rest. You worry about getting a chest infection and also how your breathing may change over time. You fear dying and struggling to breathe. You have also been worried about asbestos and whether this could have damaged your lungs as well.

Impression ☐ I'm afraid your airway disease does seem to have worsened.

Experience ☐ What do you know about the term COPD? Or chronic airways disease?

Explanation ☐ It is a long-term condition of the airways which have been damaged over time. Smoking is the usual cause, but you're right that asbestos can affect the lungs too.

Empathy ☐ I can imagine it is frightening to notice that your breathing does not allow you to do what you used to, and fear that soon you will not be able to reach the shops.

Recommend ☐ There are things we can try which should help. I would like to swap your capsule inhaler for a stronger one. I suggest an inhaler called Anoro Ellipta. It contains a medicine like your capsule inhaler but also a long-acting version of your blue inhaler. You may also find a spacer helps you take your blue inhaler. I will ask our pharmacist to demonstrate the new inhaler and spacer.

InCludE ☐ It's not easy to know if the asbestos has contributed, but let's do a CXR to look for signs.

Empower ☐ Are you interested in our stop smoking service? Stopping can help to slow the disease and make the biggest difference in the long term. I could refer you to our rehab service which aims to get your lungs working as well as possible? We often give patients with COPD rescue packs containing antibiotics and steroids to start should you become unwell. You take prednisolone 30 mg daily (steroid) if your breathing gets worse, with amoxicillin (antibiotic) if you get more phlegm or it changes colour. Would it be reassuring to have these medications at home? How do these options sound?

Future ☐ Can we talk again in 1 month to talk about what might happen to your breathing over time? We could create a care plan where we talk through different scenarios and what you might like doctors to do. I'd also like to talk more about how you are generally.

Specifics ☐ I will also ask our COPD nurse to see you, to check you are getting on well with the new inhaler, in about 6 weeks. I will also request a CXR for you as your breathing has deteriorated and you're worried about asbestos.

Safety net ☐ If you are more breathless, in pain or unsure please speak to a doctor straight away.

Respiratory Health – 3

Doctor's notes	Chao Lin, 82 years. PMH: COPD. Medications: salbutamol and tiotropium. Smoker. Consultations: 1 year ago, COPD review with PN. Sats 96%. MRC 2. Letter to patient: COPD review now due.
How to act	Breathing initially fast but this settles after a short while.
PC	*'Hello, Doctor. I had a letter asking me to call for a check-up.'*
History	You don't like to bother the doctor. Apart from your breathing you are well and you have no significant PMH. You are compliant with your tiotropium and use the salbutamol twice daily. You have no allergies. You remember your grandparents were heavy breathers. You never knew your father and your mother died when you were small. You believe you are 82 years old but don't know exactly. Your breathing hasn't been very good for the past 6 months. You started to wheeze about 3 years ago. You wheeze when walking to the shop but you are okay in your home although occasionally wheeze after a shower. You have no orthopnoea and sleep on two thin pillows. You have no fluid collecting in the legs. You have no cardiac symptoms. Where you grew up, your grandparents used to light fires throughout the day to keep you warm. You had no siblings. You had three infections last winter and once you were in hospital overnight. This was a frightening experience as you had never been in hospital.
Social	You moved to the UK when you were 36 years old and worked in the shipyards. You live alone and find life tiring. You walk to the local shop a couple of hundred yards away and stop for a rest midway. You use a shopping trolley to wheel your food back to the house but this is getting harder. You do not drive. Your son owns the local garage in the next village and he always offers to help you and you see him twice a week. He takes you wherever you need to go. You lost your wife to bowel cancer 3 years ago. You feel quite lonely but feel you should not complain. Your mood is a little low but you have no thoughts of not wanting to be alive and generally you feel grateful for life. Your faith (Buddhism) is important to you. You continue to smoke and would like to stop. The surgery is on the next street to your home so convenient if needed. You have no problems within your bungalow.
ICE	You worry about an infection or whether you will one day struggle with your breathing. Is it likely you will die of not being able to breathe? You also worry about asbestos as you have heard about old colleagues who have been affected by this from working on ship repairs. You have no expectations from the consultation and would follow any advice that the doctor gives. However, a preference would be to avoid any risk of infection if possible. If the doctor can help reduce your worries about asbestos you would appreciate this.
Examination	Chest – air entry and wheeze throughout. No accessory muscle use. Saturations 94%. HS normal. HR 72 bpm regular. No leg oedema or raised JVP. Weight 72 kg. BP 130/70. Peak flow 20 L/min. No supraclavicular lymphadenopathy. No clubbing.

CompleteMRCGP
RCA/CSA revision course

Advice below is based upon GOLD (Global Obstructive Lung Disease) Guidelines.[1]

Diagnosed using spirometry. Post-bronchodilator FEV1/FVC <0.7. Exclude asthma/reversibility – see reversibility in the Learning Points of Asthma Diagnosis (Chapter 2, Case 3). Why? – It is dangerous to prescribe a LABA without a steroid in asthma.

Assessment of severity: mMRC dyspnoea score + CAT (COPD assessment test) + number of exacerbations over last 12 months. Use to categorise as GOLD A, B, C or D group (see reference for grid).

- GOLD A – mMRC <2, CAT <10, 0–1 exacerbations (not leading to admission).
- GOLD B – mMRC ≥2, CAT ≥10, 0–1 exacerbations (not leading to admission).
- GOLD C – mMRC <2, CAT <10, ≥2 exacerbations or 1 leading to admission.
- GOLD D – mMRC ≥2, CAT ≥10, ≥2 exacerbations or 1 leading to admission.

Without exact scores to hand, roughly equates to – few symptoms and few exacerbations = A, few exacerbations but symptomatic = B, exacerbations but minimal interval symptoms = C, symptomatic and frequent exacerbations = D.

FEV1 – indicates severity of airflow limitation but doesn't directly impact management.

Initial therapy	Group A – PRN SABA. All other groups can start with LAMA or if symptomatic LAMA/LABA. Steroids are associated with pneumonia risk so limit use. Generally only Group D (i.e. symptomatic and frequent exacerbations) or if eosinophil count >0.3 or if asthma/COPD overlap. Avoid if recurrent pneumonia episodes. NB: some evidence to suggest benefit from starting LABA/LAMA if SABA PRN insufficient, so many areas have adopted this as first-line treatment. This approach is supported by NICE.[2]
Pulmonary rehab	Offer if mMRC ≥3 or recent hospitalisation.[2]
Home oxygen	Consider referral for LTOT if Sats <92% on air, cyanosis, polycythaemia, peripheral oedema, raised JVP, severe or very severe airflow obstruction.[2]
Health promotion	Smoking cessation. Flu and pneumococcal vaccine.
Carer support	Involve the carer in the management plan.
Self-management plan	For exacerbations – when to step up inhalers and take rescue medications.

Example inhalers (refer to own local formulary)

The patient should receive an explanation of how to use their inhaler. Following this, prescribe the same brand:

- SABA – salbutamol. Good practice to prescribe a spacer device as well.
- LAMA – Incruse Ellipta, Seebri Breezhaler.
- LAMA/LABA – Anoro Ellipta, Ultibro Breezhaler, Duaklir Genuair often first line after SABA.
- ICS/LAMA – Relvar Ellipta, Fostair 100/6.
- ICA/LABA/LAMA – Trelegy Ellipta, Trimbow (MDI – prescribe with spacer, good for those who struggle with poor inspiratory effort or difficulty using inhalers).

Doctor's Notes

Patient	Brian West	49 years	M
PMH	Hypertension		
	Obesity		
Medications	Ramipril 7.5 mg OD		
Allergies	No information		
Consultations	No information		
Investigations	No information		
Household	Patricia West	47 years	F

Open ☐	Oh dear, what has she told you about the snoring?
ICE ☐	What are your thoughts about the snoring? Does it worry you in any way? Any thoughts on how I could help?
History ☐	Is this something you have struggled with for a while? How do you feel in the daytime? What do you do for a living? So it's really important for you to be wide awake at work.
Impact ☐	Have you noticed tiredness or poor concentration? Have you ever nodded off unexpectedly in the day? Has the snoring affected your relationship with your wife?
Curious ☐	How do you think this tiredness might cause problems at work?
Flags ☐	Have you ever nodded off whilst driving? Any near misses in the car or lorry? Have you suffered any nosebleeds? Blocked nose? Change in your voice? Breathlessness? Or cough?
Risk ☐	I can see from your records that you have a history of high blood pressure and struggle with your weight. Do you have any other health problems? Do you smoke? Do you drink alcohol? How often do you drink alcohol? Have you noticed if this affects the snoring?
Experience ☐	Have you known anyone with snoring or breathing problems at night before?
Sense ☐	I sense you aren't particularly worried about the snoring but are worried about being able to continue working, is that right?
O/E ☐	Have you weighed yourself or checked your BP recently? Which shirt collar size do you wear?
SummarICE ☐	So you have always been a 'snorer' but it has gradually become worse and is now impacting your wife's sleep. She has noticed that you hold your breath at night and then can gasp. You have been feeling a lot more tired during the day and even nodded off in a meeting which is unlike you. You aren't worried about the snoring but need to keep earning for your family.
Impression ☐	I think you may have a condition where your breathing stops and starts whilst you are asleep called obstructive sleep apnoea syndrome.
Explanation ☐	In some people their airway becomes floppy during deep sleep which causes the airway to block. Your body then rouses you so your muscles wake up and you can breathe normally again. This disrupted sleep can make you very tired in the day. OSAS is more common in men who are carrying extra weight and can be made worse by drinking alcohol.
InCludE ☐	As you were thinking this was simple snoring, this must be a shock. I understand you're worried about how this will impact your job when you enjoy it so much and need the money.
Recommend ☐	May I text you a questionnaire called The Epworth Sleepiness Questionnaire? Please complete this honestly as it's really important. I suspect I may need to refer you to a sleep clinic to be diagnosed formally. They can measure your sleep and oxygen levels overnight. In the meantime, I must advise you to stop driving. This is the last thing you want to hear, but road traffic accidents are common in people with untreated OSAS. Of course, we need you and other people to be safe. I can refer you to the clinic urgently so you can be assessed and treated quickly. Would a fit note for your employer be helpful? Could I arrange some blood tests to check your cholesterol and for diabetes? What do you think?
Empower ☐	There are things you can do to help yourself. Losing some weight will make your neck lighter and help prevent the airways collapsing whilst you sleep. Also avoiding alcohol in the evenings will help. Can you think of ways you could improve your diet or increase exercise? Perhaps, longer term, could you take healthier foods with you when driving?
Future ☐	Please could I see you next week after your bloods and with your completed questionnaire so I can examine your throat and nose? We can then decide on the referral. If you have OSAS, treatment is usually with a breathing machine you wear at night which keeps your airway open. You should then get a more restful night's sleep and be able to function normally in the daytime.
Specifics ☐	I will ask reception to book you in for your bloods and with me next week.
Safety net ☐	If you notice any new symptoms or start to feel unwell please contact me straight away.

Doctor's notes	Brian West, 49 years. PMH: hypertension, obesity. Medications: ramipril 7.5 mg OD.
How to act	Relaxed
PC	*'Hi Doc, the Mrs has told me to phone you. I keep waking her up with my snoring.'*
History	For several months your snoring has been disturbing your wife. You've always been prone to snoring, particularly after a drink, but it has become worse. Your wife says you can make grunting noises and seem to hold your breath whilst asleep. You have been feeling more tired during the day and fell asleep at a morning team briefing at work, much to your boss's annoyance. Your weight has been steadily climbing over the years. You don't have much time for exercise and have a sedentary job being a lorry driver. You rely heavily on takeaway food and fast food from service stations whilst you are working. You work for a big company and drive all over Europe. You enjoy your job and you are the bread winner of the family so it is very important to you.

You don't have any nasal obstruction or nose bleeds. You have not noticed any changes to your voice. Your blood pressure has been reasonably well controlled recently, you have your own machine: it was 134/78 last Sunday. No urinary symptoms. You are not aware of waking in the night. |
| Social | Married to wife Patricia for 29 years. Two grown-up children who live in London. You no longer smoke, having quit 5 years ago. You enjoy drinking craft ales during the evenings of your days off. You love your job as a long-distance lorry driver and rely on the income. |
| ICE | You believe you are just a 'snorer' and wonder if you could get some nasal strips on the NHS. You are a little concerned that your concentration has been poor recently and it's not like you to fall asleep in meetings. You expect a lecture about losing weight and stopping drinking.

If the doctor mentions stopping driving become quite upset *'It's only snoring.'* Calm down if the doctor explains the condition and what happens next. |
| Examination | Neck circumference 44 cm. BMI 45. BP 143/87. ENT – NAD. Chest examination – NAD. Collar size 45 cm. Last weight 144 kg about a month ago. Height 177 cm. |

CompleteMRCGP
RCA/CSA revision course

Terminology	Obstructive Sleep Apnoea/Hypopnoea Syndrome (OSAHS) – irregular breathing at night with collapsing of the upper airway resulting in interrupted sleep and excessive daytime sleepiness, reduced concentration and alertness.[1]
	OSAH – as above but without the daytime sleepiness/poor concentration.
	Obstructive Sleep Apnoea Syndrome (OSAS) – term used interchangeably with OSAHS.
Prevalence	4% middle-aged men, 2% middle-aged women, 1–2% children (associated with obesity).

Risk factors

Smoking	Obesity	Neck circumference > 43 cm	Family history
Alcohol	Male sex	Hypothyroidism	Acromegaly
Craniofacial abnormalities		Sleeping supine	Deviated septum

Children: Obesity, adenotonsillar hypertrophy, congenital conditions, e.g. Down, Prader–Willi.

Complications	Hypertension, stroke, road traffic accidents.
	In children – behavioural problems, faltering growth in severe cases.
Symptoms	Excessive daytime sleepiness, poor concentration, behavioural changes, unrefreshed from sleep, snoring, pauses in breathing (noted by partner/parent), choking noises, nocturia.
Assessment	Check red flags for alternative diagnoses (e.g. head and neck cancers), unilateral epistaxis, severe nasal obstruction, hoarseness, dysphagia, rapid onset of symptoms without rapid weight gain.
	Epworth Sleepiness Questionnaire:[2] >10 abnormal. 11–14 mild, 15–18 moderate, >18 severe.
	Examine: throat, nasal obstruction, BMI, neck circumference (collar size), BP, chest – ?COPD/respiratory failure/cor pulmonale.
Management	Lifestyle advice: reduce alcohol, stop smoking, weight loss if BMI raised, sleep on side, advice to STOP DRIVING until have been assessed if sleepiness whilst driving. Group 2 licence (bus, lorry)/pilot – stop immediately.[3]
	Cardiovascular disease assessment bloods, HbA1c. Regular BP checks.
	Refer to sleep clinic:

- Urgent: sleepiness whilst driving or high-risk occupation, signs of respiratory or heart failure, symptoms suggest coexisting severe OSAS + COPD.
- Routine: Snoring + Epworth sleepiness questionnaire score >10.

Refer children to ENT if adenotonsillar hypertrophy + snoring + symptoms OSA.

Treatment from secondary care is usually CPAP or intraoral devices.

Doctor's Notes

Patient	Doris Ripley	76 years	F
PMH	COPD		
Medications	Anoro Ellipta OD		
	Salbutamol PRN		
Allergies	No information		
Consultations	Chronic cough, sputum, sometimes containing streaks of blood. Feeling more SOB. Diagnosis: IE-COPD. Management: Abx + steroids, will arrange CXR due to haemoptysis.		
Investigations	Coin lesion right upper lobe, suggestive of malignancy. Forwarded to lung MDT.		
Household	Peter Ripley	78 years	M

Open ☐	How can I help? That must be worrying, I'm sure together we can find the answers.
ICE ☐	What has been going through your mind? What is your biggest fear? There are clearly questions which need answering but were you hoping for anything else today?
Explanation ☐	Unfortunately the CXR has shown something unexpected. There is a shadow on your right lung. It is possible this is a patch of pneumonia but it could be something more serious. To better understand the CXR, it would be helpful to know a little more about you and the symptoms you have been having.
History ☐	Could tell me what led to the CXR being suggested? Can you tell me anything more about the cough? Have you had any chest pain? Any fever or sweats? Do you feel short of breath? Have you brought anything off your chest?
Flags ☐	Have you coughed up any blood? Have you noticed any weight loss?
Impact ☐	How has the cough been affecting you? Has it stopped you from doing anything?
Risk ☐	Do you smoke, or have you been a smoker in the past? Is there any family history of lung problems? What did you used to do for a living?
Experience ☐	Have you known anyone with similar chest problems? Or an abnormal CXR?
Curious ☐	That must have been a difficult time, how is Peter now? Has he come with you today?
O/E ☐	Would it be possible for me to have a listen to your chest and check your heart, oxygen levels and temperature?
SummarICE ☐	So you have had a cough for about 12 weeks. You initially thought it was your COPD playing up but when you coughed up blood you were more worried. You are also concerned that the usual antibiotics and steroids haven't done the trick this time. You've noticed yourself being more breathless and have experienced some weight loss. You've just had a CXR and been told by the hospital you need to see a specialist. You'd like to know what this all means and what the next steps are. Is there anything else?
Impression ☐	Unfortunately, you have some worrying symptoms which suggest the shadow on your lung could be lung cancer. (Pause about 10 seconds).
Empathy ☐	I'm sorry, this must be a shock, what's going through your mind?
Options ☐	Would you like to talk about what happens next? It's good news that you have an appointment with the lung specialist so soon. The sooner these things are investigated the better the chance of successful treatment. When you see the specialist, they will likely arrange a detailed scan of your body to get a better idea of the cause of the shadow. They may offer you a test to put a small flexible camera into your lung so a sample of any lump there can be taken. If it did turn out to be lung cancer, possible treatment options are surgery, radiotherapy or chemotherapy. What are your thoughts? I would like to arrange some blood tests to help the lung specialist decide which scans and possible treatments would be best. Is this okay?
Empower ☐	To help yourself, try to keep your strength up by eating regularly. There will be support groups and information you could access should it turn out to be bad news.
Future ☐	I would really like to see you again after your hospital appointment next week? Could I book you an appointment here?
Specifics ☐	Please make an appointment for blood tests at reception. I will see you again on Tuesday, after your appointment with the lung specialist. If you have any more questions or problems please give me a call.
Safety net ☐	If you're unable to make your appointment, start feeling more poorly, particularly with fever or breathlessness, please call us straightaway.

Doctor's notes	Doris Ripley, 76 years. PMH: IE-COPD. Medication: Anoro Ellipta OD, salbutamol PRN. Recent CXR results: coin lesion right upper lobe, suggestive of malignancy. Forwarded to lung MDT.
How to act	Upset. Push the doctor for the X-ray result. Be shocked if cancer is mentioned.
PC	*'I've had a phone call from the hospital saying I need to see a specialist next week. What is going on?'*
History	You visited the doctor 2 weeks ago with a cough which had been going on for 12 weeks. Initially you thought it was just your COPD, so you ignored it. However, when you started to notice blood in your spit you went to the doctor. The doctor was nice and said it was probably a chest infection, so you were given antibiotics and steroids, but wanted a CXR to be on 'the safe side'. You then received a phone call from the hospital stating your CXR was abnormal and you had been booked into a '2-week wait' appointment next week. You don't know what this means and are worried. You don't feel much better after the antibiotics and steroids. You are still short of breath and occasionally see blood when you cough. Some right-sided chest pain, sharp in nature. You have noticed a 2 stone weight loss over the last few months but put this down to lack of appetite. No fevers or night sweats. No foreign travel. The cough has been keeping you awake at night and the breathlessness has made your weekly shop more difficult. You are able to get yourself dressed without being too breathless but have to walk slower than you used to due to shortness of breath.
Social	You live with your husband. He is reasonably fit and well, although he has been unable to attend with you today as he is at home with a bad cold. You have two children but they are grown up and live 'down South'. You are an ex-smoker – you gave up 6 years ago, previously smoking 20 a day since you were 15. You don't drink alcohol. You are a retired seamstress.
ICE	You presume the CXR was looking for pneumonia so are worried why there is a fuss. You were given antibiotics anyway. *'Is it pneumonia? Should the antibiotics have cleared it?'* Your husband Peter had pneumonia a few years back and was quite poorly. You expect the doctor to explain the CXR results. You would like the doctor to explain why you have been referred to the hospital and what is likely to happen when you get there.
Examination	Temperature 36.6 °C. HR 84 bpm. RR 16. Sats 94%. Normal chest examination. BMI 18.

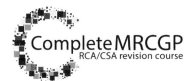

Causes of coin lesions[1, 2]:

- Malignancy: primary lung tumour or metastases.
- Infections: pneumonia, TB, abscess, hydatid cyst.
- Benign disease: granuloma (e.g. sarcoidosis), rheumatoid nodule, AV malformation.

Lung Cancer 2WW Criteria[1]

- Refer people using a suspected cancer pathway referral for lung cancer if they:
    - Have CXR findings that suggest lung cancer or
    - Are aged 40 and over with unexplained haemoptysis.
- Offer an urgent CXR (to be performed within 2 weeks)[3] to assess for lung cancer in people aged 40 and over if they have two or more of the following unexplained symptoms, or if they have ever smoked and have one or more of the following unexplained symptoms:
    - Cough
    - Fatigue
    - Shortness of breath
    - Chest pain
    - Weight loss
    - Appetite loss.
- Consider an urgent CXR (to be performed within 2 weeks)[3] to assess for lung cancer in people aged 40 and over with any of the following:
    - Persistent or recurrent chest infection.
    - Finger clubbing.
    - Supraclavicular lymphadenopathy or persistent cervical lymphadenopathy.
    - Chest signs consistent with lung cancer.
    - Thrombocytosis.

'Unexplained' is defined as symptoms or signs that have not led to a diagnosis being made by the healthcare professional in primary care after initial assessment (including history, examination and any primary care investigations).

	Normal	Obstruction	Restrictive
FEV1/FVC (FEV1%)	>0.7	<0.7	>0.7
FEV1	>80% predicted	<80%	<80%
FVC	>80% predicted	Normal/low	<80%

If overweight the spirometry may suggest they have a restrictive airway disease.

Must check relaxed VC as well as FVC. If VC > FVC then should calculate FEV1/VC.

Reliability: three consistent readings (within 5% or 150 mL).

Obstructive

Obstruction which is non-reversible confirms COPD. Severity of airway obstruction is classified below:

- Mild   FEV1 50–80%
- Mod   FEV1 30–49%
- Severe   <30%

Reversibility testing

Reversibility testing can be performed before and 20 minutes after 2–4 puffs salbutamol.

Or before and after a steroid trial (prednisolone 30 mg) for 14 days.

Always interpret the results of reversibility testing with the clinical history.

Restrictive

E.g. Fibrotic lung disease: extrinsic allergic alveolitis (farmer's lung), sarcoidosis, silicosis, pneumoconiosis and cryptogenic fibrosing alveolitis. Obesity, muscular weakness, curvature of spine.

	COPD	Asthma
Smoker or ex-smoker	Nearly all	Possibly
Symptoms under age 35 years	Rare	Often
Chronic productive cough	Common	Uncommon
Breathlessness	Persistent and progressive	Variable
Night time waking SOB/wheeze	Uncommon	Common
Variability	Uncommon	Common

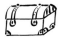

See the Link Hub at CompleteMRCGP.co.uk for useful links to
Flow volume and time volume curves
A guide to how to use and interpret spirometry in the GP practice
A flow chart – interpreting spirometry

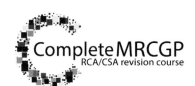

CHAPTER 20 OVERVIEW

Sexual Health

	Cases in this chapter	Within the RCGP 2020 curriculum: Sexual Health	Learning points in this chapter include:
1	Erectile Dysfunction	'Male sexual dysfunction, including erectile dysfunction due to organic causes (such as diabetes, drug induced (including smoking), neurological disease and vascular disease) and psychological causes'	ED investigations and management The Well Man check
2	Contraception – Combined	'Be aware of the key legal precedents, guidelines, and ethical issues that influence sexual healthcare provision especially regarding patients under 16 years of age in relation to consent and confidentiality' 'Female contraception including: hormonal contraception: combined oral/patch/ring contraception, progesterone-only methods including oral, depot injection, subdermal implant, intrauterine systems (IUS)' 'Consent and confidentiality in respect of under 16s accessing sexual health services (Fraser Guidelines)'	Fraser Guidelines Missed pill rules UKMEC guidelines Evra patch NuvaRing
3	Pelvic Inflammatory Disease	'Common and important conditions – pelvic inflammatory disease' 'Be able to take a concise sexual history that enables risk assessment for STI' 'Vaginal swabs: use of 'self-taken' samples (vulvo-vaginal and urine) for chlamydia and gonorrhoea; indications for clinician-taken swabs'	IMB PID
4	LARC and Sterilisation	Other important content – long-acting reversible contraception sterilisation	Implant Injection IUS/IUD
5	Gender Dysphoria	'Recognises that gender, gender identity, gender dysphoria and sexual orientation are all different facets of a person's health and that issues relating to these may present in childhood, adolescence or adulthood and have a wide influence on wellbeing' 'Feelings and behaviours related to gender dysphoria'	Terminology Helping patients with gender identity issues
Extra Notes	Emergency Contraception Stopping Contraception	'Female contraception including ... emergency contraception'	Emergency contraception Stopping contraception

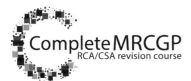

CompleteMRCGP
RCA/CSA revision course

CHAPTER 20 REFERENCES

Erectile Dysfunction

1. http://www.njurology.com/_forms/shim.pdf
2. http://patient.info/doctor/erectile-dysfunction. Apr 2016.
3. https://www.relate.org.uk/
4. NICE Guideline NG12. Suspected cancer: recognition and referral. Jan 2021.

Contraception – Combined

1. British Medical Association (BMA). Consent Toolkit. London, UK: BMA, 2019.
2. http://www.fsrh.org/pdfs/ceuGuidanceYoungPeople2010.pdf. May 2019.
3. https://www.fsrh.org/standards-and-guidance/documents/fsrh-ceu-guidance-recommended-actions-after-incorrect-use-of/. Mar 2020.
5. https://www.fsrh.org/standards-and-guidance/documents/ukmec-2016-summary-sheets/. Sep 2019.
6. https://www.fsrh.org/documents/combined-hormonal-contraception/. Nov 2020.
7. Killick S.R., Eyong E., Elstein M. Ovarian follicular development in oral contraceptive cycles. *Fertil Steril* 1987; 48: 409–13.
8. Schwarz J.L., Creinin M.D., Pymar H.C., Reid L. Predicting risk of ovulation in new start oral contraceptive users. *Obstet Gynecol* 2002; 99: 177–82.
9. Danforth D.R., Hodgen G.D. 'Sunday start' multiphasic oral contraception: ovulation prevention and delayed follicular atresia in primates. *Contraception* 1989; 39: 321–30.
10. https://www.fsrh.org/standards-and-guidance/fsrh-guidelines-and-statements/quick-starting-contraception/. Apr 2017.
11. http://patient.info/health/contraceptive-patch. Oct 2017.
12. http://patient.info/health/contraceptive-vaginal-ring. Apr 2018.

Pelvic Inflammatory Disease

1. http://patient.info/doctor/intermenstrual-and-postcoital-bleeding. Aug 2020.

LARC and Sterilisation

1. https://www.fsrh.org/standards-and-guidance/fsrh-guidelines-and-statements/method-specific/progestogen-only-implants/. Feb 2021.
2. http://www.fsrh.org/pdfs/CEUGuidanceProgestogenOnlyInjectables.pdf. Oct 2020.
3. https://www.fsrh.org/standards-and-guidance/documents/ukmec-2016-summary-sheets/. Sep 2019.

Gender Dysphoria

1. https://www.stonewall.org.uk/help-advice/glossary-terms
2. https://www.nhs.uk/conditions/body-dysmorphia/
3. https://gids.nhs.uk/
4. https://gids.nhs.uk/parents-and-carers#how-can-i-help-my-teenager

Emergency Contraception

1. http://www.fsrh.org/pdfs/CEUguidanceEmergencyContraception11.pdf. Dec 2020.
2. Piaggio G., Kapp N., von Hertzen H. Effect on pregnancy rates of the delay in administration of levonorgestrel for emergency contraception: a combined analysis of four WHO trials. *Contraception* 2011; 84: 35–9.
3. HRA Pharma UK Ltd. ellaOne: Summary of Product Characteristics (SPC). 2010.
4. http://www.medicines.org.uk/emc
5. Wilcox A.J., Dunson D., Baird D.D. The timing of the 'fertile window' in the menstrual cycle: day specific estimates from a prospective study. *Br Med J* 2000; 321(7271): 1259–62.

Stopping Contraception

1. https://www.fsrh.org/documents/fsrh-guidance-contraception-for-women-aged-over-40-years-2017/. Sep 2019.
2. http://www.fsrh.org/pdfs/MaleFemaleSterilisation.pdf

Information taken from NICE guidelines with kind permission. Please note the guidelines change frequently and you should ALWAYS check for the latest updated guidance. Remember that NICE guidance is only applicable to patients in the UK.

Doctor's Notes

Patient	Kevin Barton	57 years	M
PMH	Hypertension		
Medications	Indapamide 2.5 mg OD		
Allergies	No information		
Consultations	No recent consultations		
Investigations	No recent investigations		
Household	No household members registered		

Open ☐	Thank you for phoning. Tell me what made you ask for a Well Man check. What did you hope we might include?
Sense ☐	Are there changes in your body you have noticed or are worried about?
History ☐	I see you have high BP but a recent reading was fine. Are you otherwise well? Do you live alone? Work? Any stress in your life? How is your mood? Do you worry about your health?
Risk ☐	Do you smoke? How much alcohol do you drink? Any family history?
Flags ☐	Any pain in your chest, legs or breathing problems? Any problems going to the toilet? Do you go at night or have problem with the flow? Dribbling at the end or needing to go again? Do you check your testes for lumps? Any problems with erections? Do you have any erections? Is this a problem maintaining erections or do you struggle to have an erection in the first place? Are you worried about anything else; for example, when you ejaculate? Do you have any erections on your own or in the morning?
Impact ☐	How has the impotence affected you or your relationship?
Curious ☐	How is your relationship? What does your husband think? Have you had any other sexual partners? When was this? Tell me more about this person? Male or female?
ICE ☐	Has this been worrying you? What has been going through your mind? What is your biggest fear? Is there anything specific you were hoping I would do today?
Impact ☐	Has anything else in your life changed since? Your mood? How are you and David?
Curious ☐	You mentioned David encouraged you to attend – is he worried about you?
Flags ☐	Do you have any symptoms that may suggest an infection?
SummarICE ☐	To summarise, you are troubled with impotence and you worry you may have an infection. You are feeling low in mood and fear this may affect your marriage.
Empathy ☐	Impotence can often be frustrating and can increase the stress in your life.
O/E ☐	It would be helpful to examine you with a chaperone present to ensure the skin of the penis is healthy, then check your BP and weight. Could you come to the surgery for this?
Experience ☐	Have you read or heard about anything that may cause impotence?
Explanation ☐	Stress or low mood or conditions that affect the vessels can cause impotence. For an erection, blood needs to flow into the vessels in the penis.
Impression ☐	Either your BP or indapamide may contribute to impotence. It's reassuring that you are sometimes able to have erections, so I think it is most likely due to your recent worries. What are your thoughts? Infections don't usually cause impotence but worry certainly can.
InCludE ☐	Given your worries, we could check for infections by getting you to come to the surgery for an appointment, doing swabs and testing your urine?
Options ☐	Or – visit the GUM clinic which will provide a thorough assessment for infections quickly. There is a walk-in clinic this afternoon. Shall I give you the details of where to go? We could try stopping indapamide to see if this helps. You could also talk to a relationship counsellor or try sildenafil (Viagra), which increases the blood flow to the penis. What would suit you best? I can give you information on Relate, relationship counsellors.
Empower ☐	Have a think if there are lifestyle changes you could make that may help your vessels. You've stopped playing squash but exercise is important. We can check your cholesterol and blood sugar, both affect vessels. You have no prostate symptoms, but we offer a blood test for prostate cancer to anyone attending with impotence. I can email you a PIL to read about the test and its limitations. I appreciate that discussing your prostate may be unexpected, but can be part of a Well Man check. We examine the prostate through the back passage, as well as arranging a blood test. Shall I go into detail about this now? Okay, let's discuss when you come to surgery.
Recommend ☐	I recommend waiting to have sex until your sexual health screen is clear and, if you do need treatment, both you and David should complete this before you have sex. Here is a prescription for 50 mg sildenafil. Take one an hour before you plan to have sex. It works for hours, so no rush. It will only cause an erection when you become aroused. Unfortunately, some men may get a headache.
Specifics ☐	Please book in to speak to me in a month to discuss your results and catch up?
Safety net ☐	If your mood deteriorates or anything else worries you, please phone me sooner.

Doctor's notes	Kevin Barton, 57 years. PMH: HTN. Medications: indapamide 2.5 mg OD. BP 2 weeks ago 134/78.
How to act	Embarrassed. You do not give much away unless pushed.
	You do not mention you have a problem with ED until the doctor asks directly.
	Then call it impotence.
PC	*'I would like to know if I can have a Well Man check please.'*
History	Your friends have had a Well Man check.
	You are unsure what this is exactly.
	You have no symptoms of bladder outflow obstruction.
	You have had problems with impotence.
	You have morning erections and find masturbation easier.
	You are well and healthy. You exercise. You do not smoke.
	You drink 1 pint of lager a night.
	You have no other medical history and no family history.
Social	You married your male partner, David, 3 years ago.
	David has encouraged you to go to the GP.
	You had an affair a year ago with a male friend from the squash club and for which you feel guilty. You do not disclose this until the doctor explores your sexual history.
	This has put stress on your marriage.
	You no longer see this friend or play squash.
ICE	You fear you have an STI and that one day your husband will discover this.
	You fear your relationship with your husband ending if he ever found out.
	You fear you have let him down and are struggling to forget what you did.
	You would like blood tests for a general check-up but don't insist on a prostate test and you would prefer time to think about prostate tests if this is mentioned.
	You would like to try Viagra.
Examination	Genitalia NAD. BP 134/78. BMI 24.

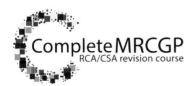

CompleteMRCGP
RCA/CSA revision course

Causes of ED

Vascular disease	Risk factors include: HTN, smoking, hypercholesterolaemia and DM.
Structural	Surgery within the pelvis. Peyronie's disease.
Skin disorders	Foreskin problems such as lichen sclerosus (balanitis xerotica obliterans).
Neurological	Tumour, spinal cord disease, MS, Parkinson's, stroke, peripheral neuropathy (DM).
Hormonal	Hypogonadism, Cushing's, thyroid, hyperprolactinaemia.
Drug induced	Diuretics, SSRIs, GnRH analogues and antagonists, antipsychotics.
Alcohol and recreational drugs	
Psychological causes	Stress, depression, anxiety, relationship difficulties, performance anxiety.
SHIM	Sexual health inventory for men[1] score may be useful.
	Tailor investigations to the likely cause depending on symptoms, age and risk factors.
	The patient may have their own terminology in a sexual health history. Use words they have chosen.
	Make no assumptions. Ask about other sexual partners and confirm their partner's gender.

Management options

Sildenafil	Generic available on NHS prescription now. CI include: already on a nitrate, unstable angina, recent MI or stroke, optic neuropathy.
	Side effects: headaches, flushing, N&V, dizziness and visual disturbances.
	Interactions: no alpha-blocker within 4 hours.
Other options	2nd line tadalafil (Cialis) with a longer duration of effect.
	Vacuum pumps. MUSE (alfraprostadil per urethra) and Caverject.[2]
	Relationship counselling[3] or a referral to psychosexual medicine may be helpful.
	Show you have recognised the opportunity for health screening and promotion.
The Well Man check	CVD RFs, prostate and testicular screening, weight and bowel changes, stress/mood.
PSA screening	Offer all men with ED PSA screening.[4]

Doctor's Notes

Patient	Gemma Briggs	15 years	F
PMH	No information		
Medications	No current medications		
Allergies	No information		
Consultations	No recent consultations		
Investigations	No recent investigations		
Household	Davina Briggs	48 years	F
	Simon Briggs	47 years	M

Open ☐	What's led to this decision? How did you meet your partner?
Flags ☐	I can help today but I need to ask a few personal questions to make sure we make the right choice for you and, as you are under 16, I have to make sure you are not at risk. Is anyone forcing you to have sex? How old is your boyfriend? As you tell me you are in no danger then what you say to me is confidential. Have you had sex already? Is there any possibility you might be pregnant now? Would you have sex if you were not on the contraceptive pill? What is your relationship like with your parents? Could you tell them? What might they say? Is there anyone else you could talk to, an older sister or auntie perhaps?
ICE ☐	Do you have any worries about starting the pill? Was there anything else you were hoping for?
History ☐	When was your last period? Do you have a regular cycle? Before we proceed, I would just like to check you have no other medical problems that would prevent you from taking the pill. Do you have any health problems? Take any medicines? Do you smoke? Can you tell me how tall you are and how much you weigh? Thank you.
Risk ☐	Have you or anyone in your family ever had a blood clot? Do you suffer with migraines? Have you ever had a headache which caused a problem with your vision or arms or legs? Has anyone in the family had breast cancer?
SummarICE ☐	So to summarise, you are in a new relationship and you'd like to start the pill. You don't have any worries about this but would like some more information.
Experience ☐	What do you know about the pill?
Explanation ☐	The OCP is taken for 21 days then you have a 7-day break when you will have your period. Side effects can include breast tenderness or mood changes. There are risks to consider when taking the pill. Rarely, women can have a stroke or a blood clot due to the pill. The COCP also slightly increases your risk of breast and cervical cancer; however, it is protective against ovarian and womb cancer. No contraception is 100% protective against pregnancy and the pill does not protect you against STIs. Can I please check I have been clear; what are the risks of the pill? That's correct.
InCludE ☐	You've indicated you would like to start the pill and that is certainly an option.
Options ☐	There are more reliable options such as a hormone implant which is like a matchstick under the skin, an injection or a coil in the womb. Are you interested in any of these? Okay.
Recommend ☐	I suggest starting the pill on the first day of your next period. Do you feel you can wait until then? If you miss one pill then that is okay, just take it when you remember, even if that means taking two in a day. However, if you miss two or more pills within the month then you will need to use condoms for 7 days. If this happens in the first week of the pill packet and you've had sex during your pill-free week, you may need EC. If this occurs in the third week of the packet, miss the break and start the next packet straightaway. Remember to use condoms for 7 days.
Empathy ☐	I know this is a lot to take in. If you're ever unsure what to do, please phone us for advice. There is a leaflet in the pill packet which can also help and you should read it now and keep it safe. Can I check I have been clear? Can you explain to me how to take the pill?
Empower ☐	I will email you a PIL so you have further information regarding what to do if you are unwell. For example, if you have vomiting or diarrhoea. Remember, only condoms protect you from STIs. You should always encourage your partner to have an STI check. Do protect yourself as STIs can cause long-term pain or infertility.
Future ☐	I will send a prescription to the chemist for you to collect; the pill is called Microgynon. There is nothing to pay: even when you become 16, the pill is free if you tick the 'free of charge contraceptive' box on the back of the prescription. You will need a pill check just before your first box runs out in 3 months. Please book in with our practice nurse or a GP. Please call if you have any questions in the meantime.
Safety net ☐	If you ever have a painful swollen leg or a severe headache, see a doctor immediately as these may be signs of the rare risks of the pill.

Patient's Story

Contraception – Combined

Doctor's notes	Gemma Briggs, 15 years. PMH: none. Medications: none. BP 1 week ago (self-check at the surgery) 90/50.
How to act	Mature and intelligent.
PC	*'I would like to go on the pill.'*
History	You have a new boyfriend. You met at school in your class.
	No one is forcing you. You have not had sex yet.
	You would also use condoms.
	You would still have sex even if you were not prescribed contraception.
	You get on well with your parents but will not tell them. It would just be too awkward.
	However, you will tell your older sister, who is 22 years. You know that your sister had to have her BP checked before she started the pill, so you have gone into the self-check area at the surgery to do this already.
	No PMH or other medication.
	Height 170 cm. Weight 55 kg. BMI 19.
	You have read a little about the pill on the internet but would like the doctor to explain again. A friend of yours has a contraceptive implant but you don't like how it feels under the skin. You aren't keen on regular injections and wouldn't like anything inserted into your womb.
	You started your periods when you were 12 – they are usually regular 7/30.
	Your LMP was 3 weeks ago, you expect to start again in about 5 days' time.
	You do not plan to have sex prior to your period and are happy to wait.
Social	In year 10 at school. Living with parents. Your older sister lives with her partner. Never smoked.
ICE	You have no concerns.

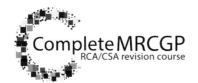
CompleteMRCGP
RCA/CSA revision course

To meet Fraser guidelines the patient:

- Will not tell her parent/carer despite encouragement from the doctor.
- Understands the advice.
- Is likely to have sex if the contraception is not prescribed.
- Her mental or physical health may be at risk if not prescribed.
- It is in her *best interests.*[1,2]
- In practice you should document all this clearly in the notes.

'Is this confidential?' A suggested answer begins with 'yes' – *'Yes … so long as you are not in danger.'*

Understanding the OCP missed pill (>24 hours) rules

'No indication for EC if the pills in the preceding 7 days have been taken consistently and correctly (assuming the pills thereafter are taken correctly and additional contraceptive precautions are used).'[3] Therefore the week prior to and following the pill-free week is the most risky time as 7 days could be extended. Although the standard advice suggests one pill can be missed anywhere in the pack, if the woman were to take her next pill late (but not missed), the risk of ovulation and therefore pregnancy is increased. The woman may choose to have a 4-day pill-break to minimise this risk.

The advice for backup contraception for 7 days following two missed pills 'may be overcautious in the second and third weeks, but the advice is a backup in the event that further pills are missed.'[3]

UKMEC guidelines[4]	Contraception cautions and contraindications.
	'Each UK category should be considered separately (it is NOT appropriate to consider categories 1 and 2 safe and 3 and 4 unsafe).'[5]
Tailored regimes	The woman does not have to have a period every month! She may prefer to tricycle 3 packets (without pill-free days) or back-to-back packets until breakthrough bleeding occurs then have 4–7 pill-free days. Some can take continuously whether they bleed or not. These regimes reduce risk of pregnancy so are supported by FSRH but may be off licence.[6]
Commencing the OCP	'COCs containing ethinylestradiol can be started up to and including Day 5 of the cycle without the need for additional contraceptive protection.'[6–9]
Risk of OCP to a fetus	Studies are limited but with no consistent data to support serious abnormalities. Read more at 'Effects of fetal exposure to steroid hormones'[10] within the reference.
Benefits	Decreased risk ovarian/endometrial/colorectal cancer.[9]
	May reduce menopausal symptoms.[9]
Thrombosis risks	>3 hour flight – 'should be advised about reducing periods of immobility'.[9]
	>7 days at >4500 m altitude – 'consider switching to an alternative method'.[9]
Increased risks	Breast and cervical cancer, thrombosis and stroke[9] – read more within the reference.
Evra patch	Weekly for 3 weeks then a patch-free week. If falls off >48 hours – apply a new patch, condoms for 7 days and ECP if sex within the previous 5 days.[11]
NuvaRing	Insert for 3 weeks then remove for 1 week.
	If it falls out, no need for condoms or ECP if replaced within 3 hours.[12]

Doctor's Notes

Patient	Stephanie Smith	24 years	F
PMH	No information		
Medications	Cilest		
Allergies	No information		
Consultations	No recent consultations		
Investigations	No recent investigations		
Household	No household members registered		

Open ☐	Tell me more about this spotting? Anything else that is new? How are your periods?
ICE ☐	What has gone through your mind as to what may be causing this bleeding? Is there anything specific that you worry is causing it? Any other thoughts? What did you think I may suggest today?
History ☐	Do you have any medical problems? Allergies? Do you remember to take your pill? Tell me more about you. Are you in a relationship? Is that long-term?
Impact ☐	How has the bleeding impacted on day-to-day life or the relationship?
Sense ☐	I can see that you are keen to get to the bottom of this and I hear how bothersome this is for you.
Risk ☐	I'm wondering about clues in your sexual history – have you ever had an STI? Could you be at risk? When did you first have sex? Have you had a check-up since restarting your relationship? Has any family member had any women's health problems? When was your LMP? Was the period due? Was it a normal period?
Flags ☐	Have you had any: fevers? Bleeding after sex? Pain during sex? Discharge? Smell? Burning passing urine? Or going more frequently? How are your bowels? How do you feel in yourself? Any stomach pain?
Curious ☐	Have you spoken to your partner about relationships you have had during your time apart?
SummarICE ☐	To summarise, spotting for 2 months is starting to impact on everyday life. You have had lower stomach pain including during intercourse. You are not sure what has caused this or what to expect today.
O/E ☐	May I examine you? I'd like to take your temperature and pulse, feel your tummy and feel the womb through the vagina, as pain may suggest an infection. May I look at the neck of the womb with a speculum, a plastic tube, which fits into the vagina? It can be uncomfortable but will allow me to check the cervix and take swabs for infection including general bacteria, thrush, chlamydia and gonorrhoea. Does this sound okay? Would you like a chaperone? May I have a urine sample for a pregnancy and infection test?
Impression ☐	I believe you may have an infection, possibly chlamydia, causing pelvic inflammatory disease.
Experience ☐	Have you come across either of these?
Recommend ☐	Before the chlamydia result returns, I would prefer to treat for what I suspect is inflammation from an infection.
Explanation ☐	If not treated, you could become unwell or have problems with fertility in the future. Two antibiotics, metronidazole and ofloxacin, are taken twice a day for 14 days. You can use paracetamol/ibuprofen for pain relief. You cannot drink alcohol during this treatment as you will be unwell due to the metronidazole antibiotic.
Empathy ☐	Do you think you will be able to tell your boyfriend? What might he say?
Empower ☐	Does this plan sound okay so far? You should both complete the sexual health screen at the GUM clinic. Please do not have sex again until you have both been assessed and completed any necessary treatment. Your smear test, which screens for cancer of the cervix, is due next year. Any questions? The risk of chlamydia is infertility so it is important to protect yourself.
Specifics ☐	Please arrange to speak to the doctor again next week about your test results.
Future ☐	If the bleeding persists then we will review your pill.
Safety net ☐	If your period is late, please repeat the pregnancy test. If you start to feel unwell, the stomach pain feels worse, you have a fever or if the symptoms and bleeding have not started to improve within 48 hours, please see the doctor straight away as infections can be serious if you don't respond to the antibiotics. I can explain any of that again if you like? So, when would you seek help from a doctor? Yes, you've got it.

Doctor's notes	Stephanie Smith, 24 years. PMH: none. Medication: Cilest.
How to act	Very pleasant.
PC	*'It's my periods. I don't bleed just during my period but other times too.'*
History	2 months of bleeding – spotting randomly throughout the month.
	Occasional PCB.
	You are very well in yourself and have no prescribed medications.
	LMP almost 4 weeks ago.
	Your LMP was a 5-day period surrounded by the spotting.
	Periods have always been regular. You are a good pill taker. No FH.
	No medicines apart from the OCP which you commenced 18/12 ago.
	You have had deep pain on intercourse but you didn't make the connection.
	You have had some lower abdominal pain and thought this may be your bowels.
	You occasionally need a Fybogel for mild constipation.
	You have no urinary symptoms.
	No PV discharge. You have never had an STI check.
	You have never had an STI or a smear test. You have never been pregnant.
	You split up from your boyfriend 8 months ago.
	The relationship restarted 3 months ago.
	During the break you both had one other sexual contact using condoms.
	Since the age of 18 years, you have had two other sexual relationships in total.
	The bleeding has been too light to comfortably use tampons and you don't like the smell of wearing liners. You have also had to avoid intercourse.
	You will tell your partner what the GP says today.
	You realise you should have both been to GUM.
Social	You did a Master of Business Administration and now you are an investment banker.
	You are enjoying your job and thrive on the pressure of the work. You are happy in your relationship. All is going well.
ICE	You have no idea why you are bleeding. It is just very irritating. You are not concerned about anything particular, only that it may continue. You have no idea what the GP will suggest.
O/E	Abdomen. LIF pain. No palpable mass. No guarding or rebound tenderness.
	PV – left adnexal tenderness and cervical excitation. No masses.
	Speculum – normal-looking cervix.
	HR 70 bpm. Apyrexial. BP 120/60. Urine dipstick negative.
	Pregnancy test negative.

Learning Points Intermenstrual Bleeding

Causes	Physiological	2% spot around ovulation.[1]
	Pregnancy	Miscarriage or ectopic.
	Smear/trauma	
	Infection or vaginitis	
	Structural/histological	Cancer, polyps or ectropion.
	Any contraception	Especially low oestrogen hormones.
	↓Contraception efficacy	Secondary to interactions, e.g. tamoxifen, steroids, SSRIs, warfarin, St John's wort.[1]
History	Menstrual history	Onset, LMP, IMB, PCB and cycle pattern.
	Gynaecological history	Smears, contraception, operations and FH.
	Obstetric history	Gravida and parity.
	Sexual history	Age became sexually active, partners and infections.
	General health	Feeling unwell or fevers, urinary/bowel symptoms.
Risk factors	Endometrial cancer	Obesity, PCOS, nulliparity and late first child.
	Cervical cancer/STI	Early sexual activity and multiple partners.
Examination	Abdomen	Tenderness and masses.
	Pelvic examination	Masses, adnexal tenderness and cervical excitation.
	Inspection and speculum	Vulva, vagina and cervix (ectropion/polyps/ulceration).
	Swab for infection	i.e. chlamydia, gonorrhoea, TV, BV, candida.
	Observations	If possibility of infection/sepsis.

Investigations Pregnancy test (ask the patient to do this at home).

If negative it needs to be repeated 3 weeks after last UPSI.

Urine dipstick. Swabs. FBC/TFT.

Consider TVUSS to assess the endometrium and, if abnormal/ongoing concern (especially if >40 years), a hysteroscopy for biopsies.[1]

Be sure the woman does not meet the criteria for a 2WW gynaecology cancer referral.

Gynaecology rule

The same rule applies to both abnormal PV bleeding or pelvic pain.

Consider/rule out pregnancy, infection and structural/histological causes.

Structural/histological causes include polyps, fibroids, cancer or ovarian cysts.

Remember no contraception is 100% so do not be reassured if they are taking a contraception.

If the cause of abnormal bleeding (especially in a young woman) is most likely secondary to her hormone Rx, you may decide to change Rx as a trial first before investigating (but do exclude pregnancy and chlamydia).

The IMB may be due to the strength of the OCP, especially if menses occurs early but remains regular.

Consider changing the progesterone or increasing the dose of the ethinylestradiol to 30–35 μg and the next step may be a triphasic OCP. Remember the ↑risk of the OCP with increasing strengths of ethinylestradiol.

PID	Symptoms may include: dyspareunia, discharge, abnormal bleeding, pain and fevers.
	Signs: adnexal tenderness ± cervical excitation ± fever or tachycardia or low BP.
	Treat immediately as per local guidance before waiting for swab results.
	Refer if systemically unwell or no improvement in 48 hours or pregnant.

Sexual Health – 3

Doctor's Notes

Patient	Fedora Baros	38 years	F
PMH	No information		
Medications	Ovranette		
Allergies	No information		
Consultations	No recent consultations		
Investigations	No recent investigations		
Household	Domenic Baros	42 years	M

Fedora telephones with her husband Domenic present. He is also registered at the practice and has no known medical history.

Open ☐	Please tell me about what has led to this decision.
ICE ☐	What are your thoughts so far?
History ☐	I'm interested to know more about you both. Fedora, do you have any medical history? Have you ever been pregnant? Do you have regular periods? Do you take any tablets?
Flags ☐	Would you mind, Domenic, if I spoke to Fedora alone for a couple of minutes? Would you be able to leave the room and close the door? Fedora, because you are my patient today, I just wanted to make sure that you have not been encouraged by anyone to make a decision you are not comfortable with.
Risk ☐	Before thinking about the coil, have you had any abnormal bleeding in between periods or after sex, or heavier bleeding or discharge? Any pain on intercourse or infections in the past 3 months? Are your periods manageable or painful?
ICE ☐	What is the right thing for you? Did you have any concerns at all? Or worries about either procedure? How would you feel if you did fall pregnant? It sounds as if this would be stressful for you. What did you expect us to decide today? Is there anything else you were wondering? Or would like to discuss today?
Impact ☐	How is your relationship? We should consider your risk of regret if your husband had a permanent procedure. You should be at peace with a vasectomy being irreversible.
Sense ☐	You were not expecting me to say that? Does this change things? Is your mood okay?
Curious ☐	How would Domenic feel if you fell pregnant? Is there anything you want to ask whilst we are alone? Would you like to finish this consultation with the two of us or invite your husband back in? Are you happy for me to share your concerns with Domenic?
SummarICE ☐	Hello Domenic. To summarise, you have both made the decision to not have children together. Fedora, you feel that this would put you under financial pressure. You are currently looking for work. You are fed up with taking the pill. Therefore, you are both happy with the plan for a vasectomy. However, Fedora you were not aware that this should be seen as irreversible. We started to discuss the risk of regret; for example, if you did find work life became less stressful and you decided you wanted children. The other option you have considered is the coil, but you do not want erratic bleeding and you feel comforted by regular periods.
Impression ☐	You would like a reliable form of contraception which you can forget about and is free from hormones, but is reversible should things change. You wondered about the coil.
Options ☐	Other options include using condoms or a diaphragm if you wish to avoid all hormones, continuing with the pill or hormones in the form of an injection or skin implant.
Experience ☐	What do you understand about how the coil works? And the risks?
Explanation ☐	There are two types of coil – the copper coil which has no hormones and usually gives regular periods but you may have heavier and longer periods. Or the hormone coil which is the one which can give erratic bleeding or no bleeding at all. As you have manageable periods you may find you tolerate heavier periods with a copper coil. No contraception is 100% but the coil is a very good form of contraception. If you did fall pregnant, however, there is an increased risk of ectopic pregnancy, a pregnancy not in the womb, which is dangerous. There is the risk of pushing an infection through to the womb and if this occurred you may become very unwell, but we minimise this risk by recommending swabs to check for infection a week before we fit the coil, and it is a sterile procedure, which means we use equipment which is very clean. There is a 1 in 20 chance the coil may fall out, especially in the first few months. When we put it in, your blood pressure may drop or you may be in pain. Usually, the pain is like a period cramp which settles. There is a 1–2/1000 chance of the coil going through the womb.
Empower ☐	Have you made a decision or may I provide you with information to explain further? I can email this to you.
Empathy ☐	It is a lot of information and a big decision. Domenic, what are your thoughts?
Specifics ☐	Would you like to call me when you have made a decision or if you have further questions? I will also email you some information on vasectomies.

Doctor's notes	Fedora Baros, 38 years. PMH: none. Medications: Ovranette.
	Husband Domenic Baros, 42 years, is also present in the call.
How to act	Very pleasant.
PC	*'We would like to discuss whether the coil or vasectomy is the best option.'*
History	You have decided not to have children.
	This is a decision you have made together.
	You have been married for 2 years.
	Domenic has three children from a previous marriage.
	Fedora has not been married before and has no children.
	You are both very well and have no medical history. You take no medicines.

Social	**Fedora**	You are currently unemployed. Money is tight and you are looking for work.
		You used to work as a cleaner. You have decided you are not able to afford having a child. You believe you are happy with this decision.
	Domenic	You are a security guard. You see your three children twice a month. You would be very happy to have children if this is what Fedora wanted. However, she has decided that with life's stressors you should not have more children.
		Neither of you smokes or drinks.

ICE	**Fedora**	You would prefer Domenic to have a vasectomy.
		You are fed up with taking the OCP. You don't want any hormones in your body. You have concerns about the coil as you have heard that it is painful.
		You expect the doctor will arrange a vasectomy for Domenic today.
		You believe that if you did change your mind the vasectomy can be reversed by putting the tubes back together. If asked about your risk of regret, you become unsure.
		Your main concern about the coil is erratic bleeding. You like monthly and regular periods.
		If the doctor explains how the coil is inserted and discusses the risks, you decide you feel comfortable to have this procedure.
	Domenic	You are happy to have a vasectomy if this is what Fedora wants.
		You decided to call the doctor together, however, to discuss all options.
		You expect the doctor will arrange a vasectomy for you today.

Contraceptive implant[1]

Implant indication	LARC or dysmenorrhoea.
How to take	Insert days 1–5 of cycle. Repeat within 3 years.
Side effects	Acne, bleeding changes, mood or libido changes and headaches reported although 'no evidence of a causal association'.[1] No osteoporosis risk.
Bleeding risk	<1/4 regular periods, 1/3 infrequent bleeding, 1/5 no bleeding, and 1/4 frequent/prolonged bleeding.[1]
Lost implant	If impalpable implant, use additional contraception and arrange an USS.
Problematic bleeding	Exclude pregnancy, chlamydia and malignancy (view cervix).
	Consider an additional hormone off licence (COCP or POP) for 3 months.[1]
	Use judgement: risk unknown with longer use and see guidance.

Injection[2]

Side effects	The same as other progesterone contraceptives and 'associated with weight gain'.[2]
Fertility	Can be delayed for up to 1 year after discontinuation.[2]
BMD	Small loss of BMD usually recovers after discontinuation. Review 2-yearly.[2]
Caution/CI	Maximum recommended age of 50 years. Caution in CVD.[2]

IUS (Mirena)/IUD (Copper)[2]

Indication	IUS = LARC, progesterone cover for HRT and menorrhagia.
	IUD = LARC and EC.
Mode of action	IUS prevents implantation. IUD prevents fertilisation and implantation.
Risks	Infection, perforation, failure rate, ectopic, expulsion and cervical shock.
Contraindications	Must be 'reasonably certain'[2] she is not pregnant.
	See also UKMEC guidance.[3]
Side effects	IUS: erratic bleeding. Small risk of systemic progesterone side effects.
	IUD may give longer/heavier periods.
	Tampons can be used.
Licensing of duration	Mirena = 5 years.
	= 4 years if the indication is endometrial protection for HRT.
	Jaydess = 3 years.
	Copper = depends on the device – 5 or 10 years so check the device.

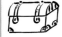 See the Link Hub at completeMRCGP.co.uk for a link to UKMEC guidance which should be followed when commencing contraception.

Doctor's Notes

Patient	Florence Wriggley	13 years	F
PMH	Nil		
Medications	Nil		
Allergies	NKDA		
Consultations	Nil		
Investigations	Nil		
Household	Michael Wriggley	40 years	M
	Veronica Wriggley	39 years	F

Veronica is phoning about Florence.

Open ☐	I'm sorry you have been worried, what changes have you noticed?
ICE ☐	What thoughts have you had about what may be going on? What worries you most? Had you had any thoughts about how I could help?
Impact ☐	This sounds like a challenging time. Has this been affecting the family?
History ☐	Did there seem to be any trigger to her change in behaviour? How are things at home generally? How has she been at school? Have you spoken to Flo about your worries? Have you noticed changes in her mood?
Risk ☐	Are you aware of any bullying at school or over the internet? Has she struggled with her mood in the past? Has she mentioned feeling very low?
Flags ☐	Any concerns about self-harm? Has she expressed any suicidal thoughts?
Empathy ☐	This must be a confusing and worrying time for you and Flo. Nobody wants to see their child unhappy.
Sense ☐	Emotionally how do you feel?
Experience ☐	Have you come across gender identity issues before?
SummarICE ☐	So since beginning her periods about a year ago, Flo's behaviour has changed, for example wearing baggy clothes and getting rid of anything girly. She seems to be self-conscious about her body and she told you that she feels that she should have been born a boy. You wonder if she is gay or possibly transgender. You were hoping I could provide some information about this and how to support her.
Impression ☐	It sounds as if Flo may be struggling with her gender identity, or this could be a sign of a mental health problem, or possibly a mixture of both.
InCludE ☐	Being 'gay' is a term which means you are romantically or sexually interested in people of the same sex. Transgender is different, this means that the person feels like they are a different gender to the one they were given at birth. As if the body is one gender but the mind is another. Gender is now thought of as a spectrum, with male and female at opposite ends but everything in between does exist.
Explanation ☐	It is completely normal for children and adolescents to explore gender and thoughts can change with time. However, if thoughts are persistent into adolescence, then help may be needed to explore the person's gender identity more formally.
Options ☐	Initially it would be really helpful if I could meet Flo so we can chat about her feelings and I can see if there are any signs of significant anxiety or depression. It may be that she needs help from our counselling team or even our children's mental health team. If needed, we could refer her to the gender identity team.
Empower ☐	In the meantime you can support her by reminding her she is normal, that you love her and that it is fine for her to take her time in discovering who she is. It may be helpful to speak to school so they can be sure to support her too.
Future ☐	Would it be possible for us to meet up in person with Flo in the next couple of weeks?
Specifics ☐	Please arrange an appointment with me at reception.
Safety net ☐	Great, we will meet soon but if you notice any evidence of self-harm, have concerns about suicidal thoughts or any other worries, please get in touch with us straight away. The Gender Identity Development Service website has lots of information you and Flo may find helpful.

Doctor's notes	Florence Wriggley, 13 years.
	You are her mother – Veronica Wriggley.
How to act	Concerned
PC	*'I'm worried about Flo; she's been acting oddly recently and seems unhappy.'*
History	Florence was always a happy child but over the last year or so she seems unhappy. Initially you thought that it was just the challenges of growing up but now you're not so sure. She has always been a 'tomboy' but last week you caught her wrapping a bandage around her chest. When you asked her what she was doing she looked embarrassed but then told you she 'should have been a boy'. Looking back, you feel that her mood changed around the time her periods started last year. Flo seems anxious a lot of the time and worries over small things. She has started refusing to do PE at school and says it's because she doesn't want to get changed in front of the other girls. She's cleared out her wardrobe and replaced anything even slightly girly with baggy T-shirts and jeans. She's started wearing trousers to school. Flo has been spending more and more time in her room. She has become distant from her friends and keeps saying that she no longer fits in. You are worried and don't know what to do.
Social	Florence is attending school and still plays football but seems less enthusiastic about going now. You are not aware of any bullying at school. Her teachers have noticed a drop in the quality of her schoolwork. She is bright – but not attaining at present. You work as a nail technician and Florence's dad is a builder. You are open minded about gender/sexual identity issues but come from a traditional family and you worry what Flo's grandparents will say.
ICE	You think Florence may be gay or possibly transgender but you aren't really sure what the difference is and if such issues can affect a child so young. You are worried that she is having a difficult time and will become depressed. You want information from the GP and advice about support and how to talk to Flo. You would like the GP to explain the difference between being gay and transgender.

CompleteMRCGP
RCA/CSA revision course

Terminology[1]

Trans – An umbrella term to describe people whose gender is not the same as, or does not sit comfortably with, the sex they were assigned at birth.

Trans people may describe themselves using one or more of a wide variety of terms, including (but not limited to) transgender, transsexual, gender-queer (GQ), gender-fluid, non-binary, gender-variant, crossdresser, genderless, agender, non-gender, third gender, bi-gender, trans man, trans woman, trans masculine, trans feminine and neutrois.

Transgender man – a person who was assigned female at birth but now lives and identifies as a man.

Transgender woman – a person who was assigned male at birth but now lives and identifies as a woman.

Non-binary – an umbrella term for people whose gender identity does not sit comfortably with 'man' or 'woman'.

Gender dysphoria – when a person experiences discomfort or distress because there is a mismatch between their gender assigned at birth and their gender identity.

Pansexual – a person whose romantic and/or sexual attraction towards others is not limited by sex or gender.

Body dysmorphia – body dysmorphic disorder (BDD), or body dysmorphia, is a mental health condition where a person spends a lot of time worrying about flaws in their appearance. These flaws are often unnoticeable to others.[2]

Helping patients with gender identity issues

Gender is now believed to be a spectrum with male on one end and female on the other. It is normal for children to explore gender and may demonstrate preferences across the spectrum. Not all these preferences will remain with the child through adolescence. However, some will continue to identify with a different gender to which they were assigned at birth. In children and adults experiencing this, it is common for mental health problems to coexist, e.g. anxiety or depression. Helping patients will need to incorporate both gender identity needs and mental health needs. Specialist gender clinics exist (Gender Identity Development Service)[3] where patients can be assessed by a specialist, and where appropriate, can be guided through gender reassignment treatments. Hormone blockers (GnRH analogues) can be used in adolescents followed by hormone treatments (testosterone or oestrogen). Ultimately, surgery can be performed to change a person's sexual characteristics. This usually takes place after 'social gender role transition' where a person is living as their chosen gender (e.g. changed name, etc.) and they have taken hormone treatments.

Ways parents can help[4]

- Remind young people that they are normal. It is normal to explore gender.
- Consider how gender identity is expressed in their family – does the child fit in? If not, they may need extra support to feel accepted. Try to avoid overtly masculine or feminine roles.
- Encourage the young person to talk about their feelings.
- Accept uncertainty about what the future holds. Encourage exploration and keep options open.
- Consider where sources of anxiety are coming from.

Levonorgestrel (LNG) 1.5 mg, e.g. Levonelle

Prevents/delays ovulation. Licence = up to 72 hours.

Efficacy demonstrated up to 96 hours[1,2] and if other EC is not an option consider prescribing up to 120 hours (off-licence use).[3]

If vomiting occurs within 2 hours of ingestion then repeat the LNG dose.[4]

Double the dose or offer a Cu-IUD if liver enzyme inducing drugs have been taken with 28/7.[1]

Ulipristal acetate (UPA) = EllaOne 30 mg

CI: pregnancy, hypersensitivity to UPA and severe asthma.[1]

Caution in hepatic dysfunction or if liver enzyme inducing drugs have been taken with 28/7.[1]

Prevents/delays ovulation. Licence = 120 hours.

If vomits <3 hours repeat UPA.[4]

Cu-IUD

CI if there is a risk that implantation has already taken place.

Licence: can be inserted up to 5 days after SI or up to 5 days after ovulation (only if regular cycles) – whichever event is the latest. If referring for Cu-IUD also provide oral EC when possible in case insertion is delayed or the patient changes her mind.

Prevents fertilisation and implantation.[1]

'All women requiring EC should be offered a Cu-IUD if appropriate as it is the most effective method of EC.'[1]

Quick-starting contraception is off licence after an emergency contraceptive pill

Advise to check a pregnancy test 3 weeks later or if there is a delayed period.

After LNG can start straight away but use condoms for 7 days with COCP, or 2 days with POP, or 9 days for Qlaira.[1]

After UPA, contraception should be delayed for 5 days as may block effectiveness of UPA. After starting use, extra protection for 7 days with COC (9 days for Qlaira), IMP, DMPA; 2 days with POP.

Case: 'I've already taken LNG this cycle'

UPA and IUD not an option as there is already a risk of implantation.

Therefore, may use second LNG.[1]

LNG 'is not thought to be harmful to the fetus if accidental exposure occurs'.[3]

Case: 'I've had UPSI earlier this month but didn't take any EC'

If requested before 5 days after expected ovulation the IUD would be recommended.[1]

>55 years presumed infertility even if still experiencing menstrual bleeding: may stop contraception.

Non-hormonal method	≥50 years – after 1 year of amenorrhoea.[1]
	<50 years – after 2 years of amenorrhoea.[1]
Progesterone only	≥50 years and amenorrhoea for a year.
	*If FSH level tests ≥30 IU/L, stop 1 year after the second raised FSH level.[1]
LNG-IUS	Inserted ≥45 years Mirena may be left for contraception and HMB until 55 years.
IUDs (copper)	Inserted ≥40 years and if Cu-IUD containing ≥300 mm² copper:

- Can retain the device 'until the menopause'.[1]
- If amenorrhoeic for 1 year consider removing the coil aged 55 years – both IUS/IUD should not remain indefinitely.[1]

Progesterone injection	≥50 years an alternative contraception is advised.[1]
COCP	≥50 years an alternative contraception is advised.[1]

The POP cannot replace the progesterone in HRT but can be used with combined HRT.[1]

'FSH is not a reliable indicator of ovarian failure in women using combined hormones, even if measured during the hormone-free interval.'[1]

*The FSRH advise FSH monitoring may be used for woman on progesterone-only methods. However, as discussed in the Gynaecology and Breast chapter, Menopause and HRT Learning Points, NICE advise GPs not to rely on FSH to confirm the menopause in women taking high-dose progesterones.

Sterilisation

What has led to this decision?

How has this decision been made?

What is the risk of regret?

Is the family complete?

Do both partners agree?

Female	If tubal occlusion is performed at the same time as a caesarean section, counselling and agreement should be given at least 2 weeks in advance of the procedure.[2]
Male	Semen sample at 12 weeks.
	A routine second sample is not required if azoospermia in the first sample.[2]

Smoking, Alcohol and Substance Misuse

Cases in this chapter		Within the RCGP 2020 curriculum: Smoking, Alcohol and Substance Misuse	Learning points in this chapter include:
1	Sleeping Tablets	'Recognise that smoking, alcohol and substance misuse are common problems in the community and understand their relationship to disease and premature death'	Benzodiazepines
2	Alcohol and Safeguarding	'Recognise and manage medical consequences of smoking, alcohol and substance misuse' 'Be aware of wider social issues, including the need to protect children and family members from the potential impact of smoking, alcohol or substance misuse, and respond to any safeguarding concerns'	Harmful drinking Hazardous drinking Alcohol dependence Safeguarding
3	Domestic Violence	'Social consequences of substance misuse, e.g. contact with the criminal justice system (including incarceration), domestic violence, homelessness, poor attendance or functioning at school or work, relationship issues, safeguarding concerns, unemployment'	Domestic violence Child protection Coercive controlling behaviour
4	Opiate Abuse	'Identify and offer interventions, including effective advice and treatment, to people who smoke or misuse alcohol or substances'	NICE Guideline CG51. Drug misuse in over 16s: psychosocial interventions. July 2007
5	Harmful Drinking	'Understand that harmful use of alcohol and other substances is often unrecognised and can take a range of forms (including excessive use, binges, and dependency)' '…Medical complications of long-term alcohol misuse'	NICE Guideline CG115. Alcohol-use disorders: diagnosis, assessment and management of harmful drinking (high risk drinking) and alcohol dependence. February 2011

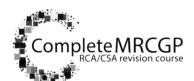

CompleteMRCGP
RCA/CSA revision course

CHAPTER 21 REFERENCES

Sleeping Tablets

1. https://www.sleepstation.org.uk

Alcohol and Safeguarding

1. NICE Public Health Guideline PH24. Alcohol use disorders: prevention. https://www.nice.org.uk/guidance/ph24/chapter/7-Glossary#harmful-drinking-high-risk-drinking. Jun 2010.

Domestic Violence

1. https://www.womensaid.org.uk/information-support/what-is-domestic-abuse/coercive-control/
2. Stark E. *Coercive Control: How Men Entrap Women in Personal Life*. New York: Oxford University Press. 2009.

Opiate Abuse

1. NICE Guideline CG51. Drug misuse in over 16s: psychosocial interventions. https://www.nice.org.uk/guidance/cg51. Jul 2007.

Useful Resources

https://www.crisis.org.uk/ending-homelessness/health-and-wellbeing/drugs-and-alcohol/
https://www.nhs.uk/live-well/healthy-body/ways-to-manage-chronic-pain/
https://livewellwithpain.co.uk/

Harmful Drinking

1. NICE Guideline CG115. Alcohol-use disorders: diagnosis, assessment and management of harmful drinking (high risk drinking) and alcohol dependence. https://www.nice.org.uk/Guidance/CG115. Feb 2011.
2. 'Note that the evidence for acamprosate in the treatment of harmful drinkers and people who are mildly alcohol dependent is less robust than that for naltrexone. At the time of publication (February 2011), acamprosate did not have UK marketing authorisation for this indication. Informed consent should be obtained and documented.'[1]
3. 'At the time of publication (February 2011), oral naltrexone did not have UK marketing authorisation for this indication. Informed consent should be obtained and documented.'[1]
4. 'All prescribers should consult the SPC for a full description of the contraindications and the special considerations of… disulfiram.'[1]
5. https://www.nhs.uk/live-well/alcohol-support/tips-on-cutting-down-alcohol/

Doctor's Notes

Patient	Ella Jones	42 years	F
PMH	Insomnia		
Medications	Zopiclone 7.5 mg – 14 tablets last prescribed 3 weeks ago.		
Allergies	No information		
Consultations	No recent consultations		
Investigations	No recent investigations		
Household	No household members registered		

Open ☐	Tell me more about your sleep disturbance … and evening routine? What have you tried?
Impact ☐	How does this affect your life? What do you think about when you can't sleep?
History ☐	Tell me about the pressures you are under. How's life at home? Do you live alone? Are you active? I see that you were given 2 weeks of tablets 3 weeks ago. You are requiring them most days?
Flags ☐	Is your mood okay? Do you suffer with anxiety? Do you drink much alcohol or caffeine? How do you feel in the morning? Do you feel groggy when you need to drive?
ICE ☐	What do you think may be causing the problem with sleeping? Has anything else happened or upset you? What worries you about this sleeping problem? Is there anything else on your mind or anything you have been wondering? Have you had any thoughts regarding what else you could try?
Sense ☐	I hear that you feel you've made an informed decision that this is the right thing for you at present.
Curious ☐	I'm thinking longer term also – what are your thoughts about the future plan for these tablets?
SummarICE ☐	To summarise, you have always struggled with sleep and, despite trying all the sleep hygiene advice, only the zopiclone 7.5 mg tablet helps. Without it you fear you cannot get through the next few months which will be stressful and require your attention. You are hoping to continue zopiclone on an infrequent basis, as required, as you feel you have no alternative.
Empathy ☐	I appreciate it must be horrible not having any sleep. This is especially difficult when you have your level of responsibility at school. You have also followed all the doctor's advice diligently.
Impression ☐	It sounds as if you suffer with insomnia, exacerbated by recent stress at work.
Experience ☐	Can you please explain to me what you know about the risks of these tablets?
Explanation ☐	If I may explain again the risks of these tablets. Even after a few weeks there is the risk your body becomes tolerant. The sleeping tablets are then no longer effective, but increase your risk of poor concentration, poor memory, poor coordination and low mood. Although the body has become tolerant, without them you cannot sleep due to the rebound effect of stopping them abruptly.
InCludE ☐	I understand that you feel you cannot be without them, but we need to prevent the pattern of tolerance then rebound withdrawal. It may take a few weeks of being free from them before your body finds its natural rhythm. What are your thoughts about this?
Options ☐	We could change the tablet to a longer-acting tablet to avoid withdrawal symptoms; however, side effects may last all day. How do you think longer-acting tablets may affect you at work? An alternative is an antihistamine used for insomnia, promethazine, in the interim.
Recommend ☐	To safely wean, I suggest zopiclone 3.75 mg for 2 weeks, then use the 3.75 mg tablets and promethazine on alternate nights for a week, then change to promethazine only when required. Is that okay? Do you feel you can try this now?
Future ☐	Okay, we could wait until after Ofsted and then try this in 2 months' time.
Empower ☐	Do you think it's reasonable to plan that sleeping tablets are not lifelong? I wonder if you may be interested in CBT… Have you come across this? It is a course designed to help change patterns of thinking and behaviour and can be effective in insomnia. You can get an NHS referral to 'Sleep Station' which is a CBT service for people with sleep problems. Should I pop the link in a text to you? Also avoid strenuous exercise in the few hours before sleep.
Safety net ☐	If you ever feel sleepy, or your coordination does not feel 100%, you must not drive. If you ever feel unwell, for example with palpitations or dizziness, this can be due to the tablets, so please see a doctor. All the best with the next Ofsted meeting.

Doctor's notes	Ella Jones, 42 years. PMH: insomnia. Medications: zopiclone 7.5 mg – 14 tablets last prescribed 3 weeks ago.
How to act	Relaxed but pushy.
	You are planning to reassure the doctor that you will be safe with the tablets.
PC	*'Doctor, I need some more sleeping tablets please. I just need them occasionally.'*
History	You have always been a terrible sleeper and over the past year it has become worse.
	You were first prescribed sleeping tablets 3 months ago.
	You were busy at work and they helped. These days, you do not sleep without them.
	You may manage 3 hours between 3 and 6 a.m. You have a healthy lifestyle and eat well.
	You tried the 3.75 mg tablets but these did nothing.
	You take the tablet every school night and just put up with the problem at the weekend.
Social	You are the headmistress of a school. You have just been given bad ratings by Ofsted and you have further reports to write and further meetings planned in 2 months' time.
	You have no children of your own.
	You have a female partner and you are both very happy.
	You go to yoga and enjoy playing hockey or going for a run in the evening.
	You don't drink alcohol or caffeine. You relax, read a book and avoid the computer.
ICE	You are concerned that without the tablets you will not be able to function.
	You especially need them at the moment due to the stress at work.
	You are worried the doctor will stop giving them to you.
	You have tried all the sleep hygiene advice GPs have suggested.
	You expect the doctor will be concerned…
	'I thought you may want to counsel me regarding the risks. I appreciate the risks of addiction but I will only take them when I need them, not every night and it's really important I have them please.'
	You are happy to negotiate with the doctor.
	Suggest after 2 months you will limit the use to twice weekly.
	However, if the doctor explains the risks and understands your situation, agree that you will try to wean off them completely.
	You cannot try a long-acting benzodiazepine as you need to drive and function through the day.

Negotiate a plan to reach a mutual agreement.

Wean benzodiazepines (zopiclone may have similar effects) gradually to prevent: anxiety, panic, depression, palpitations, malaise and seizures.

Withdrawal symptoms may commence up to a week after stopping longer-acting benzodiazepines. This consultation requires patient education and negotiation after gaining an understanding of the person's individual circumstances.

Converting shorter-acting benzodiazepines (e.g. nitrazepam, temazepam and lorazepam) to longer-acting benzodiazepines (e.g. diazepam) may be required before initiating a gradual weaning process over a period of weeks to months depending on the dose. Note some patients may be concerned with using longer-acting benzodiazepines due to side effects and therefore potential restrictions of driving.

The BNF contains information regarding withdrawing benzodiazepines (hypnotics and anxiolytics chapter) including the approximate equivalent doses when compared with diazepam.

Sleep Station[1] – CBT for insomnia (CBTi). Patients can register for an NHS referral online and then their GP completes a form for the patient to access this service free of charge.

 See the Link Hub at CompleteMRCGP.co.uk for a useful link to Dose conversions of benzodiazepines

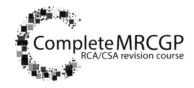

Doctor's Notes

Patient	Kirsty West	38 years	F
PMH	No known medical history		
Medications	No current medications		
Allergies	No information		
Consultations	No recent consultations		
Investigations	No recent investigations		
Household	Simeon West	42 years	M
	Rose West	11 years	F
	Toby West	6 years	M

Example Consultation

Open ☐ — Please tell me the story from when this began.

History ☐ — How is your husband's health? How is his mood? And how about you? Do you work? Do you have any close family or friends? Are they aware? Do you drink any alcohol? What has made you come today; has something happened?

Flags ☐ — Is there any violence in the home? How have the children reacted? Does your husband drive? Does your husband take care of the children alone? Does he ever take drugs?

Impact ☐ — What impact has his drinking had on you? Your relationship? The children? How are you coping financially?

Sense ☐ — I can hear how exhausting this is for you.

ICE ☐ — What has been going through your mind? What makes you feel most upset? Did you have any hopes of what we may decide today?

Curious ☐ — You haven't asked your family for help – I'm wondering why that is. (Pause) Are you close to them? How may they react? Do you feel there is risk of violence if your husband knew you were speaking to me?

SummarICE ☐ — To summarise, you are very concerned about the amount your husband is drinking and the impact this is having on your family. You are worried he won't find work and that home life will continue to be stressful. You are aware the children are having to make their own meals and you have felt too embarrassed to inform your parents.

InCludE ☐ — You were hoping I could speak to your husband. You don't know what else to do.

Empathy ☐ — Kirsty, I can hear this is a really difficult situation. You feel the pressure of running the home is on you and you recognise your husband may be depressed and you want to seek help for your family.

Impression ☐ — It sounds as if your husband is drinking a harmful amount; he may be depressed too.

Options ☐ — To begin with, I could call your husband. You have done the right thing seeking help. There is much that we can do to help your husband: support, medication, counselling and advice. As a couple, you may also wish to go to relationship counselling. I wonder if your children need someone to talk to? I am concerned that the children are having to make their own meals. When any children are involved, I have a duty to inform the safeguarding team, social services. I can hear you are upset; what is going through your mind?

Experience ☐ — What do you know about social services?

Explanation ☐ — I appreciate this is not what you were expecting but I believe this would be a positive step toward moving forward. This team will be able to provide you with support during this time of crisis. Social services aim to help families through difficult times and not take children from their parents. Your husband sounds unwell and it seems you would welcome additional help. Do I have your support to inform this team so they can contact you to make their assessment and offer help?

Empower ☐ — Would you be able to discuss our conversation with your husband? What do you think he'll say? If he will not talk to me on the phone, I could visit. As well as involving your parents, I wonder if you need a work note so you can either leave work early or have time off work if you feel you need to relieve this pressure. We have identified many options today. Out of these options can you summarise how you would like to proceed? Good!

Specifics ☐ — We should talk again with your husband within the week. Which day would suit you? Let's book the appointment now.

Safety net ☐ — If ever you feel there is a risk to anyone, including your husband, contact the police or your GP.

Doctor's notes	Kirsty West, 38 years. PMH: none. Medication: none.
How to act	Concerned. Articulate. You are mentally and physically well.
PC	*'Doctor, I want to talk about my husband's drinking.'*
History	He is in good health but has started drinking half a bottle of whisky every night.
	He was made redundant last year and can't find a job. You are worried and angry.
	Your life has changed as he has stopped interacting with the children and you feel the pressure. Your relationship is strained as you are often angry with him.
	There is no violence in the home. You think he is depressed.
	You are looking after the children, running the home as well as bringing in the income.
	You are not depressed, *'just fed up with it'.*
	Last night he fell over. He was not injured but the children started to cry.
Social	You work full time in a pharmacy as an assistant and return home at 7 p.m. You drink no alcohol. Your children are 6 and 11 years old. You have no time for hobbies.
	Your family are close by. You've felt too embarrassed to tell your parents about the problem.
ICE	*'I don't know what to do.'*
	You are worried he will never get a job now and you can't see life getting better.
	'Will you come to the house to see him? He may listen to you.'
	If the doctor asks to arrange a phone call with your husband, you think this may be helpful.
	If asked, you feel the children are starting to become withdrawn and spending more time in their rooms.
	He is not violent. He is home alone with the children after school and on Saturdays.
	He does not drive. The children return home on the school bus.
	He sometimes makes their tea but often the older child is making them beans on toast.
	If the doctor mentions contacting social services, start to cry. Tell the doctor the children are safe. Then suggest you will inform your parents who can look after the children.
	Plead with the doctor not to inform social services and be angry – you have asked for help!
	If the doctor asks what you are thinking, say: *'We are not bad parents.'*
	If the doctor makes suggestions, a work note for altered hours for you whilst your husband seeks help or explains why he or she is informing social services, agree you need help. You accept any suggestions offered. You believe your husband will accept help when he is aware of how serious this is.

Harmful drinking 'A pattern of alcohol consumption that is causing mental or physical damage.'[1]

Hazardous drinking 'A pattern of alcohol consumption that increases someone's risk of harm. Some would limit this definition to the physical or mental health consequences (as in harmful use). Others would include the social consequences. The term is currently used by WHO to describe this pattern of alcohol consumption. It is not a diagnostic term.'[1]

Alcohol dependence 'A cluster of behavioural, cognitive and physiological factors that typically include a strong desire to drink alcohol and difficulties in controlling its use. Someone who is alcohol dependent may persist in drinking, despite harmful consequences. They will also give alcohol a higher priority than other activities and obligations. For further information, please refer to: 'Diagnostic and statistical manual of mental disorders' (DSM-IV) (American Psychiatric Association 2000) and 'International statistical classification of diseases and related health problems – 10th revision' (ICD-10) (World Health Organization 2007)'.[1]

Safeguarding

This case requires the doctor to negotiate speaking to the husband and the safeguarding referral. It can be difficult to decide when social services should be involved. If you are considering it, it is likely that a referral is required and, if safe to do so, make your thoughts known to the patient. You may signpost that you will seek advice from your safeguarding lead and be in touch with the patient/relative again.

Safeguarding teams ask that you gain consent from the parent before making the referral. You can also proceed without consent if this is not forthcoming.

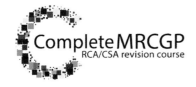

CompleteMRCGP
RCA/CSA revision course

Doctor's Notes

Patient	Isabel Forster	33 years	F
PMH	Fracture of thumb 1 year ago		
Medications	No known medical history		
Allergies	No information		
Consultations	No recent consultations		
Investigations	No recent investigations		
Household	No household members registered		

Open ☐	Okay, what are your thoughts about this?
ICE ☐	Have you had thoughts about what may be delaying a pregnancy? Are you worried? What would you like to happen?
Sense ☐	I am sensing David is more concerned about this than you. Is that right?
Curious ☐	What discussions have you had as a couple? Do you argue? Do you want to have a baby?
History ☐	Are you worried about your health? Do you: take any medicines? Work? Have regular periods? How often do you have sex? Have you ever had an STI? When were you last checked? What made you have an STI check? How is your relationship now? What else do you argue about? Do you ever feel unsafe at home? Are you able to tell me more about that? Do you have any support from family/friends? Can you confide in them? Do you feel isolated? Do you drink alcohol? Or take drugs? Do you own your house? Do you have your own access to money? What do you enjoy doing? Would you like to investigate your fertility? Thank you for sharing this with me.
Flags ☐	Questions about David… Does he work? Does he hit you? Has he used objects to hurt you? Does he force himself on you sexually? Is anyone else aware? Does he spend time with children? What is he capable of? Do you feel that your life is at risk? Has he ever been arrested? Has he threatened to kill you or someone else? Does he have any mental health problems? How much alcohol does he drink? What about drugs? Thank you for telling me. I appreciate it must be upsetting to talk about. Is the abuse getting worse? Do you feel he is controlling you? How is your mood? Do you ever have thoughts that life is not worth living? Have you ever tried to self-harm or commit suicide? Have you ever made plans to? Do you have any other injuries? Has he harmed himself? Have you tried to leave before?
Impact ☐	How do the violence and unkind words you receive affect you?
SummarICE ☐	To summarise, David is keen for a family but because of the violence in the relationship you are taking the Depo injection to give you time to think about your options.
Impression ☐	It sounds like you do not feel safe in your home and David's behaviour could be described as coercive and controlling.
Explanation ☐	Violence in the home is just as illegal as violence in the streets.
Empathy ☐	This must be very difficult for you to talk about. It can also be frightening telling someone.
ICE ☐	What are your thoughts about your options? What would you like to happen? Are you starting to think about planning to leave? What frightens you? What do you need? Have you thought about telling the police?
Experience ☐	Have you heard of any support groups? Are there family/friends who may be able to help?
Recommend ☐	I recommend that I see you. Could you tell David you are attending the surgery for an examination or blood test if I booked an appointment for you? I can give you information about sources of help. If you are thinking of leaving there are a lot of people who can help: Domestic Violence helpline, Women's Aid, Freedom Programme, Recovery Toolkit, Sanctuary Scheme.
Empower ☐	We need to give you control back. Have a think about what steps you would like to take.
Future ☐	Would you like to meet tomorrow? I could give you a sticker which looks like a barcode which has a crisis number on it – put it on something like a lipstick. What will you tell David?
Safety net ☐	If you ever feel you need help you could call this number, us, 111 or the police.

Doctor's notes	Isabel Forster, 33 years. PMH: fracture of thumb 1 year ago. Medications: none.
How to act	Very quiet. You have a concern that you have not shared with anyone else.
PC	*'Doctor, we've been trying for a baby for over a year now.'*
History	You are well. Fracture of the thumb after you tripped 1 year ago.
	You have regular periods. No STIs and smears are up to date.
	You have had no other sexual relationships since this relationship with David.
	'David thought I should call. He is at work.'
	'He thinks something must be wrong.'
Social	You met David 4 years ago. You work in the kitchen of the local primary school.
	David is a building manager for large corporation sites. He has no children.
	You drink no alcohol and take no drugs. David drinks *'too much'* alcohol.
ICE	You tell the doctor it is likely that you haven't fallen pregnant because David is often at work or you have been busy around the time of ovulation.
	'I'm not worried. I know it takes time. I'm not sure now is the right time anyway.'
	'We argue about it.' If asked why, say you feel you should wait until you have bought a house.
	'I thought maybe have some blood tests, that is what David would like.'

If the doctor responds to cues or senses that there is more you want to tell him or her...

'David sometimes hurts me.' You have been taking the contraceptive injection every 3 months at family planning since your coil was removed 1 year ago. You would like to leave the relationship but you are waiting for the right time. You have no concerns about your health. You had a GUM check 6 months ago because you were concerned David may have had an affair. It was normal. David drinks large amounts after work.

He says hurtful things, e.g. that you are fat and ugly. He has never used a weapon and has never hurt another person or animal. He sometimes apologises and can be very loving. He takes no drugs. He has no access to children. He has never been involved with the police. He doesn't drink and drive. You do not feel he would kill anyone including yourself. You want to start thinking about ending the relationship. You tried before and he got very angry then very remorseful and loving. You were scared and you stayed. He is controlling.

He pushes himself on you for sex but you do not resist. You need time to think about how and when to leave.

One year ago, you broke your thumb after he pushed you into a radiator. Your mood is okay. You have lived with his aggression for years. You have never had suicidal thoughts. You have a best friend whom you may now tell. You have no money. You don't know where you would go or how you would pay for rent if you lost your job. You will lie to him and say you have an appointment next week for blood tests.

Opportunities to discuss domestic violence

Asking about relationships is part of any social history. The doctor should always be prepared to sensitively ask about DV if there are any concerns or it crosses the doctor's mind.

There are many opportunities to ask about DV: injury, pregnancy, contraception, pain (e.g. abdominal) and repeated minor illness.

Raising DV   *'Tell me more about your relationship. Do you often argue?'*
                  'Does he/she ever say or do anything that upsets you?'
                  'Do you ever feel threatened by anyone at home?'
                  'Is there any violence at home?'

Be aware of your local support groups for DV.

Child protection

Establish whether there was a child protection concern:

'Does he/she have any contact with children?'
'Do any children witness the violence?'
'Has a child been hurt?'
'How are the children getting on?'
'How are they getting on at school?'
'Is there any pet abuse?'

Ensure immediate reporting to the local safeguarding team if another adult or child is at risk. When children are in the home, even if the parent/guardian feels the children are not affected by the violence, they almost always are in some way and so reporting to the local safeguarding team should be discussed.

Suggestions of how to approach a consultation if the person presenting is the perpetrator, not the victim:

'You have honestly explained when you feel angry you …'
'And recognise this is serious.'
'It sounds as if you would like to receive help for this?'
'What thoughts have you had?'
'We have local teams… e.g. Give Respect – here is their number.'
'May I ask you to see me again and follow this up …?'
'Could you bring your husband/wife with you next time?'

Do not collude or offer relationship counselling

Coercive controlling behaviour (CCB)[1]

As well as asking about DV, the doctor should be aware of the possibility of CCB – which is emotional abuse that is damaging to the mental health of the victim and is illegal in the UK. In the above consultation, there is evidence of CCB as well as DV. David says hurtful things, he is controlling, he became angry when Isabel wanted to leave and he forces sex. Some features of CCB include:

- Controlling aspects of another's life – where they go, who they can meet.
- Repeated 'put-downs' – 'You're fat and ugly'.
- Controlling finances or access to money.
- Humiliating or degrading behaviour.
- 'Gaslighting', e.g. hiding things, denying something that's been said, telling lies so that the victim starts to question their own reality and even thinks they are losing their mind.

'The victim becomes captive in an unreal world created by the abuser, entrapped in a world of confusion, contradiction and fear.' Professor Evan Stark.[2]

Doctor's Notes

Patient	Michaela Butt	32 years	F
PMH	2 NVDs – 2 and 3 years ago		
	Postnatal depression		
	Sciatica		
	Referred to the spinal team and now discharged to physiotherapy.		
	MRI 6 months ago showed minor degenerative changes only.		
	DNA last physiotherapy appointment.		
Medications	Morphine sulphate M/R 30 mg BD. Last issued 60 tablets 20 days ago.		
	Oramorph 10 mg/5 mL		
	Codeine 30 mg		
Allergies	No information		
Consultations	No recent consultations		
Investigations	No recent investigations		
Household	Neil Butt	38 years	M
	Jasmine Butt	3 years	F
	Joseph Butt	2 years	M

Open ☐	Tell me more about the pain from when it began. And the nature of the pain? Have you noticed any other symptoms? Tell me exactly how and when you take each of your medicines.
Impact ☐	What impact has the pain had on life? What can you no longer do?
History ☐	What makes the pain worse? Looking at your history, I see you had depression? How is your mood now? How do you spend your days? Who is at home with you? What can you do yourself? Do you drink alcohol? Have your symptoms changed over recent months?
Flags ☐	Have you injured your back? Does the pain wake you? Is there weakness in your legs? Do you lose control of going to the toilet? Have you lost weight? Are you running any fevers?
ICE ☐	What are your thoughts regarding the cause of your back pain? How can we make progress? What do you think stops your back from recovering? What are you most worried about? What did you think we may decide?
Experience ☐	What is your understanding of what they found on the MRI?
Sense ☐	Do you feel angry? Tell me more about why.
Curious ☐	Do you see things getting better in the future? Did you enjoy being able to do more in the past? Why would going to work make you depressed? Do you fear becoming depressed again? What stress do you have in your life?
SummarICE ☐	It sounds as if you have made great progress with your mood but your back prevents you from living an active life. You fear that going back to work would make your back worse and make you ill again with depression. You haven't done the exercises and didn't attend your physiotherapy as this all increases the pain.
Impression ☐	You have a small amount of wear and tear in your back, as seen on the MRI. However, it seems you have developed chronic pain relating to this.
Explanation ☐	Chronic pain is pain which lasts many months when it would be expected that the tissue should have healed and pain improved. It tends to involve different processes in the brain and spinal cord compared with acute pain such as twisting your ankle. Research shows tablets for chronic pain aren't that effective and can do harm. It's a worry how much pain relief you require. We obviously need to change how we help you. I am concerned you have become addicted to your medication and this has led you to take more. Do you think this is possible?
Empathy ☐	You are in a lot of pain and have had a difficult couple of years. I want to help you today but also aim to get you better in the long term. Is this something you could work towards with me?
Recommend ☐	I recommend we prescribe you tablets on repeat but 2 weeks at a time and you will not be able to collect the tablets early. This will help to prevent you taking too many. Over time I would like you to start weaning off your medication, particularly as you feel they haven't been that effective. Does that sound okay? You should not be on both codeine and morphine. To help I will add paracetamol. I appreciate that paracetamol alone doesn't help but it works with the morphine. Have you tried an anti-inflammatory – ibuprofen or naproxen? Did you try an additional tablet with this called omeprazole to help avoid side effects? Would you like to try that again but with omeperazole? It may help reduce any inflammation. May I text you a link to a website which helps people with chronic pain? It helps you to understand how chronic pain happens and how you can beat it? It's called 'live well with pain'.
Empower ☐	It is important to keep your back moving. What steps could you take towards getting back to your previous activities? Could you try the exercises half an hour after you have taken some Oramorph? They may make you feel stiff at first but then you should start to see an improvement. Don't be frightened of the pain, it is unlikely you will make your back worse. Do you think you could try yoga or Pilates which will help your core muscle strength, flexibility and aid relaxation? Would you be interested in therapy which helps you feel stronger when you have been worried, called CBT?
Future ☐	Can you call me in 1 month? If we are not winning, we could consider referring you to the pain team? May I refer you back to physiotherapy? Please attend, otherwise this is an appointment which someone else could have.
Safety net ☐	If you ever lose control of the bowels or bladder, you need to see a doctor straight away. With the plan you have made I'm confident we will make progress.

Doctor's notes	Michaela Butt, 32 years. PMH: 2 NVDs – 2 and 3 years ago. Postnatal depression.
	Sciatica. Referred to the spinal team and now discharged to physiotherapy. MRI 6 months ago showed minor degenerative changes only. DNA last physiotherapy appointment.
	Medications: morphine sulphate M/R 30 mg BD. Last issued 60 tablets 20 days ago, Oramorph 10 mg/5 mL, codeine 30 mg.
How to act	Demanding.
PC	*'I need more tablets. I lost the others.'*
History	You stopped working in the local care home when you had children.
	During your pregnancy you suffered with sciatica and pelvic pain.
	You have had no injuries. There are no back pain red flags.
	'Lifting the kids' makes it worse.
	You have an uncomfortable bed and can't afford a new one.
	You suffered with postnatal depression. You were seen by the postnatal depression team and you were discharged after your medications stopped.
	You are feeling mentally well now.
	Your sciatica pain was ongoing after the delivery and you have gradually had to increase your pain relief. The pain radiates down both legs.
	You have no neurological symptoms.
	You're annoyed the MRI scan didn't show anything.
	'No one knows what is causing it.'
	You had an appointment with the spinal team who discharged you to physiotherapy.
	You do not do the exercises at home as they hurt your back.
	You take occasional codeine.
	You take your Oramorph twice a day and sometimes take an additional morphine tablet.
	You missed your last physiotherapy appointment.
Social	Your husband doesn't work. He has to look after the 2 children.
	You are both on income support. You do not smoke or drink alcohol.
	Your husband does the housework. You make the meals.
ICE	You would like more morphine tablets.
	You believe the doctors don't know what the problem is.
	You are not worried, only that the doctor may tell you to stop taking so many tablets.
	Refuse any NSAID – they don't work and make you feel sick.
	You did not try it with a PPI and agree to this if offered.
	You can't see your back getting better.
	You will have to spend your life on these tablets.
	You can't do anything due to the pain.
	If the doctor tells you not to take extra morphine, say: *'I obviously need more.'*
	If the doctor asks about work, the thought of going back to work fills you with dread. Having to get up on cold mornings with a painful back.
	'If you make me go back to work, I will become depressed again.'

During every contact it is important to build a rapport and work together towards set goals. NICE stresses the importance of respecting the patient and offering continuity of support. Also take every opportunity to provide education for the services available.

Using a motivational interview strategy may be helpful. NICE encourages the patient to identify vulnerable situations where they may be at risk of substance misuse and equips the patient with coping strategies for these challenges. Consider Read Coding the patient as a vulnerable adult and enquire if there are safeguarding concerns in the home.

Coping strategies include self-help (which may be from CBT) as well as help from agencies. Make sure ongoing support is available as well as support in times of crisis.

If patients are asking for more tramadol or codeine tablets than the maximum allowed dose try… *'I cannot prescribe more than eight tablets a day as I would be prescribing an overdose. Instead, we need to decide together whether this is the correct medication for you.'*

Consider a different working diagnosis and psychosocial reasons why the amount of pain the patient is experiencing seems disproportionate to the suspected cause. Consider a referral to the pain clinic or the drug and alcohol team if you feel there is drug misuse or abuse. There are some tactics you can employ to help keep control of opiate prescribing in patients where there is a concern regarding opiate abuse (e.g. drug-seeking behaviour or PMH of illegal drug use). Prescribe in small quantities, e.g. weekly scripts. This will help you monitor use, reduce the risk of overdose and, when patients claim to have 'lost' a prescription, they will only have to wait a few days before another can be issued – rather than twisting your arm as they can't manage 3 weeks without the medication. Avoid using long-acting opiates in patients who may still be using intravenous drugs. These increase the risk of overdose as a patient may forget they are wearing a patch or have taken M/R oral opiates when they use drugs intravenously. Always get help from an experienced drug/alcohol team as such patients are notoriously difficult to manage. Using patient warnings/pop-ups on the electronic record can also highlight risk of opiate misuse to colleagues who may be unfamiliar with the patient.

Know your local services. Mentioning these services in your consultation skills exam will enhance your management plan.

'Ensure that maintaining the service user's engagement with services remains a major focus of the care plan.'[1]

For example, in Oxford, services include:

- GPs with training in drug and alcohol management
- Alcoholics Anonymous (AA)
- Evolve for young people
- FRANK
- Narcotic Anonymous (NA)
- Oxfordshire DAAT (Drug and Alcohol Action Team)
- SMART or SMART (DIP)
- SWOP Scheme
- The Women's Service or Women's Initiative on Street Health

Find out if you have social prescribing coordinators locally to help guide patients in the right direction for community and professional support. Ask them to send you their directory of local services for you to peruse at your leisure – an investment in time!

If you do not have this service, are you struggling to think of a quality improvement project (QIP)? Why not research local services and ask your colleagues for services they use, form a directory and email it to local practices and the PCN with a social prescribing proposal for your practice. *Voilà!*

Doctor's Notes

Patient	Katherine Knight	68 years	F
PMH	No medical history		
Medications	None		
Allergies	No information		
Consultations	No recent consultations		
Investigations	No recent investigations		
Household	Barry Knight	63 years	M

Open ☐	What's prompted calling me today? Tell me about your drinking pattern. How do you feel about it?
History ☐	Do you drink in the morning? Alone? Are you in good health? Any medicines? Any physical symptoms? Tremors? Stomach changes? Sleep problems? What do you do each day? Tell me about home life. Have you ever not done something expected of you due to drinking? Have you ever started drinking and felt you couldn't stop?
Impact ☐	How has this affected your life? Or relationships? Or hobbies?
ICE ☐	What do you think has led to this? What else have you been wondering? Have you known anyone else who struggled with alcohol? What worries do you have? What did you think we may decide today?
Sense ☐	You seem very sad. I'm interested to know why. Are there people you are close to?
Risk ☐	Do you feel isolated? Have you had any mental health problems/depression? Do you take any drugs?
Flags ☐	Are there any dangers you can see associated with drinking? Any injuries? Are you down? Any thoughts of life not worth living? Have you acted on them? Do you have plans to end your life? Are either of you violent or unkind? Have you had thoughts of hurting another person? Do you eat well and look after yourself? Do you drive?
Curious ☐	What does your husband think about the alcohol? And the relationship? Has it had an impact on him?
Empathy ☐	You've taken a big step today. It must seem like a difficult journey ahead.
Empower ☐	We can help. How would life be different without alcohol? Do you think you can stop? What steps could you take? Why might it be difficult? Who could help? What is your aim? When would you like to achieve that by?
SummarICE ☐	To summarise, you've been increasing your consumption of alcohol over 6 months. You feel low and this is due to being alone and bored. You hope to cut down and spend more time with your husband.
Impression ☐	It sounds like you have alcohol dependence and depression.
Experience ☐	What do you know about why alcohol is dangerous?
Explanation ☐	Alcohol affects most parts of the body. As well as damage to the liver it can cause problems with the nerves and the functioning in the brain. Sometimes people can suffer with a dementia-like illness because of alcohol. Alcohol keeps you awake at night. Alcohol is a false friend; it makes you more depressed.
Options ☐	There are things that you can do. It is actually dangerous to stop drinking straight away. We should either cut down gradually or provide support through a detox programme. What are your thoughts about these options?
Recommend ☐	Reducing your alcohol intake by 2–3 units (a large glass of wine) per day is a good starting point. Others can help with your recovery. Your husband, the alcohol team or Turning Point can support you through the process and afterwards. Would you be interested in seeing these teams? I would also suggest that I see you in the surgery to examine your tummy, to check the size of your liver, and look for any other sign of alcohol affecting your body. Would that be okay? We could also arrange some blood tests to look for harm as well – specifically your blood count and liver tests? I would like to give you some vitamin tablets – thiamine – which will prevent you becoming confused and unwell. The dose is one 100 mg tablet daily. How does this sound?
Future ☐	I will ask reception to call you back with an appointment for your blood tests then I will see you in surgery to discuss the results and examine you, is that okay? You may also want to attend AA for ongoing support. There is also Relate which offers relationship counselling – you may find this helpful. What are your thoughts? I can write down these contacts.
Safety net ☐	If you ever feel you are muddled, or start vomiting or feel shaky or generally unwell, or have thoughts of wanting to hurt yourself or anyone else, please see a doctor straight away. I'm looking forward to seeing you next week.

Patient's Story

Doctor's notes	Katherine Knight, 68 years. PMH: none. Medication: none.
How to act	Speak quietly. Do not be forthcoming with information.
PC	*'My husband thinks I'm drinking too much.'*
History	You started to drink one bottle of wine every night about 6 months ago.
	You just enjoyed it and the amount gradually increased.
	You are bored and don't have anything else to do!
	As well as the wine, you sometimes also have a brandy or two, usually starting to drink at lunchtime. If you don't drink, you feel shaky and you drink every day. You take no drugs.
	Your health has always been good and you take no medicines. You have no physical symptoms that you know of and your bowels are fine but your appetite is reduced. You often wake through the night.
	When others mention the alcohol, you feel upset. You drink alone and your husband has stopped drinking *'to make me feel guilty'*.
Social	You spend the day watching TV or you may wander to the supermarket.
	You eat quick meals these days and don't feel like cooking.
	You have never driven a car.
	Your husband is still working as a caretaker. *'He is too busy to notice.'*
	You have lost touch with friends. You missed a catch-up with a friend as you'd been drinking and fell asleep on the sofa.
ICE	Your husband told you to speak to your GP.
	Your relationship is not good. He is becoming upset.
	He is polite and kind to you but you feel very alone. You regret not having children.
	You wanted to talk to the GP today but are unsure what you want from the meeting.
	You are worried that you rely on the alcohol and you don't know how to cut down.
	Although you would like to cut down, boredom may prevent it.
	However, overall, you believe you can and know your husband will help you.
	You think you are depressed but want no medication.
	You have occasional thoughts that life is not worth living but no plans and you would not attempt suicide.
	You would like to get out of the house more. You would like to do more things together.
	You agree with the doctor's advice about your relationship and self-help measures.
	You understand that alcohol is bad for the liver.
Examination	The examination is normal.

Learning Points

Perform a risk assessment   Self (neglect, harm, suicide, injury)

Others (the public, children/vulnerable adults)

Assess psychological and social problems

e.g. mental health problems, work issues, housing issues, driving, criminal activity, relationship problems.

Investigations   U&E, LFT, GGT, FBC and clotting

Questionnaires   AUDIT, SADQ and APQ

Divide who can help into self, GP and others (friends, professionals or support groups: AA or SMART recovery). Involve families and carers in the recovery process with the patient's consent.

Consider the addition of acamprosate[2] or naltrexone[3] to psychological therapy if this therapy alone has not been successful in mild alcohol dependence.[1] In practice, for most GPs, this will require a referral to the local drug and alcohol team.

When to offer community detox programmes

For those who 'drink over 15 units of alcohol per day and/or who score 20 or more on the AUDIT, consider offering: an assessment for and delivery of a community-based assisted withdrawal, or assessment and management in specialist alcohol services if there are safety concerns… '[1]

When to consider inpatient or residential assisted withdrawal[1]

15–30 units/day   and 'significant psychiatric or physical comorbidities…

or a significant learning disability or cognitive impairment'[1]

SADQ score   >30

History of: epilepsy

withdrawal-related seizures

delirium tremens

consuming alcohol and benzodiazepines.

'Consider a lower threshold for inpatient or residential assisted withdrawal in vulnerable groups, for example, homeless and older people.'[1]

'After a successful withdrawal for people with moderate and severe alcohol dependence consider offering acamprosate[2] or oral naltrexone[3] in combination with an individual psychological intervention **or** (3rd line) disulfiram[4] after explaining the risks.'[1]

Advise patients wanting to cut down that this should be done slowly to prevent withdrawal symptoms and explain the importance of this to patients. If withdrawal symptoms start to develop, the patient can drink 2 units of alcohol and wait 30 minutes to see the response.[5]

Remember driving – the law requires all dependent drinkers to inform the DVLA.

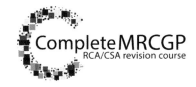

CompleteMRCGP
RCA/CSA revision course

CHAPTER 22 EXAMINATION CHECKLISTS
Examinations

Informed Consent

To gain informed consent explain what you would like to do and why it would be helpful.

'I would like to examine your chest by bringing you to the examination couch. It would be helpful if you could please remove your top (keeping your bra on) and then I'd like to take your temperature, feel your pulse and have a listen to your chest to see if there are any signs of infection. Would that be okay?'

If an intimate examination is required then either **state** you need a chaperone or, if you feel comfortable without, **offer** a chaperone. (In real consultations always document this discussion.)

Simulated cases' assessment

You need to inform the patient of everything you would like to examine just in case you do not have the opportunity to carry out the examination. Do not turn to look at the examiner to ask if you should examine!

Presume you are proceeding with the examination (even if an intimate examination) and **move** after gaining consent to either a chair or couch as appropriate. You may be stopped and given information (by card, on the iPad or verbally) at this point.

Be aware you may be signposted to a second page on the iPad with further information.

Candidates often ask:

1. Should I examine in the chair or on the couch?

   The chair is acceptable if you can obtain all the information you require without cutting corners, e.g. for a thyroid assessment. However, this is your higher level exam and therefore we recommend you demonstrate excellent skills. E.g. on the couch for a cardiovascular assessment.

2. Should I complete a thorough and formal examination of a system?

   The extent to which you examine should be appropriate and guided by the history, e.g. if a patient presents with angina, we suggest a formal/full approach to the cardiovascular examination.

When examining, always use the phrase a 'good look' not a 'quick look'.

Recorded consultation assessment (RCA)

In a face-to-face consultation, examine the patient when it is clinically appropriate to do so. Remember the 'rules', already described in Chapter 1.

- Be sure that you are examining for the benefit of the patient, not the examiner. Never 'stage' an examination that is not necessary.

  Examine behind the curtain, off camera, if removing clothing, or if the examination requires exposure in the 'swimsuit area', i.e. the area normally covered by swim shorts for males ≥ 2 years, bikini area for females ≥ 2 years and nappy area for an under 2-year-old.

- Describe what you are doing, for the benefit of the patient, and the examiner will also be able to hear this commentary. Be sure that you use language that the patient will understand.

- Do not stop or edit the tape.

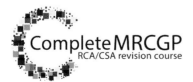
CompleteMRCGP
RCA/CSA revision course

Example description

'I'd like to **thoroughly** *examine your chest and heart by asking you to come over to the couch and take off your top, please. I will then feel your pulse, take your blood pressure and listen to your heart. This will help me to check the heart and blood vessels. Is that okay?'*

Checklist

- 'I'd like to start by measuring your blood pressure and checking your pulse.'
- 'Now may I feel both pulses together?'
- 'May I see your hands?'
- 'And now just the one pulse and I will lift your arm.' (Collapsing pulse.)
- 'Look up to the ceiling for me… and stick out your tongue.' (Anaemia.)
- 'Now please turn your neck to the side.' (JVP – if appropriate from history.)
- 'May I feel your heart?' (Apex, thrills and heaves.)
- 'Now I'll listen.' (Apex with bell for mitral stenosis.)
- 'And now please roll slightly to your left.' (Mitral regurgitation.)
- 'Please roll back.' Switch to diaphragm to check the other valves.
- 'I will now listen to the arteries in your neck.' (Carotid bruit.)
- 'Now please sit forward.' (Listen for aortic regurgitation at left lower sternal edge.)
- 'I will now listen to your lower lungs.' (Pulmonary oedema – if appropriate from history.)
- Consider checking for liver edge and leg swelling. (Right-sided heart failure.)
- Consider checking for AAA and peripheral pulses. (Depending on age and history.)

Example description

'I'd like to **thoroughly** *examine your chest and lungs in the chair and will ask you to take off your top, please. I'd also like to feel your pulse, check your breathing rate, oxygen levels, take your temperature and check a blowing test called the peak flow. This will help me look for signs of infection and check the airflow into lungs. Is that okay?'*

Checklist

- 'I'd like to start by checking your pulse and oxygen saturations.'
- Then check breathing rate.
- 'Please may I see your hands and fingers?'
- 'Can you please stick out your tongue?' (Cyanosis.)
- 'I'm going to feel for lumps in the neck.' (Lymphadenopathy.)
- 'Big breath in for me.' (Expansion.)
- 'And say 99.' (Vocal resonance in quadrants.)
- 'And now some deep breaths in and out please.' (Auscultation.)
- 'I'm going to tap on your chest.' (Percussion.)
- 'Can I just check your legs for pain and swelling?' (DVT.)
- Consider temperature.
- Consider PEFR.
- Consider inhaler technique.

Example description

'I'd like to **thoroughly** *examine your abdomen, by asking you to lie on the couch and lift up your top to under the breasts and undo the button on your trousers to look at your lower tummy. I would also like to take your pulse and temperature. This will help me to find the reason for your pain. Is that okay?'*

Checklist

- Consider taking: pulse, temperature and blood pressure. (Are they systemically unwell?)
- 'May I see your hands and fingers?' (E.g. liver disease.)
- 'I'm just going to have a close look at your face and eyes for colour change.'
- 'May I look in your mouth?'
- 'I'm just going to feel for any lumps above your collar bone.'
- 'Can you please lift your head off the bed and cough?' (Hernia.)
- 'Can you suck your tummy in?' (Peritonism.)
- 'Please tell me if you have any discomfort whilst I feel your tummy.' (Watch their face.)
- Check for rebound tenderness, McBurney's and Rovsing's signs.
- Palpate for hepatosplenomegaly.
- Then percuss for hepatosplenomegaly and consider shifting dullness for ascites.
- Auscultate.
- Consider offering: inguinal hernia, perineum, pelvic and rectal examinations.
- Consider requesting a urine sample for a pregnancy or urine dipstick test.

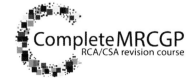

Example description

'*I'd like to* **thoroughly** *examine the nerves in your brain by asking you to make some actions. I will sit opposite you. Is that okay?*'

Checklist

II	'Can you read this chart covering each eye at a time.' (Snellen for acuity.)
	'Look at my finger at a distance and now close to your nose.' (Accommodation.)
	'Now I'll shine a light in your eye.' (Then the opposite eye for efferent/afferent pathway testing.)
	'Covering the left eye with your hand, look at my nose. Say *yes* when you see my fingers move.'
	'And now cover the other eye.' (Visual fields.)
	'Now with both eyes open how many fingers do you see?' (Double vision/4 quadrants.)
	Fundoscopy: 'Now I'd like to look at the back of your eyes. This involves shining a bright light into the eye. I will need to get close to your face, please try to keep looking straight forward – imagine you can see through me, and remember to breathe away normally.'
III, IV, VI	'Now keep your head still and follow my finger with your eyes.' (Eye movements and nystagmus.)
V	'Checking for sensation now: can you feel this on both sides?' (Upper, middle and lower face.)
VII	'Now I'm going to test the muscles. I will test the strength by resisting your movements.'
	'Please raise your eyebrows… now shut your eyes tight…'
	'Open your eyes and puff out your cheeks… and a big smile for me.'
VIII	'Can you hear me whisper a number?' Block the opposite ear, test each side at 1 m whisper.
	If not heard, try 1 m voice… if not heard try voice next to ear.
	Rinne/Weber if difficulty hearing (see ENT examinations).
IX	'Please swallow.'
X	'Open your mouth and say ah.' (Palatal rise.)
XI	'Shrug your shoulders and keep them up… and push your face against my hand' (Check sternocleidomastoid muscle strength.)
XII	'Please show me your tongue.'

Cerebellar acronym – DANISH: Dysdiadochokinesia. Ataxic gait. Nystagmus. Intention tremor. Slurred speech 'baby hippopotamus' and heel–shin test (coordination).

Example description

'I'd like to **thoroughly** *examine the nerves in your arms and legs by checking sensation and doing some movements. Is that okay?*

Do you have any pain that I should be aware of when I examine you?'

Decide bed or chair – what do you do normally? Think about the exposure of the patient. It may be appropriate to leave clothes on if sensation can be tested easily through thin clothing.

Checklist

- 'Are you able to stand up without using your hands?... Now please walk across the room and back.' ('Get up and go' in the elderly to assess falls risk, gait and strength.)
- 'Can you stand feet together and then shut your eyes.' (Romberg's for proprioception – be ready to steady the patient should they lose balance!)
- 'And now with your feet comfortably apart again, close your eyes and touch your nose.'
- 'Can you walk heel–toe?... And now please lie down on the bed facing upwards.'
- Check arms +/– legs for wasting, scars, fasciculation.
- 'I'm going to check the tone by moving your arms.'
- 'Can we now check power... and reflexes?'
- 'And now your legs.'
- 'A scratch test on your feet now.' (Plantar reflexes and check clonus.)
- 'I'm going to test your sensation.' Demonstrate pins and cotton wool on the chest and then check all dermatomes.
- Test coordination – finger nose ataxia/heel against shin.
- Consider vibration sensation. (Peripheral neuropathy secondary to diabetes.)
- Consider cerebellar signs (DANISH – see CN examination.)
- Consider testing for parkinsonism features: micrographia, each finger to thumb, hands open and closing for bradykinesia.

Example description

'I'd like to **thoroughly** *examine your thyroid gland, which is in the neck, and also look at your hands and legs which can be affected by the thyroid, if I may?'*

Patient in sitting position and expose neck fully.

Checklist

- 'May I start by looking at your hands?' (Tremor, warmth, palmar erythema, dry skin, clubbing.)
- 'And check your pulse?'
- 'Looking at your eyes now, can you look straight ahead… follow my finger up and down? (Exophthalmos, lid retraction, lid lag, chemosis.)
- 'And now looking at your neck.' (Look from the front and side for scars and a visible thyroid.)
- 'Can you please stick out your tongue… and now swallow?'
- 'I'm going to feel your thyroid… and, if you can, please swallow again.' (Stand behind. ?Asymmetry.)
- 'I'm going to listen.' (Bruit.)
- 'Now looking at your ankles for swelling. (Pre-tibial myxoedema.)
- 'And finally testing your reflexes.' (Slow relaxing reflexes.)
- 'May I check your weight now please?'

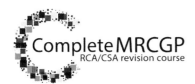

CompleteMRCGP
RCA/CSA revision course

- Look → feel → move → power → sensation → function.
- Always examine the joint above and below for swelling, tenderness and ROM.

Example description

'I'd like to **thoroughly** *examine your shoulders, neck and elbow. May I ask you to take your shirt off please? Is that okay?'*

Checklist

- 'Can you please point to where you feel the pain?'
- Look for asymmetry, deformity, wasting, swelling or redness.
- 'Please tell me if you are tender or in pain when I examine you.' (Warmth/tenderness over C-spine, shoulder and elbow.)
- 'Can you move your neck and copy me?' (Test for full ROM of the neck.)
- Keeping your arms straight, can you lift the arms up in front of you… and now move the arms out to the sides and lift the arms into the air?' (Painful arc or frozen shoulder?)
- 'Put your arms out to the sides but just a little in front of you. Now imagine you are holding a can and emptying it onto the floor. Now please hold your arm in that position whilst I try to push your arm down.' (Jobe's test/empty can test = supraspinatus test.)
- 'Now glue both elbows into your waist but with your hands push my hands out to the sides.' (External rotation for teres minor test.)
- 'Can you hold your hand out so your thumb is up and tilted away from you? Now can you try and turn your hand further away from you against my resistance?' (Infraspinatus test.)
- 'Hands behind your back and push my hands backwards.' (Subscapularis test.)
- Then finally test power throughout the upper limb.
- Consider a neuro exam. 'Can you feel me touch your skin?' (Test all dermatomes.)
- 'How high up your spine can you reach there?' (Function.)
- 'Can you touch your head with both hands as if washing your hair?' (Function.)
- 'Any issues checking your blind spot when driving?' (Function.)

- Look → feel → move → power → sensation → function.
- Always examine joint above and joint below for swelling, tenderness and ROM.

Example description

'I'd like to **thoroughly** *examine your elbow as well as your shoulder and wrists. If I may ask you to remove your shirt – is that okay?'*

Checklist

- 'Please can you point to where you feel the pain?'
- 'Let's look at your elbow… and the other elbow.' (Swelling, redness, deformity.)
- 'Please tell me if you feel any pain when I examine your elbow now.' (Heat or tenderness over the epicondyles.)
- 'Now can you move your hands to touch your shoulder and straighten both your arms?'
- 'Can you place your palms up to the ceiling… and now down to the floor?' (Pronation/supination.)
- 'Now hold my hand as if you are going to shake it. Turn your hand as if twisting a handle and I will try to resist you.' (Use both of your hands to prevent injury to yourself!)
- 'And turn the other way.'
- 'Now with your arm outstretched, bend your wrist back towards you; if I resist you does that cause pain in your elbow?' (Lateral epicondylitis.)
- 'Now can you bend your wrist toward the floor? Does it hurt your elbow if I resist this movement?' (Medial epicondylitis.)
- 'Can you feel me touch you at the elbow?'
- 'Can you reach both hands onto your head? Now can you reach your back?' (Function.)
- 'I want to have a look at the shoulder… and now feel your shoulder; is this painful? Keeping your arms straight, can you move the arms out to the sides and lift the arms into the air?'
- 'Now looking at your wrists, is there any tenderness? Can you move your wrists?'

- Look → feel → move → power → sensation → function.
- Always examine joint above and joint below.

Example description

'I'd like to **thoroughly** *examine your hands, wrists and elbows. If you could please roll your sleeves above the elbow. Is that okay?'*

Checklist

- 'Let's put a pillow on your lap for your hands to rest on.'
- 'Please point to where you feel the pain.'
- 'Now let's look and see if there is any swelling or changes.'
- 'May I feel your skin for heat?... And now, as I feel each joint in turn, let me know if you have any pain.' (Feel each finger joint, metacarpal, wrist and elbow joint in turn.)
- 'Are you able to copy the following movements?' (Make a fist, open and close hands, wrist full ROM and elbow full ROM.)
- 'Can you squeeze my fingers?'
- 'Now stretch your fingers out and keep them out.' (Ulnar.)
- 'Lift your thumb to the ceiling and press against me.' (Median.)
- Test sensation in ulnar and median distribution.
- 'Can you touch each finger against your thumb?' (Function.)
- 'Please copy me and place your hands like this. Hold the hands there and let me know if you feel any tingling.' (Phalen's test for carpal tunnel syndrome.)
- 'Now I will tap over your wrist. Tell me if you feel any tingling in the hand.' (Tinel's test for carpal tunnel syndrome.)

Example description

'*I'd like to* **thoroughly** *examine your back and hips, if I may, to find the cause of this pain.*'

Checklist

- 'Please point to where you feel the pain.'
- 'Please walk across the room.'
- 'Now with four fingers holding onto my hands, if you can please lift your right knee so you are standing on your left foot only. And now the other leg please.' (Trendelenburg's test.)
- 'Now please turn away from me and I'll look at your spine.' (Posture, lordosis, kyphosis.)
- 'As I feel your spine, please tell me if this is painful.' (Spine then paraspinal muscles.)
- 'Back to face me now… (step away) can you keep your legs straight and touch your toes?'
- 'And try leaning down each side and back.' (Flexion, extension, lateral flexion, rotation.)
- 'Now lift each leg out to each side.' (Hip abduction.)
- 'And leg behind you.' (Hip extension.)
- 'Onto the couch now; are you tender where I press on your hips?' (Greater trochanters.)
- 'Keep your leg straight and raise the leg one at a time.' (Hip flex and SLR – sciatica.)
- 'Can you bend your knee to your chest now?'
- 'Can I see if I can take that further? Now I'm going to check your hips.' (Int/ext rotations.)
- Consider lower limb neurology testing.

Trendelenburg test: 'The sound side sags' when weight bearing on weak gluteals, i.e. if unable to hold pelvis level standing on one leg, the standing leg is the affected side.

Causes include: dislocated hip, # greater trochanter, subluxation of the upper femoral epiphysis (SUFE), muscle-wasting diseases – although can be positive in any painful hip condition.

Example description

'I'd like to **thoroughly** *examine your knees as well as your hips and ankles as sometimes there is a problem with the adjacent joint. If I may ask you to remove your trousers/skirt (keep shorts on). Is that okay? If at any point you are in pain, please let me know.'*

Checklist

- 'Facing me now, please, point to where you feel the pain.'
- Look for valgus/varus positioning of knees/ankles, deformity, wasting and swelling in the lower limb.
- 'Please turn to the side, now turn away from me, turn again and now back to face me.'
- 'Please walk across the room.'
- 'Now with four fingers, hold my hands and lift one knee up at a time.' (Trendelenburg test.)
- 'Lift each leg out to each side' (Hip abduction.) 'And leg behind you.' (Hip extension.)
- 'Please come over to the couch and lie facing upwards… with your knees slightly bent.'
- 'I'm just going to check for heat and tenderness now in the hip (greater trochanter), knee (joint lines and ankle (malleolus).'
- 'Now straighten your leg and I will test for fluid.' (Patellar tap and fluid test for effusion.)
- 'Left side now, can you make this leg as straight as possible?' (Hyperextend knee.)
- 'Now lift your leg straight into the air.' (Hip flex). 'Bring your knee to your chest.' (Knee flex.)
- 'Now can I do the same and see if I can take that further?' (Feeling for crepitus.)
- 'I'm just going to test your hip movement.' (Internal and external rotation.)
- 'And now can you point your toes up and down, left and right?' (Ankle ROM.)
- 'Please bend your knee and I will pull and push, to test the ligaments in your knee.' (Anterior and posterior draw test for cruciates.)
- 'And now you will feel some pressure on the sides of the knees.' (Collateral ligaments.)
- 'And now as you straighten your knee, I will move your ankle.' (McMurray's for meniscus tear.)

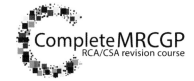

Example description

'*I'd like to* **thoroughly** *examine your foot and ankle as well as your knees as sometimes there is a problem with the adjacent joint. If I may ask you to remove your trousers/skirt (keep shorts on). Is that okay? If at any point you are in pain, please let me know.*'

Checklist

- 'Facing me now, please, point to where you feel the pain.'
- Look for valgus/varus positioning of knees/ankles, deformity, wasting and swelling in the lower limb.
- 'Please turn to the side, now turn away from me, turn again and now back to face me.'
- 'Please walk across the room... now walk on your tiptoes... and on your heels.'
- 'Please come over to the couch and lie facing upwards... with your knees slightly bent.'
- 'I'm just going to check for heat and tenderness now in the knee (joint lines), ankle (malleolus) and foot (metatarsals).'
- 'Left side now, can you make this leg as straight as possible for me?' (Hyperextend knee.)
- 'Now lift your leg straight into the air.' (Hip flex.)
- 'Bend your knee to your chest.' (Knee flex.)
- 'Now can I do the same and see if I can take that further?' (Feeling for crepitus.)
- 'And now can you point your toes up and down, left and right?' (Ankle ROM.)
- 'Right side now please.' (Repeat.)
- 'Can you now turn over so you are facing the bed? I'm just going to squeeze your calf muscles.' (Achilles test.)
- 'And feel for pain under the foot.' (Plantar fasciitis.)
- 'Can you feel me touch your skin on the feet and toes?'

Example description

'I'd like to **thoroughly** *examine your ears, nose and throat… is that okay?'*

Checklist

- 'First let's look at your ears.' Is there redness/swelling?
- 'Is it tender when I press on this bone?' (Mastoiditis.)
- 'Or pull slightly at your ear?' (Otitis externa.)
- 'What about when I press here?' (Tragus.) 'Now let's look inside the ears.'
- Ensure you hold the otoscope like a pen in the same hand as the ear which you are examining.
- 'Let's test your hearing.' (At 1 m whisper, then if required 1 m voice, then next to ear voice.)
- Weber's test: 'I'm going to place this tuning fork (512 Hz) on your forehead. Can you tell me where you hear the sound – in the middle or to one side?'
  - Conductive deafness: localises to the affected side.
  - Sensorineural deafness: localises to the unaffected side.
- Rinne's test: 'Now I'm going to place the tuning fork behind your ear and then in front. Which is louder?'
  - Normal = air conduction (AC) > bone conduction (BC).
  - Conductive deafness = BC > AC.
  - Sensorineural deafness: AC > BC.
- 'Now can you tilt your head back? I'm going to look into the nose.'
- 'Now let's look at your throat.'
- 'And finally, I want to see if you have any tenderness or lumps in your neck.'

Example description

'I'd like to **thoroughly** *examine your vessels in your tummy and legs. If I may ask you to remove your trousers so that I can feel your pulses. I'd also like to take your blood pressure if I may. Please lie on the couch facing up.'*

Checklist

- Inspect legs for hair loss, colour change and look around the feet for tissue damage/ulceration.
- 'I'm now going to feel your vessels.'
- 'May I start with your large vessel in your tummy?' (AAA.)
- 'And now the pulses starting in the groin please.'
- Femoral, popliteal, posterior tibial and dorsalis pedis.
- 'Now I'd like you to lift this leg up; we are going to hold it (in reality for 45 seconds but not in the exam!) and watch for any colour change (pallor)… And now can you drop the leg over the edge of the bed.' (Reactive hyperaemia of Buerger's test.)
- Consider examining the heart, BP, lower limb sensation, offering a urine glucose test and ankle brachial pressure index (ABPI) checks.

If varicose veins are present, check with patient standing.

- Feel for tenderness in thrombophlebitis.
- Look for signs of DVT, oedema, tenderness along the greater saphenous vein (inner thigh).
- Measure calves from 10 cm below the tibial tuberosity.

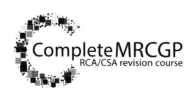

APPENDIX 1

Mandatory Cases for the RCA

At the time of writing, as well as submitting no more than two cases from any single curriculum area for the RCA, you must also evidence at least one from each of the following groups:

Children and young people – a case involving a child aged 16 years or younger. This can be by proxy – for example, a parent speaking about the child. The consultation should reflect the fact that the patient is a child, rather than the age being immaterial to the consultation.

Older adult – a case where the patient is 65 years or older.

Acute problem – a case where there is an acute problem that needs urgent investigation or referral. This means that there is a new presentation, or change in an existing condition, that needs immediate assessment or urgent (immediate or 2WW) investigation or referral.

Maternal and reproductive health – This is a broad area covering not just all maternity care, physical and mental, but also gynaecological problems, sexual health, contraception and infections – including all genders. Breast lump cases (other than lumps found in the postnatal period) are not eligible for this mandatory group.

Mental health condition – all areas covered by an ICD or DSM classification.

A long-term condition, e.g. cancer, multimorbidity or disability – this means a condition that cannot currently be cured but can be managed using, for example, medication or other therapies. Note that this MUST be an established diagnosis, not a new one. A patient with established heart failure coming for a review would count, but a consultation where you make a new diagnosis of heart failure would not.

Many cases throughout the book evidence these mandatory areas, and we have grouped these together below. Some cases cover more than one area, for example, Joshua Middleton, aged 11, with angioedema would cover both 'children and young people' and also 'acute problem'. Chloe Livingstone-Smith, with postnatal psychosis, covers three areas – 'acute problem', 'maternal health' and 'mental health condition'. We have marked these cases with an asterisk in the table.

A note of caution, however – if a case were to be disallowed by the RCGP, perhaps for technical reasons, then you could be doubly penalised if that particular case showcased more than one area. For example, if you were using Chloe Livingstone-Smith as your ONLY evidence in the above three areas, and if there was a technical breach, then as well as scoring no marks for that case you may also be penalised for not having submitted a case that fulfilled three mandatory areas. If there are two or more omitted criteria, then your whole RCA submission may be declined, meaning you need to reapply, with all-new cases and no refund of your exam fee. It may therefore be better to select the 'best' mandatory criterion for a particular case and evidence the other areas in different cases.

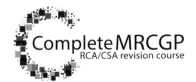

CompleteMRCGP
RCA/CSA revision course

Mandatory area	Name, age and gender of patient	Chapter and case number	Problem
Children and young people (13 cases)	Joshua Middleton 11 M*	2.1	Angioedema
	Peter Atkins 12 M	2.3	Asthma diagnosis
	Arthur Miller 12 M*	4.4	Eczema
	Sarah Smith 5 F	5.2	Acute otitis media
	Amena Khalil 4 F	6.2	Squint
	Connor McGowen 9 M	10.4	Anaemia
	Holly Forsyth 5 F	10.5	Henoch–Schönlein purpura
	Kalpesh Khan 6 M	11.1	Recurrent UTI
	Jayden Hall 13 months M	11.3	Viral illness
	Eleanor Cartwright 15 F*	13.5	Eating disorder
	Bhakti Shukla 12 months F	18.1	Immunisation refusal
	Gemma Briggs 15 F*	20.2	Contraception – combined
	Florence Wriggley 13 F	20.5	Gender dysphoria
Older adult >65 (19 cases)	Brendon Philips 74 M*	3.2	Heart failure
	Elizabeth Alderton 65 F*	3.3	Atrial fibrillation
	Hibiki Hayashi 75 M	3.5	Angina
	Paul Robson 65 M*	4.1	Skin lesion
	Maureen Staples 70 F*	4.5	Psoriasis
	Abida Khan 70 F*	6.3	Acute glaucoma
	Fred Scott 81 M	6.4	AMD and cataract
	Emmanuel Adebayo 71 M*	7.4	Change in bowel habit
	Raymond Styles 86 M	10.1	Suspected DVT
	William Jefferies 65 M	10.2	Myeloma
	Alexander Dickens 78 M	12.1	Acute kidney injury
	Bob Riley 67 M*	12.2	Chronic kidney disease
	Angus McLaughlin 72 M	12.5	Overactive bladder
	Shirley Warner 72 F	15.3	Osteoporosis
	Maggie Freestone 72 F	17.1	Peripheral neuropathy
	Lionel Moore 84 M*	17.2	Normal pressure hydrocephalus
	Lionel Morgan 82 M	19.1	Pneumonia
	Chao Lin 82 M*	19.3	COPD
	Katherine Knight 68 F*	21.5	Harmful drinking
A. Acute problem (15 cases)	Joshua Middleton 11 M*	2.1	Angioedema
	Mary Jones 45 F	3.1	Chest pain of recent onset
	Elizabeth Alderton 65 F*	3.3	Atrial fibrillation
	Paul Robson 65 M*	4.1	Skin lesion

Mandatory Cases for the RCA

Mandatory area	Name, age and gender of patient	Chapter and case number	Problem
	Mike Williams 55 M	5.1	Facial nerve palsy
	Abida Khan 70 F*	6.3	Acute glaucoma
	Eric Johnson 61 M	6.5	Retinal detachment
	Rosie Carpenter 40 F	7.1	Abdominal pain
	Emmanuel Adebayo 71 M*	7.4	Change in bowel habit
	Hilda Rowland 53 F	9.3	Post-menopausal bleeding
	Chloe Livingstone-Smith 28 F*	13.4	Postnatal psychosis
	Mary Owen 35 F	14.1	Hyperglycaemia
	Lionel Moore 84 M*	17.2	Normal pressure hydrocephalus
	Ahmed Hidad 58 M	17.4	TIA
	Daisy Fitton 24 F	19.2	Acute asthma
B. Reproductive and maternal health	Jennifer Adeyemi 27 F	2.4	Varicella in pregnancy
(13 cases)	Francesca Reece 32 F	4.3	Melasma
	Heather Mumford 33 F	8.1	Down syndrome
	Olivia Wales 29 F	8.2	Cystic fibrosis
	Jacqui Mason 24 F	9.1	Heavy menstrual bleeding
	Juliet Perkins 27 F	9.2	Polycystic ovary syndrome
	Chloe Livingstone-Smith 28 F*	13.4	Postnatal psychosis
	Jayne Smith 37 F	14.5	Diabetes in pregnancy
	Chloe Atherton 25 F	18.2	Cervical screening
	Kevin Barton 57 M	20.1	Erectile dysfunction
	Gemma Briggs 15 F*	20.2	Contraception – combined
	Stephanie Smith 24 F	20.3	Pelvic inflammatory disease
	Fedora Baros 38 F	20.4	LARC and sterilisation
C. Mental health problem (10 cases)	Stephen Harper 42 M	13.1	Anxiety
	Jessica Miller 24 F*	13.2	Depression
	Andrea Lockwood 36 F	13.3	Personality disorder
	Chloe Livingstone-Smith 28 F*	13.4	Postnatal psychosis
	Eleanor Cartwright 15 F*	13.5	Eating disorder
	Justin Walton 17 M	16.3	Autism and transition process
	Janine Paton 33 F	16.4	Mental health and intellectual disability
	Ella Jones 42 F	21.1	Substance use
	Michaela Butt 32 F	21.4	Opiate abuse
	Katherine Knight 68 F*	21.5	Harmful drinking

Mandatory Cases for the RCA

Mandatory area	Name, age and gender of patient	Chapter and case number	Problem
D. People with LTC	Brendon Philips 74 M*	3.2	Heart failure
(10 cases)	Arthur Miller 12 M*	4.4	Eczema
	Maureen Staples 70 F*	4.5	Psoriasis
	Anthony Carlisle 26 M	7.5	Inflammatory bowel disease
	Louise Barker 33 F	9.4	Cervical cancer
	Bob Riley 67 M*	12.2	Chronic kidney disease
	Jessica Miller 24 F*	13.2	Depression
	Fatima Sayed 47 F	14.4	Hyperthyroidism
	Yasmin Small 23 F	17.3	Migraine
	Chao Lin 82 M*	19.3	COPD

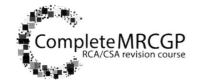

CompleteMRCGP
RCA/CSA revision course

Mandatory Cases for the RCA

APPENDIX 2
Useful Resources

Updated at the Link Hub at CompleteMRCGP.co.uk

Information for GPs	Patient.co.uk and GP Notebook
PILs in different languages	https://www.cntw.nhs.uk/resource-library/
DermNet	http://www.dermnetnz.org/
Primary care dermatology	http://www.pcds.org.uk/
Translated dermatology PILs	https://www.skinhealthinfo.org.uk/a-z-conditions-treatments/
Medicines in pregnancy	http://www.medicinesinpregnancy.org/
Medications in breastfeeding	https://www.ncbi.nlm.nih.gov/books/NBK501922/
DVLA at a glance	https://www.gov.uk/government/publications/assessing-fitness-to-drive-a-guide-for-medical-professionals
Fitness to fly	https://www.caa.co.uk/passengers/before-you-fly/am-i-fit-to-fly/guidance-for-health-professionals/assessing-fitness-to-fly/
Travel clinic	http://www.fitfortravel.nhs.uk/home.aspx
Drug monitoring requirements	http://www.bucksformulary.nhs.uk/docs/sc/
Parent advice	http://www.whenshouldiworry.com/
	The Incredible Years by Carolyn Webster-Stratton.

Oxford antimicrobial guidelines

Adults and children	https://clinox.info/local-guidelines-and-pathways/antimicrobial-guidelines-adults/58134

Useful guidance		
	Contraception	www.fsrh.org
	Green-Top Guidelines	https://www.rcog.org.uk/guidelines
	SIGN	http://sign.ac.uk/
	NICE	https://www.nice.org.uk/guidance
	BTS	https://www.brit-thoracic.org.uk/quality-improvement/guidelines/

Mental health	http://www.oxfordmindfulness.org/about-mindfulness/
	http://www.fearfighter.com/
	https://moodgym.com.au
	http://www.mind.org.uk/
Antidepressant switches	https://www.mims.co.uk/table-antidepressants-guide-switching-withdrawing/mental-health/article/1415768

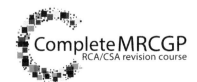

Prescribing in psychiatry	Taylor D.M., Paton C., Kapur S. (2015) The *Maudsley Prescribing Guidelines in Psychiatry,* 12th edition. Oxford: Wiley-Blackwell.
CBT book for the keen reader	Williams M., Penman D. (2011) *Mindfulness: A Practical Guide to Finding Peace in a Frantic World.* London: Piatkus Books.
CBT – if struggling to concentrate	Black A. (2012) *Living in the Moment: With Mindfulness Meditations.* London: Ryland, Peters & Small.
Joint exercises	https://www.versusarthritis.org/
Back screening tool	https://www.keele.ac.uk/search/?q=back+screening+tool
Osteoporosis assessment	https://www.sheffield.ac.uk/FRAX/
Physiotherapy websites	http://www.sheffieldachesandpains.com/
Vitamin D guidelines – adults	http://www.ouh.nhs.uk/osteoporosis/useful-info/documents/VitaminDSupplementationinprimarycarev16.pdf
Vitamin D guidelines – children	https://www.nuh.nhs.uk/vitamin-d-deficiency-in-children/
Alcohol – useful information	https://www.who.int/health-topics/alcohol#tab=tab_1
Intellectual disability PILs	https://www.nhsinform.scot/translations/formats/easy-read http://www.fairadvice.org.uk/free-downloads.php
Cardiovascular risk	http://qrisk.org/
Institute of Blind People	https://rnib.org.uk/
Deaf Association	http://www.bda.org.uk/
BMJs Easily Missed Series	http://www.bmj.com/specialties/easily-missed
	We recommend this exercise – for each 'easily missed' condition:
	1. Consider what symptoms the patient may have presented with.
	2. Then for each symptom think about what are the most likely diagnoses (common things are common!) and what is 'easily missed'?
E learning	http://elearning.rcgp.org.uk/
	http://www.pulse-learning.co.uk/
	http://www.gponline.com/education
Courses not to miss!	http://www.gp-update.co.uk/The-GP-Update-Course
	https://www.nbmedical.com/courses/subject/hot-topics-gp-update
	http://www.rcgp.org.uk/learning/one-day-essentials.aspx
RCGP curriculum	https://www.rcgp.org.uk/training-exams/training/gp-curriculum-overview.aspx
Conference not to miss!	https://www.rcgp.org.uk/learning/rcgp-annual-conference.aspx
Consultation skills	Moulton L. (2016) *The Naked Consultation: A Practical Guide to Primary Care Consultation Skills,* 2nd edition. Boca Raton: CRC Press.
Time out from revision…	Watch a TED Talk for inspiration!

Index

in acute COPD, 466
in acute otitis media, 128
in blepharitis, 148
in Lyme disease, 276
in pelvic inflammatory disease, 492
in pneumonia, 462
in prostatitis, 306
in sinusitis, 136
after splenectomy, 254, 256
anticoagulation
in atrial fibrillation, 82, 93–4
risk factors for bleeding, 93
in VTE, 248, 265
antidepressants, 324
antihyperglycaemics, 359–60
metformin, 226, 342, 358
antimuscarinics, 310
antisocial personality disorder, 328
anxiety, 76, 318–20
aortic aneurysm, 172
apixaban, 82, 265–6
appendicitis, 172
apraxia, 414–16
ARBs (angiotensin receptor blockers)
in heart failure, 80
in hypertension, 96
AREDS2, 160
aspirin
in angina, 92
in TIA, 424
asthma
acute, 464–6
diagnosis, 58–60, 479
asylum seekers, 152, 440–2
atopic eczema, 112–14
atrial fibrillation (AF), 82–4
cardiology referral, 94
stroke risk management, 93–4
atrioventricular septal defect (AVSD), 195, 196
autistic spectrum disorder, 394–5
and MMR, 434
autoimmune hepatitis, 189
autosomal-dominant disorders, 213–14
autosomal-recessive disorders, 214
autosplenectomy, 256
avoidant personality disorder, 328
azelaic acid, 106

B
B12 deficiency, 260
'baby blues,' 332
back pain, 302, 364–6

bad news, 196
bariatric surgery, 450
Becker muscular dystrophy, 214
Bell's palsy, 122–4
benign paroxysmal positional vertigo (BPPV), 138–40
benign prostatic hypertrophy (BPH), 313
benzodiazepines, 320
weaning, 510
beta-blockers
in AF, 86
in angina, 92
in heart failure, 80
in hypertension, 96
bicalutamide, 313
biliary colic, 172
bisphosphonates, 372, 374
bladder outflow obstruction, 302
bladder overactivity, 308–10
blepharitis, 146–8
blood pressure targets
in CKD, 298
in TIA/stroke, 424
blurred vision, 162–4
body dysmorphia, 502
borderline personality disorder, 328
bowel cancer screening, 454
bowel habit, change in, 182–4
bowel obstruction, 172
BRCA1, BRCA2, 208
breast cancer
family history of, 206–8
risk from HRT, 240
screening programme, 454
breasts, gynaecomastia, 232–4
breathlessness
COPD, 466, 468–70
heart failure, 78–80
pneumonia, 460–2
see also asthma
Buerger's test, 541
bulimia nervosa *see* eating disorders
bunions, 378

C
CA125 testing, 230
calcium channel blockers
in AF, 86
in angina, 92
in heart failure, 80
in hypertension, 88
calcium supplementation, 374